Perinatal Cardiology

Part 1

Edited by

Edward Araujo Júnior

Department of Obstetrics, Discipline of Fetal Medicine,
Federal University of São Paulo (EPM-UNIFESP),
São Paulo-SP,
Brazil

Nathalie Jeanne M. Bravo-Valenzuela

Department of Obstetrics, Discipline of Fetal Medicine,
Paulista School of Medicine,
Federal University of São Paulo (EPM-UNIFESP),
São Paulo-SP,
Brazil

Alberto Borges Peixoto

Discipline of Gynecology and Obstetrics,
University of Uberaba (UNIUBE),
Uberaba-MG,
Brazil

Perinatal Cardiology

Part # 1

Editors: Edward Araujo Júnior, Nathalie Jeanne M. Bravo-Valenzuela and Alberto Borges Peixoto

ISBN (Online): 978-981-14-4680-1

ISBN (Print): 978-981-14-4678-8

©2020, Bentham Books imprint.

Published by Bentham Science Publishers Pte. Ltd. Singapore. All Rights Reserved.

need for a court order if at any point you breach any terms of this License Agreement. In no event will any delay or failure by Bentham Science Publishers in enforcing your compliance with this License Agreement constitute a waiver of any of its rights.

3. You acknowledge that you have read this License Agreement, and agree to be bound by its terms and conditions. To the extent that any other terms and conditions presented on any website of Bentham Science Publishers conflict with, or are inconsistent with, the terms and conditions set out in this License Agreement, you acknowledge that the terms and conditions set out in this License Agreement shall prevail.

Bentham Science Publishers Pte. Ltd.
80 Robinson Road #02-00
Singapore 068898
Singapore
Email: subscriptions@benthamscience.net

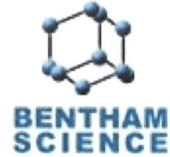

BENTHAM SCIENCE

CONTENTS

FOREWORD

In *Perinatal Cardiology,* Edward Araujo Júnior, Nathalie Jeanne M. Bravo-Valenzuela, and Alberto Borges Peixoto have compiled a concise textbook, encompassing the fascinating, and demanding, study of the developing human heart. Malformations and disorders affecting the cardiovascular system are both the most commonly occurring in fetuses and neonates, and the most frequently missed in prenatal scanning. They contribute significantly to neonatal morbidity and mortality and impact on all stages of obstetric and neonatal management. Prenatal diagnosis of congenital heart disease (CHD) can improve neonatal and later outcomes. With the ongoing improvements in perinatal and pediatric care of patients with congenital heart defects, their impact will be evinced in later life stages, in reproductive care of women with CHD as well as genetic counseling for affected families.

Perinatal Cardiology comprises all these aspects of CHD, not overlooking the development of the uteroplacental circulation and the placenta itself, integral parts of the fetal cardiovascular system. The editors have enlisted an international cast of contributing authors who offer their expert guidance on fetal echocardiographic evaluation, and the particular nuances of fetal echocardiography performed early in gestation. Chapters are also devoted to the genetic investigation necessary in CHD, as well as the environmental factors that may be associated with CHD. This volume provides an overview of the anatomic malformations and disordered cardiovascular function that clinicians might encounter, and the pre- and post-natal interventions that can be offered.

Perinatal Cardiology will be of interest to everyone, including obstetricians, midwives, maternal-fetal medicine specialists, pediatric cardiologists, sonographers, and others dedicated to improve health and wellness of mothers and their babies.

Prof. Simcha Yagel
Division of Obstetrics and Gynecology
Hadassah-Hebrew University Medical Centers
Jerusalem
Israel

PREFACE

This first edition of the *Perinatal Cardiology* book is the culmination of concerted efforts of experts in the field of fetal cardiology. Congenital heart disease (CHD) accounts for the most common birth defects and is the leading cause of mortality associated with birth defects in infants. Critical CHD is defined as a condition that necessitates surgical intervention during the first year of life and accounts for approximately 25% of all CHD cases. Advances in prenatal diagnosis and surgical interventions/therapeutic *in utero* have improved the management and outcomes of CHD. Rapid technological advances in fetal echocardiography and prenatal cardiac ultrasonography (US) screening facilitate the early and accurate diagnosis of CHD, thereby ensuring prompt and optimal treatment. In accordance with the concepts and themes associated with this field, *Perinatal Cardiology* provides a comprehensive overview of the key learning points with regard to CHD. The authors have outlined strategies to improve prenatal diagnosis and management of this condition, which would benefit the following specialties: obstetricians, perinatal and pediatric cardiologists, general cardiologists, sonographers, and other allied health professionals. This book highlights the features of cardiac development, fetal cardiovascular hemodynamics, genetic factors associated with CHD, and fetal echocardiography/cardiac US evaluation, focusing on the prenatal diagnosis and perinatal management of CHD. The introductory chapters describe in detail the development of the cardiovascular and uteroplacental circulation, beginning with early gestation. This anatomical background will provide a better understanding of the pathogenesis/pathophysiology of cardiac malformations. The authors have described the US/echocardiographic features that would aid in the prenatal diagnosis of CHD and also highlighted features of fetal cardiac dysfunction correlated with their clinical applicability. Environmental exposures that can lead to cardiovascular malformations and the genetic aspects of CHD, including chromosomal abnormalities and extracardiac anomalies are discussed, for enhancing parental counseling. Additionally, this book provides updated information regarding *in utero* management and treatment of CHD, as well as postnatal clinical and surgical approaches to the management of most commonly occurring conditions categorized as CHD. Furthermore, the book describes interesting aspects of the cardiac rhythm *in utero* following the development of the cardiac conduction system, the characteristics of regular and irregular heart rhythms, and the important features of the different types of arrhythmias observed in these patients, as well as their perinatal management. The chapters in this book have been added after careful consideration and are subdivided into sections after thoughtful deliberation. These include various topics such as fetal cardiology, including the classification of prenatal CHD, cardiovascular and uteroplacental circulation development, fetal echocardiography evaluation, normal cardiac rhythm and arrhythmias, structural and functional defects, prenatal cardiac interventions, extracardiac cardiac defects in fetuses with CHD, genetic and environmental factors associated with cardiac defects, parental genetic counseling in cases of CHD, prenatal management and planned delivery of a fetus with CHD, and a systematic postnatal approach to the management of CHD. The anatomical classification of CHD is subdivided into the following topics: malpositions and abnormal situs, septal defects, right heart malformations, left heart malformations, conotruncal anomalies, aortic arch anomalies, myocardial and pericardial diseases, fetal cardiac tumors, and ventricular inflow anomalies. In recent years, significant technological progress in fetal echocardiography has enabled the diagnosis of various types of CHD, and it is possible to evaluate cardiac function in fetuses with CHD and in those without anatomical malformations. The following conditions (among several others) may affect fetal cardiac function: functional cardiac malformations such as premature closure of ductus arteriosus and foramen ovale and extracardiac conditions, such as maternal diseases (diabetes mellitus and chronic hypertension), fetal tumors, twin-to-twin transfusion syndrome, and fetal anemia. The Cardiovascular Profile Score is a useful tool for the assessment of fetuses with heart failure (HF). This tool utilizes US markers to monitor fetal cardiovascular unwellness based on univariate parameters, which are correlated with perinatal mortality. This instrument is used to record the "heart failure score" and is potentially useful in much the same way and in combination with the biophysical profile score. The chapters discussing fetal heart function comprise one of the differential topics of this book in the field of fetal cardiology. These chapters describe objective and important information regarding the clinical parameters for the evaluation of cardiac function. Chapters explaining the analysis of cardiac function discuss hemodynamic and cardiovascular fetal adaptations that enable optimization of outcomes and prediction of the risk in a fetus with HF or the one at risk of HF. Currently, the role of contemporary fetal cardiologists is not limited to the diagnosis and management of CHD *in utero*. These specialists also predict the risk of CHD in the newborn after delivery and participate in planning potential treatment after birth. Thus, a new classification system of prenatal CHD has been proposed based on risk stratification to identify an appropriate level of care. Critical CHD may progress *in utero*, and fetal echocardiography is an important tool to identify high-risk fetuses of mothers who require obstetric care at specialized centers to ensure optimal perinatal, obstetric, cardiology, and cardiothoracic surgery services. In conclusion, we hope this book serves as a comprehensive compendium of the latest optimal clinical approaches to the diagnosis, management and delivery planning for fetuses with CHD.

Edward Araujo Júnior
Department of Obstetrics, Discipline of Fetal Medicine
Federal University of São Paulo (EPM-UNIFESP)
São Paulo-SP
Brazil

Nathalie Jeanne M. Bravo-Valenzuela
Department of Obstetrics, Discipline of Fetal Medicine, Paulista School of Medicine
Federal University of São Paulo (EPM-UNIFESP)
São Paulo-SP
Brazil

&

Alberto Borges Peixoto
Discipline of Gynecology and Obstetrics
University of Uberaba (UNIUBE)
Uberaba-MG
Brazil

List of Contributors

Agata Wloch Department of Obstetrics and Gynecology, Woman's Health Chair, Medical University of Silesia, Katowice, Poland

Alberto Borges Peixoto Discipline of Gynecologyy and Obstetrics, University of Uberaba (UNIUBE), Uberaba-MG, Brazil
Department of Gynecologyy and Obstetrics, Federal University of Triângulo Mineiro (UFTM), Uberaba-MG, Brazil

Alberto Galindo Department of Obstetrics and Gynaecology, Fetal Medicine Unit-Maternal and Child Health and Development Network (SAMID), Hospital Universitario 12 de Octubre, Instituto de Investigación Hospital 12 de Octubre (imas12), Faculty of Medicine, Universidad Complutense de Madrid, Madrid, Spain

Aline Wolter Division of Prenatal Medicine & Fetal Therapy, Justus-Liebig University Giessen, Giessen, Germany

Cecilia Villalaín Department of Obstetrics and Gynaecology, Fetal Medicine Unit-Maternal and Child Health and Development Network (SAMID), Hospital Universitario 12 de Octubre, Instituto de Investigación Hospital 12 de Octubre (imas12), Faculty of Medicine, Universidad Complutense de Madrid, Madrid, Spain

Daniel L. Rolnik Department of Obstetrics and Gynaecology, Monash Womens, Monash Health, Clayton, Victoria, Australia

Darren Hutchinson Department of Cardiology, Fetal Cardiology Unit, Royal Women's Hospital, Melbourne, Australia

Edward Araujo Júnior Discipline of Fetal Medicine, Department of Obstetrics, Paulista School of Medicine –Federal University of São Paulo (EPM-UNIFESP), São Paulo-SP, Brazil
Medical Course, Municipal University of São Caetano do Sul (USCS), Bela Vista Campus, São Paulo-SP, Brazil

Enery Gómez Montes Department of Obstetrics and Gynaecology, Fetal Medicine Unit-Maternal and Child Health and Development Network (SAMID), Hospital Universitario 12 de Octubre, Instituto de Investigación Hospital 12 de Octubre (imas12), Faculty of Medicine, Universidad Complutense de Madrid, Madrid, Spain

Gabriele Tonni Department of Obstetrics and Gynecologyy, Prenatal Diagnostic Service, Guastalla Civil Hospital, Istituto di Ricerca a Carattere Clinico Scientifico (IRCCS), AUSL di Reggio Emilia, Reggio Emilia, Italy

Ganesh Acharya Department of Clinical Science, Division of Obstetrics and Gynecologyy, Intervention and Technology, Karolinska Institutets, Stockholm, Sweden
Center for Fetal Medicine, Karolinska University Hospital, Stockholm, Sweden
Department of Clinical Medicine, Women's Health and Perinatology Research Group, UiT-The Artic University of Norway, Tromsø, Norway

Gianpaolo Grisolia Department of Obstetrics and Gynecology, Maternal Fetal Unit, Carlo Poma Hospital, Mantua, Italy

Ignacio Herraiz
Department of Obstetrics and Gynaecology, Fetal Medicine Unit-Maternal and Child Health and Development Network (SAMID), Hospital Universitario 12 de Octubre, Instituto de Investigación Hospital 12 de Octubre (imas12), Faculty of Medicine, Universidad Complutense de Madrid, Madrid, Spain

Jader Cruz
Fetal Medicine Unit, Centro Hospitalar Universitário de Lisboa Central, Lisboa, Portugal

Jesus Rodríguez Calvo
Department of Obstetrics and Gynaecology, Fetal Medicine Unit-Maternal and Child Health and Development Network (SAMID), Hospital Universitario 12 de Octubre, Instituto de Investigación Hospital 12 de Octubre (imas12), Faculty of Medicine, Universidad Complutense de Madrid, Madrid, Spain

Jon A. Hyett
RPA Women and Babies, Royal Prince Alfred Hospital, Sydney Institute for Women, Childrenand their Families, Sydney, Australia
Discipline of Obstetrics, Gynaecology and Neonatology, Central Clinical School, Faculty of Medicine, University of Sydney, Sydney, Australia

Judy A. Jones
London Health Sciences Centre, London, Ontario, Canada

Kersti K. Linask
Department of Pediatrics, USF Morsani College of Medicine, Tampa and St. Petersburg, FL, USA

Laudelino M. Lopes
London X-Ray Associates, London, Ontario, Canada
Department of Obstetrics & Gynaecology, Maternal Fetal Medicine, Schulich School of Medicine & Dentistry - University of Western Ontario, London, Ontario, Canada

Leonor Ferreira
Fetal Medicine Unit, Centro Hospitalar Universitário de Lisboa Central, Lisboa, Portugal

Luciane Alves da Rocha
Postgraduate Program in Health Sciences, Medical School, Federal University of Amazonas (UFAM), Manaus-AM, Brazil

Maciej Słodki
Faculty of Health Sciences, The State University of Applied Sciences, Plock, Poland
Department of Prenatal Cardiology, Polish Mother's Memorial Hospital Research Institute, Lodz, Poland

Maria Respondek-Liberska
Fetal Malformations and Prevention Department, Medical University of Lodz, Poland
Cardiology Department Research, Institute Polish Mother's Memorial Hospital, Lodz, Poland

Maria Virgina Lima Machado
CardioFetal Clinic – Centro de Cardiologia e Ecocardiografia Fetal, São Paulo – SP, Brazil

Maya Reddy
Department of Obstetrics and Gynaecology, Monash Womens, Monash Health, Clayton, Victoria, Australia
Department of Obstetrics and Gynaecology, Faculty of Medicine, Nursing and Health Sciences,Monash University, Clayton, Victoria, Australia

Michael Tartar
London X-Ray Associates, London, Ontario, Canada

Nathalie J.M. Bravo-Valenzuela
Department of Obstetrics, Discipline of Fetal Medicine, Paulista School of Medicine-Federal University of São Paulo (EPM-UNIFESP), São Paulo-SP, Brazil
Discipline of Pediatrics (Pediatric Cardiology), Department of Medicine, Federal University of Rio de Janeiro (UFRJ), Rio de Janeiro-RJ, Brazil

Oliver Graupner
Division of Prenatal Medicine & Fetal Therapy, Justus-Liebig University Giessen, Giessen, Germany

Ricardo Palma-Dias
Department of Obstetrics and Gynaecology, Department of Ultrasound, Royal Women'sHospital, University of Melbourne, Victoria, Australia

Ritu Mogra
RPA Women and Babies, Royal Prince Alfred Hospital, Sydney Institute for Women, Childrenand their Families, Sydney, Australia
Discipline of Obstetrics, Gynaecology and Neonatology, Central Clinical School, Faculty of Medicine, University of Sydney, Sydney, Australia

Roland Axt-Fliedner
Division of Prenatal Medicine & Fetal Therapy, Justus-Liebig University Giessen, Giessen, Germany

Sheldon Bayle
College of New Caledonia Prince George, Prince George, British Columbia, Canada

Travis Kowlessar
London Health Sciences Centre, London, Ontario, Canada

CHAPTER 1

Classification of Prenatal Congenital Heart Diseases

Maciej Słodki[1,2,*] and **Maria Respondek-Liberska**[2,3]

[1] *Faculty of Health Sciences, The Mazovian State University in Plock, Poland*

[2] *Department of Prenatal Cardiology, Polish Mother's Memorial Hospital Research Institute, Lodz, Poland*

[3] *Department of Diagnoses and Prevention of Fetal Malformations, Medical University of Lodz, Poland*

Abstract: The *in utero* progression of congenital heart diseases (CHDs) can be observed in almost all CHDs during the first, second, and third trimesters of pregnancy. The progression of a cardiac disease can be associated with worsening of structural defects, new onset of foramen ovale restriction, decreased ventricular inflow or outflow, or worsening arch obstruction. The role of contemporary fetal cardiologists is to not only diagnose CHDs but also foresee the condition of the newborn after delivery and plan potential treatment in the first hours-or even minutes-of life. For this reason, pregnancy and delivery management of newborns with a prenatal diagnosis of CHD requires a multidisciplinary team composed of fetal and pediatric cardiologists, obstetricians and maternal–fetal specialists, neonatologists, and other pediatric specialists. The potential progression of CHD severity *in utero* and changes occurring during the transition from fetal life to infancy led to the creation of new classifications of CHDs dedicated to fetuses only. Severest heart defects are defined as CHDs in fetuses whose treatment results in death in nearly all cases, and potential treatment is needed immediately after birth; severe urgent heart defects are defined as CHDs in fetuses who need to undergo an invasive cardiologic treatment or cardiologic surgery within the first hours of postnatal life; severe planned heart defects are defined as CHDs in fetuses who need to undergo cardiologic surgery within the first month after birth, usually with ductal-dependent circulation and prostaglandin infusion to prolong prenatal physiology; and planned heart defects are defined as CHDs in fetuses who do not need to undergo cardiologic surgery within the first month after birth (usually surgery may be postponed to infancy). The only tool for the proper qualification of fetuses to one of the groups in the new classification system is fetal echocardiography.

Keywords: Classification, Fetal echocardiography, Planned and urgent congenital heart disease.

* **Corresponding author Maciej Słodki:** Faculty of Health Sciences, The Mazovian State University in Plock, Poland; Tel: +48 243665420, E-mail: maciejslodki@op.pl

Edward Araujo Júnior, Nathalie Jeanne M. Bravo-Valenzuela and Alberto Borges Peixoto (Eds.)

INTRODUCTION

Congenital heart diseases (CHDs) are the most common congenital defects in fetuses and neonates. They are responsible for the mortality and morbidity of newborns in 3 of 10 cases [1 - 3]. CHDs develop in fetuses three times more often than in neonates; prenatal CHDs are more complex and frequently coexist with chromosomal abnormalities, extracardiac anomalies (ECAs), and extracardiac malformations (ECMs) [4 - 8]. Fetal cardiologists performing fetal scanning must be aware of this association with ECMs, especially the defects that may affect the management of pregnancy or prognosis for surgery [9]. Recent studies have shown that infants with a prenatal diagnosis of high-risk CHD and adequate postnatal management have better preoperative outcomes compared with those diagnosed postnatally, especially in areas with limited pediatric resources [10 - 14]. Prenatal cardiologists have three main clinical aims that go beyond parental counseling: (1) diagnose the specific cardiac defect; (2) plan perinatal management by identifying the fetuses at risk of postnatal hemodynamic instability, which may require medical intervention in a delivery room (DR) or within the first days of life; and (3) identify fetuses who may benefit from fetal cardiac interventions [14 - 16]. The aim of prenatal cardiology consultation is to provide perinatologists, neonatologists, cardiologists, and parents with the right information rather than provide fetuses with medical therapies [9]. Several studies have proved the high sensitivity of prenatal diagnosis in referral centers and almost 100% correlation with postnatal diagnosis [2, 17, 18]. The specificity of prenatal cardiology results in pediatric cardiology classifications is useless in terms of managing and observing fetuses with CHDs. For example, tetralogy of Fallot (TOF) and dextro-transposition of the great arteries (d-TGA) are cyanotic diseases developing in the neonatal period. Without the differentiation between these CHDs in fetuses, the condition of newborns after delivery could be extremely different. TOF is usually a planned CHD that requires surgery in the first 6 months of life, whereas d-TGA is a CHD that requires surgery in the first days of life. Sometimes an invasive procedure needs to be performed in the first hours of life. The classification based on ductal-dependent lesions was useful before the era of prenatal cardiology. Nowadays, with prenatal detection of CHDs and prostaglandin administration immediately after birth, only ductal-dependent lesions are not critical anymore. In the case of a CHD that is additionally foramen ovale (FO) dependent, prostaglandin administration may be insufficient to stabilize the newborn. None of the pediatric cardiology classifications differentiate this malformation. Nor do they consider the changes occurring during the transition from fetal life to infancy, which is one of the most important aspects of CHDs in fetuses. All these dimensions have led to the creation of new classifications of CHDs dedicated to fetuses only (Table **1**) [8, 17, 19 - 21].

Table 1. New classification system of congenital heart disease (CHD) dedicated only for fetuses.

Classification					
	Berkeley *et al.*, 2009	**Respondek-Liberska and Słodki, 2012**	**Donofrio *et al.*, 2013**	**Pruetz *et al.*, 2014**	
Low risk	Care plan 2	Planned CHD	LOC 1	ENCI 1	Shunt lesions, Mild valve disease, TOF, AVSD Cardiology consultation and telemedicine, with outpatient cardiology evaluation
Medium risk	Care plan 3	Severe planned CHD	LOC 2	ENCI 2	Mostly ductal-dependent lesions Neonatologist in the DR: PGE if indicated and transport to the cardiac center for catheterization/surgery
High risk	Care plan 3 and 4	Severe urgent CHD	LOC 3	ENCI 3	HLHS with restricted FO D-TGA with restricted FO Critical AS Referral center, ready for urgent intervention
Extremely high risk	Care plan 5	Severest CHD	LOC 4	ENCI 4	Ready for immediate intervention in DR HLHS with IAS TGA with severe RAS and abnormal DA shunt Obstructed TAPVR Severe Ebstein's anomaly or TOF/APV with hydrops

ENCI, emergent neonatal cardiac intervention; LOC, level of care; TOF, tetralogy of Fallot; AVSD, atrioventricular septal defect; DR, delivery room; PG, prostaglandin; HLHS, hypoplastic left heart syndrome; FO, foramen ovale; AS, aortic stenosis; IAS, interatrial septum; TGA, transposition of the great arteries; RAS, restrictive atrial septum; DA, ductus arteriosus; TAPVR, total anomalous pulmonary venous return; APV, absent pulmonary valve.

In 1998, Wald and Kennard presented their classification, which is similar to those independently suggested by the Royal College of Obstetricians and Gynaecologists Working Party on Ultrasound Screening for Fetal Abnormalities. They specified four groups: (A) major abnormalities (death inevitable); (B) abnormalities associated with long-term handicap; (C) abnormalities potentially amenable to intrauterine treatment; and (D) fetal conditions that require immediate postnatal investigation and/or treatment. For each abnormality, screening detection and false-positive results need to be estimated together with the medical and financial costs of screening, particularly those arising from findings of uncertain or mild medical consequence that may lead to worry and further unnecessary obstetric intervention [22].

In 2004, Allan and Huggon suggested grading cardiac lesions on a scale of 1 to 10, with 1 being the least severe (ventricular septal defect [VSD], mild pulmonary stenosis [PS]) and 3 and 6 being lesions where the heart structure can be restored, although with difficulty, to a "normal" or near normal anatomy, for example, d-TGA, coarctation of the aorta (CoA), and double outlet right ventricle (DORV). Then, most "one-ventricle repairs" would fit in the 7 to 10 range, depending on the precise anatomy (hypoplastic left heart syndrome [HLHS], hypoplastic right heart syndrome, tricuspid atresia (TvA), and mitral atresia). Alternatively, they also divided CHDs into "good," *i.e.*, those that are easily treated and will not affect the child in the long term; "intermediate," *i.e.*, those that can be successfully repaired surgically but are likely to affect long-term survival; and "bad," *i.e.*, lesions likely to manifest themselves in childhood and have a profound impact on the chances of reaching healthy adulthood. This classification focuses mainly on the short- and long-term prognosis and lifespan after surgery [9].

In 2009, Berkeley *et al.* presented one of the first classifications guiding delivery management in pregnancies complicated with CHD. They proposed five care plans depending on the level of references of the hospital: (1) comfort care, (2) delivery at the local hospital, (3) delivery at a tertiary neonatal intensive care unit (NICU) with medical support, (4) delivery at a tertiary NICU with planned delayed surgery at a tertiary cardiac center, and (5) maternal transport with delivery at a quaternary cardiac center. They conclude that a prenatal diagnosis of CHD may lead to better coordination of care and improved emotional and psychosocial support for the family. Prenatal diagnosis may also improve neonatal surgical and neurological outcomes, and they proved that fetal echocardiography was highly accurate in guiding delivery planning [17].

In 2011, in Poland, Respondek-Liberska presented her classification in a book titled "Atlas of congenital heart diseases" [19]. She described 24 different cases of CHD with different requirements in terms of management after birth. In her book, Respondek-Liberska discussed a greatly important problem of fetuses with critical CHDs requiring procedures in the first hours of life. In 2012, Słodki, drawing upon her study, expanded the classification to six groups, adding fetuses with coexisting ECAs and ECMs [8]. This classification considers different postnatal treatment and coexistence of ECAs and ECMs. ECAs are defined here as problems that do not require surgical interventions after delivery and are usually markers of a genetic syndrome, *e.g.*, hypoplastic nasal bone, micrognathia, single umbilical artery, ventriculomegaly, choroid plexus cysts, shortening long bones, and pyelectasis. ECMs are defined by Słodki as problems requiring surgical interventions after delivery or lethal malformations, *e.g.*, duodenal atresia, hydrocephalus, Dandy–Walker syndrome, spina bifida, cleft lip and palate, pulmonary hypoplasia, diaphragmatic hernia, acranius, holoprosencephaly, and renal agenesis. The percentage of the coexistence of CHD and ECM and/or ECA was 37%, and this association has a significant influence on postnatal outcomes [23 - 27]. In fetuses with CHD and ECM, only 14% of infants were discharged home after surgery. Infants who were not required to undergo two separate surgeries had the chance to survive [8]. Atrioventricular septal defects (AVSDs) usually coexist with ECAs, ECMs, and genetic syndromes [8, 28 - 30]. Moreover, the presence of ECAs that do not require surgery after delivery affects the outcome. Hypoplastic nasal bone, micrognathia, single umbilical artery, ventriculomegaly, choroid plexus cysts, and shortening long bones are not directly life-threatening, but their presence increases the risk of genetic syndromes or complications after delivery. The survival rate in fetuses with CHD + ECA was 60% and lower than that in fetuses with isolated CHD (p = 0.075504) [8].

Słodki defined four groups of isolated CHD and two additional groups for ECA and ECM [8]:

1. Severest heart defects – isolated CHD in fetuses whose treatment results in death in nearly all cases.
2. Severe urgent heart defects – isolated CHD in fetuses who need to undergo an invasive cardiologic treatment or cardiologic surgery immediately after birth, *i.e.*, within the first hours of postnatal life.
3. Severe planned heart defects – isolated CHD in fetuses who need to undergo cardiologic surgery within the first month after birth, usually with ductal-dependent circulation and prostaglandin infusion to prolong prenatal physiology.
4. Planned heart defects – isolated CHD in fetuses who do not need to undergo cardiologic surgery within the first month after birth (usually surgery may be postponed to infancy).
5. Heart defects coexisting with ECMs.
6. Heart defects coexisting with ECAs.

In 2013, Donofrio *et al.* presented their study on the accuracy of fetal echocardiography in predicting the need for specialized DR care and determining the effectiveness of care protocols for the treatment of patients with critical CHD. The anticipated level of care (LOC) was assigned by fetal echocardiography: (1) LOC 1, nursery consultation/outpatient follow-up; (2) LOC 2, stable in the DR with transfer to a cardiac hospital; and (3 and 4) LOC 3 or 4, DR instability/urgent intervention needed. They concluded that fetal echocardiography can predict the need for specialized DR care in fetuses with critical CHD [20].

In 2014, Pruetz *et al.* presented their emergent neonatal cardiac intervention (ENCI) classification system and management guidelines based on a four-level classification system for prenatally diagnosed CHD that considers both the level of postnatal clinical acuity and need for an emergent postnatal intervention [21].

In the past 15 years, several authors have created highly similar guidelines for the management of high-risk patients with CHD who may require emergent treatment in the newborn period [16, 31] (Table 1). These classification systems, which in particular focus on the most critical forms of CHD in fetuses and newborns, change the definition of critical CHD to that which requires urgent intervention in the first 24 h of life to prevent death. Such cardiac interventions may not only be life saving for the infant but also decrease subsequent morbidity. Fetuses with critical CHD may require delivery at specialized centers that can provide perinatal, obstetric, cardiologic, and cardiothoracic surgery care. Fetuses diagnosed in mid-gestation require detailed fetal diagnostics and serial echocardiography monitoring during the prenatal period to assess ongoing changes and identify progression to a more severe cardiac status. Critical CHD may progress *in utero*, and there is still much to be learned on how to best predict those that will require urgent neonatal interventions [16, 31, 32].

PLANNED CHD

Low-risk CHD: LOC 1 [20], ENCI 1 [21], and Care Plan 1 or 2 [17]

Cardiovascular defects that are expected to be hemodynamically stable at birth include left-to-right shunt lesions such as atrial or VSD or mild valve abnormalities and benign arrhythmias (*i.e.*, premature atrial contractions) with normal cardiac function. In the absence of additional fetal abnormalities, the delivery plan for fetuses diagnosed with these CHDs using fetal echocardiography should be determined according to the presence or absence of maternal or obstetric complications or levels of maternal care. Newborns with low-risk CHD can usually be delivered at or near term *via* a normal mode of delivery. They require inpatient consultation or telemedicine confirmation of the diagnosis with outpatient cardiology follow-up within the first weeks of life [8, 16, 17, 19 - 21, 31].

Low-risk CHDs frequently have normal four-chamber view (4CH) (69.4%) and three-vessel view (3VV) (44.9%) [8], which results in low detection because of the suspicion of CHD in screening examinations. This is probably the CHD group with the lowest prenatal detection rate [8]. The prognosis for newborns delivered at term is exceptionally good although coexisting ECMs influence the mortality rate, which is significantly higher in the CHD + ECM group than that in the isolated low-risk CHD and CHD + ECA groups [8]. The most common prenatally diagnosed low-risk CHDs are VSD, atrioventricular defects, TOF, and mild aorta stenosis, (AS) and pulmonary stenosis (PS).

VSD is a CHD with exceptionally good prognosis, ECMs being the only factor that complicates the outcome [8]. Minor VSD usually closes itself in the prenatal period or the first month after birth [33]. If this does not occur, neonates are qualified for surgery, mostly between the 6th and 12th months of life.

AVSDs frequently coexist with other cardiac malformations or ECMs and genetic syndromes, that is why highly precise examinations are required to exclude additional problems. In the case of isolated AVSDs, the prognosis is exceptionally good, and 10 years of survival after cardio surgery is achieved in 80% of the cases. Complex AVSDs with additional cardiac malformations are classified as high-risk CHD. Isolated AVSDs require routine care, delivery in a local hospital, telemedicine consultation, and outpatient cardiology follow-up and do not need specialized care in a DR. Isolated AVSDs have 100% of survival, whereas AVSD + ECM has only 18% (p = 0.002) [8]. This is why consultations in referral centers, after prenatal detection of AVSDs are required in all fetuses.

TOF exists in 2–3 of 10,000 live births [34, 35]. TOF is usually characterized by normal 4CH, except for TOF with pulmonary atresia (PvA), but this type of TOF is classified as a high-risk CHD. Medium-risk TOF can be detected prenatally on the basis of 3VV, which is abnormal in nearly 98% of fetuses with TOF [8]. Increasing gradient of the pulmonary valve between the 21st and 36th weeks of pregnancy causes growing disproportion between the aorta and pulmonary artery sometimes observed in 3VV only in the third trimester. It is highly important for obstetricians to check the 3VV in both second and third trimesters. The delivery plan is based on the prediction of infants with TOF who will be cyanotic after ductal closure. Medium-risk TOF has mild PS with peak systolic velocity <140–160 cm/s and usually does not require prostaglandin infusion or cardio surgery in the neonatal period [36]. Another study by Donofrio *et al.* shows that, in fetuses with TOF, the presence of reversed flow in the ductus arteriosus (DA) has a sensitivity of 100% and specificity of 97% in the prediction of the need for PGE1 at birth and subsequent neonatal surgery [37, 38]. This TOF is classified as high-risk CHD. Pulmonary stenosis in TOF can progress during the fetal period, which means that serial echocardiography and monitoring of the growth and gradient of the pulmonary valve and presence of the reversed flow in DA should be performed every 4 weeks until delivery [38, 39]. The final qualification of the fetus with TOF to the group with low or medium risk should be performed after 35 weeks of pregnancy.

PS and AS are CHDs that are characterized by fast progression during the fetal period [40, 41]. Appropriate management in DRs can assure exceptionally good prognosis for low- and high-risk fetuses with PS and AS [8, 20]. Low-risk stenosis usually has normal 4CH and 3VV; the only feature that can be observed is high flow (Fig. **1**), which in low-risk stenosis is usually <200 cm/s [8]. Detection of stenosis in the early fetal period can be crucial as it provides the chance to consider prenatal therapy; otherwise, we can have an infant with HLHS at term.

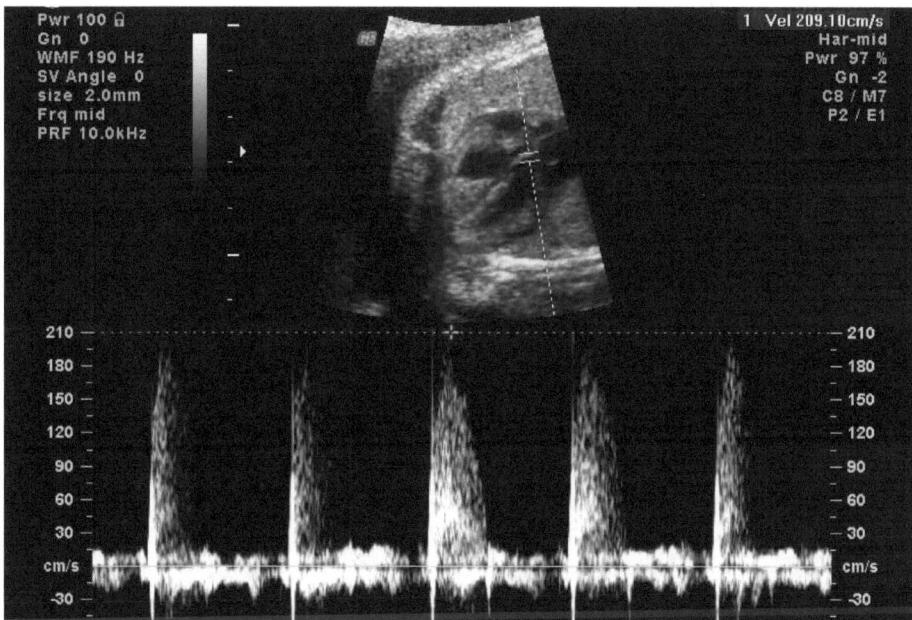

Fig. (1). Mild aortic stenosis in fetuses at 25 weeks of pregnancy. Normal 4-chamber view, abnormal aortic flow, and Vmax of 200 cm/s.

SEVERE PLANNED CHD

Medium-risk CHD: LOC 2 [20], ENCI 2 and 3 [21], and Care Plan 3 [17]

Medium-risk CHDs form the largest group of CHDs diagnosed prenatally (66%). They are usually ductal-dependent lesions and require prostaglandin infusion (84%) [8]. The mode and time of delivery should be planned ≥39 weeks, with a neonatologist in the DR and transport to a cardiac center for catheterization/surgery, if required. In the medium-risk group, we can also find AVSD and TOF, but in these cases, the hemodynamic changes result in the classification as the medium-risk group (unbalanced AVSD, TOF with reversed flow in DA). The mortality rate in medium-risk CHD is approximately 15% but increases to 35% with presence of ECAs (p = 0.087) [8]. The most common prenatally diagnosed medium-risk CHDs are HLHS, d-TGA, DORV, CHD with single ventricle, CoA, TvA, PvA, interrupted aortic arch (IAA), and truncus arteriosus. Classified as medium-risk CHDs, these usually require cardio surgery in the first weeks of life [8, 16, 17, 19 - 21, 31].

CoA and IAA are extremely difficult to detect and differentiate prenatally [42, 43], and still many cases diagnosed prenatally have false-positive diagnoses, probably due to the umbilical cord around the neck, which was frequently observed with disproportion in 4CH. This clinical observation from Poland requires a prospective study on a larger group of fetuses [44, 45].

AVSD is classified as a medium-risk CHD coexisting with other cardiac problems, usually DORV, CoA, or TOF. Sometimes, we can have unbalanced AVSD, which may require cardio surgery in the first week of life [8].

TOF as a severe planned CHD coexists with PvA and major aortopulmonary collateral arteries [8, 46].

HLHS is one of the CHDs that are most often diagnosed prenatally [47]. Improvements in prenatal diagnosis and cardio surgery allow several patients to survive, with the survival rate reaching 80% [8, 48 - 51]. Prognosis for fetuses with HLHS depends on many factors such as ECA, tricuspid regurgitation, and prenatally detected FO restriction [8, 51, 52]. The difference in mortality between fetuses with HLHS with and without risk factors is statistically significant [8, 51, 53]. Of all evaluated Doppler parameters, a forward/reverse velocity time integral ratio (VTIf/VTIr) of pulmonary vein flow >5 (Fig. **2**) is a sensitive predictor that emergent postnatal atrial septectomy is unnecessary [53]. Owing to the potential for disease progression in fetuses with HLHS, pregnant women carrying fetuses with HLHS should have serial echocardiographic examinations with the final study conducted late in the third trimester, 2 to 3 weeks before delivery, to assess pulmonary vein flows and changes in right ventricular function and the presence or increase of tricuspid insufficiency [52 - 54].

d-TGA exists in 7% of fetuses with CHD and is one of the most common ductal-dependent defects. It is also extremely difficult to detect because of normal 4CH and remarkably rare coexistence with ECMs and genetic syndromes [8]. 3VV is greatly helpful in detecting d-TGA prenatally [55]. Prenatal detection is crucial in planning the treatment and affects short- and long-term outcomes [56, 57]. Detecting d-TGA prenatally is just the first step, and the second step, which is even more difficult, is to differentiate severe planned and critical d-TGA. d-TGA is not only ductal dependent but also FO dependent. Sometimes prostaglandin administration is insufficient, so it is greatly important to assess both connections, especially near the delivery [58], to differentiate severe planned and critical d-TGA [8]. Severe planned d-TGA is characterized by wide FO, patent DA, and maximum velocity "s" wave <41 cm/s in pulmonary vein Doppler (Fig. **3**), proximal to the left atrium [58 - 61].

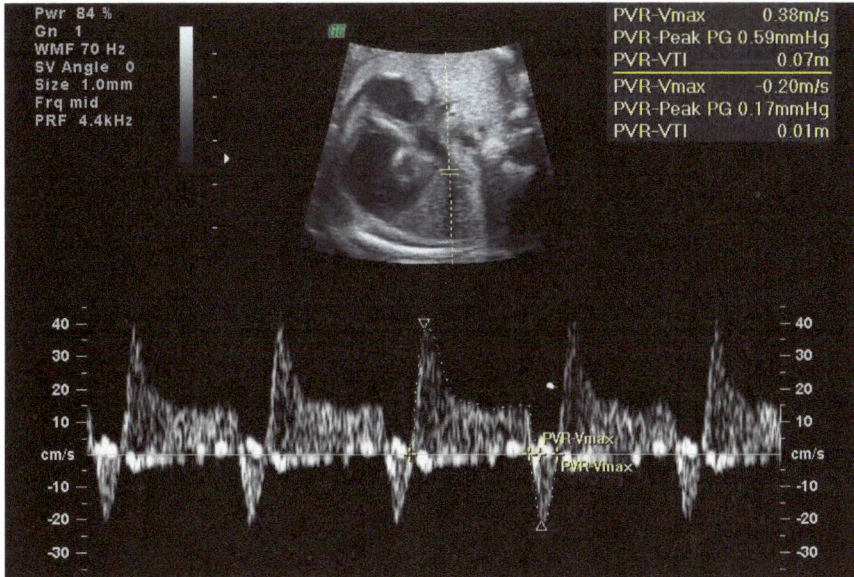

Fig. (2). Fetus with severe planned hypoplastic left heart syndrome with velocity time integral index >5.

SEVERE URGENT CHD

High-risk CHD: LOC 3 [20], ENCI 3 and 4 [21], and Care Plan 3 or 4 [17]

Severe urgent CHDs are lesions that usually require treatment in the first day of life. The typical severe urgent CHDs are HLHS with restricted FO, d-TGA with restricted FO, critical AS, and totally abnormal pulmonary venous connection. In fetuses with HLHS, FO is crucial for pulmonary circulation during the fetal period; its normal flow assures normal pulmonary vessel development. Restricted FO is diagnosed in 6–20% of fetuses [8, 62 - 64]. Restricted FO sometimes requires balloon valvuloplasty before the first stage of surgery. To improve outcomes in fetuses with HLHS with restricted FO, a number of centers worldwide perform balloon valvuloplasty in the first hours after delivery [54, 62, 64]. Therefore, it is greatly important to detect these groups of fetuses and organize the delivery in referral centers that are prepared to perform catheterization a few hours after delivery [54]. This requires exceptionally effective cooperation among obstetricians, neonatologists, and cardiologists [14 - 16, 31].

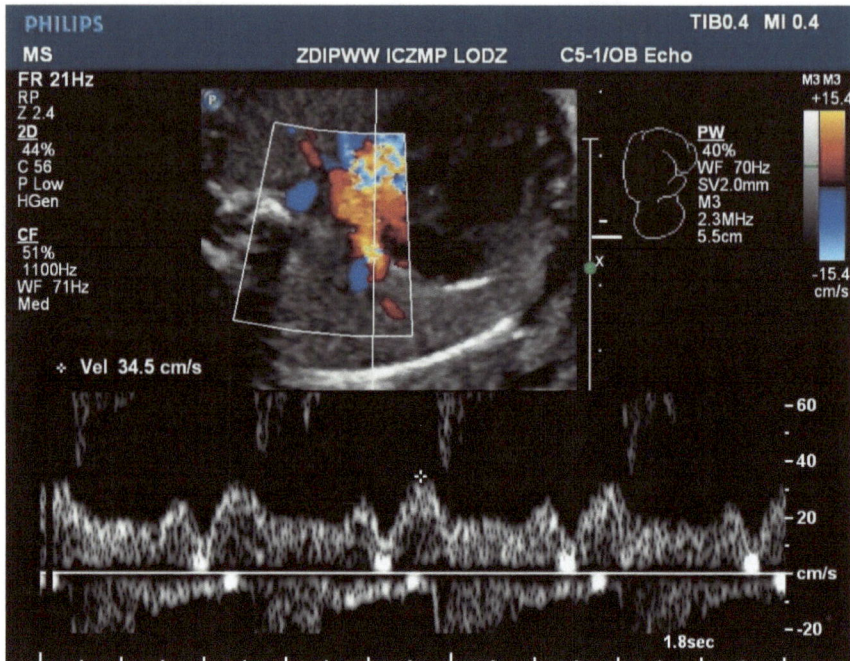

Fig. (3). Fetus with severe planned dextro-transposition of the great arteries with maximum pulmonary vein flow <41 cm/s.

It is greatly important to monitor fetuses with **HLHS** and check their FO status. Direct assessment of FO is difficult and hardly accountable. The only factor that has become accountable is its width, but it has no relationship with the condition of the infant after birth [65, 66]. Increased A-wave flow in systemic veins reflects high pressure in the right atrium [67, 68]. It has been proved that, in assessing FO restriction, we only need to check pulmonary vein flow [65, 66, 69, 70]. The outcome of fetuses with FO restriction improves after immediate catheterization after delivery [71].

The classification of prenatally diagnosed HLHS can be based on the study presented by Michelfelder *et al.* and Divanovic *et al.* [53, 72]. They predict urgent Rashkind procedure after delivery, assessing pulmonary vein flow. They have proved that the best factor is the ratio of forward/reverse flow of VTI (Fig. **2**). Forward/reverse VTI ratio <5 could be an indication of urgent Rashkind procedure after delivery [53]. In 2011, Divanovic *et al.* revealed that a VTI ratio <3 is the most predictable factor (Fig. **4**). On the basis of their study, prenatally diagnosed HLHS can be classified as severe planned if the VTI ratio is >5 and urgent if the VTI ratio is <5. If the ratio is <3, a prenatal intervention should be considered [72]. All fetuses with HLHS require regular monitoring every 4 weeks because the restriction and pulmonary vein flow can change during pregnancy and the VTI ratio can deteriorate.

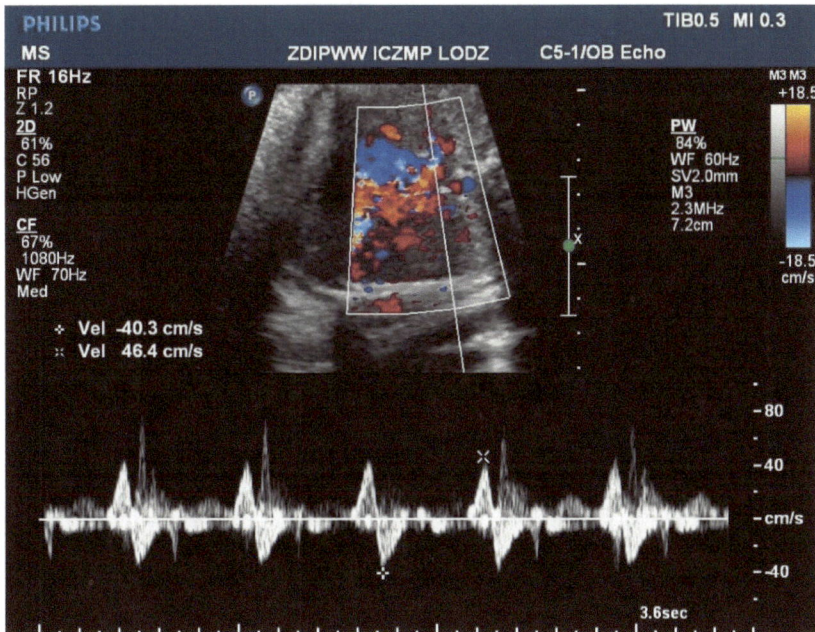

Fig. (4). Fetus with severe urgent hypoplastic left heart syndrome with velocity time integral index <3.

To classify **d-TGA** as severe planned or urgent, we need to assess FO, DA, and pulmonary vein flow [58, 61]. Prenatal FO restriction in the normal heart anatomy is extremely rare [73, 74], but in the case of CHD, the restriction may occur more often and have a crucial meaning in terms of prognosis and outcomes [14, 58, 59]. In fetuses with d-TGA, cardiac output to the DA is approximately 20% and differs from the normal heart-approximately 30–40%. Frequently, this causes prenatal restriction of the DA [75, 76]. We need to regularly monitor fetuses with d-TGA, especially near term. Several studies address the problem of false-positive classification to severe planned d-TGA [14]. The reason could be extremely long interval between fetal echocardiography examination and delivery [8, 14]. Fetuses with d-TGA need to be monitored every 4 weeks and even every week after 38 weeks of pregnancy [31]. The factors that cause FO restriction are numerous and complex. As presented in 2017, one of these factors is pulmonary vein flow. Two centers' retrospective studies revealed an extremely high risk of urgent Rashkind procedure after birth in fetuses with maximum pulmonary vein flow >41 cm/s (Fig. **5**), regardless of FO status [61].

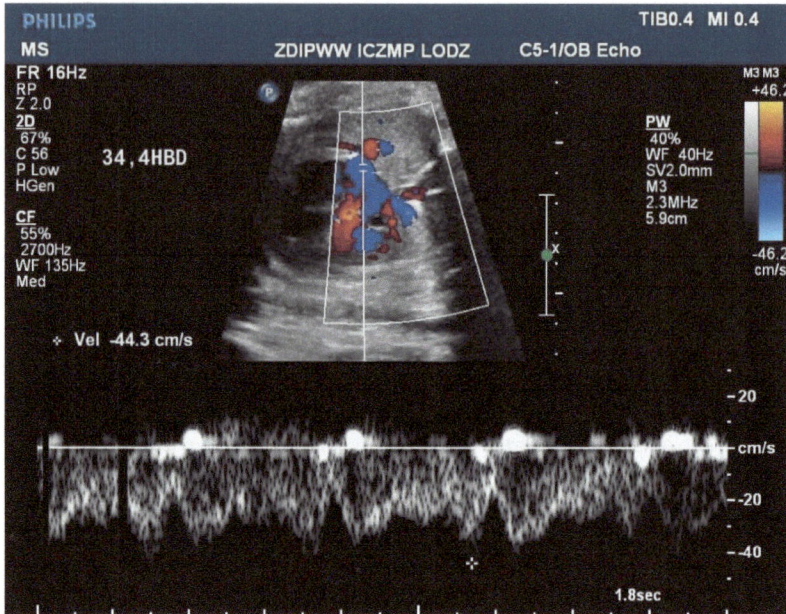

Fig. (5). Fetus with severe urgent dextro-transposition of the great arteries with maximum pulmonary vein flow >41 cm/s.

AS is a CHD that can progress extremely quickly during pregnancy [40, 41]. AS can be classified in all groups of the new classification depending on the hemodynamic status. Usually, it is a low-risk CHD, but these cases are rarely detected during pregnancy because they have normal 4CH and 3VV. In many cases, the progression leads to HLHS, and consequently, a prenatal intervention is considered [77 - 79]. In critical AS, which was a lethal condition in 1996, urgent catheterization after birth is crucial in terms of saving the newborn's life [80, 81]. In some cases of critical AS, transplacental digoxin therapy can help the fetus reach maturity and enable immediate catheterization after delivery at term [81 - 83].

SEVEREST CHD

Extremely High-risk CHD: LOC 4 [20], ENCI 4 [21], and Care Plan 5 [17]

Fetuses with severest isolated heart defects are usually those with AS, HLHS, and Ebstein's anomaly accompanied by cardiomegaly (HA/CA > 0.6). In the case of HLHS, the critical point is an intact atrial septum that causes abnormal pulmonary vascular development. Changes in the vessel structure are irreversible and lead to neonatal demise [63]. These fetuses usually die after delivery, with no urgent intervention [8, 54]. For these fetuses, *in utero* septal valvuloplasty is seen as a chance to improve the survival rate [71, 84]. The best effect was achieved after the procedure was performed between 28 and 30 weeks of pregnancy [84]. In the case of the severest forms of AS and Ebstein's anomaly, the main cause of infant death was pulmonary hypoplasia associated with serious cardiomegaly (HA/CA > 0.6) in the fetal period. In this heart defect group, the death rate was 100% [8]. The only chance to survive for fetuses with severest CHD is immediate stabilization in the DR. In such infants, immediate cardiac interventions in the DR after delivery, such as cardiac catheterization, pediatric cardiothoracic surgery, or initiation of extracorporeal membrane oxygenation, must be available [14].

CONCLUSION

The *in utero* progression of CHD can be observed in almost all CHDs during the first, second, and third trimesters of pregnancy. The progression of cardiac disease can be associated with worsening of structural defects, such as worsening of hypoplasia, new onset of FO restriction, decreased ventricular inflow or outflow, and worsening arch obstruction. We can also observe new onset or progressive valvular regurgitation, diminution or closure of a VSD, and development of congestive heart failure with high risk for poor perinatal outcomes such as Ebstein's anomaly and TOF with absent pulmonary valve. The potential progression of CHD severity *in utero* supports sequential evaluation to detect a potential change in the qualification of the fetus to one of the groups of the new classification. The only tool for the proper qualification of fetuses with HLHS, among others, to one of the three groups of the new classification system is fetal echocardiography. The role of contemporary fetal cardiologists is not to diagnose CHDs but to foresee the condition of the newborn after delivery and plan potential treatment in the first hours-or even minutes-of life. For this reason, pregnancy and delivery management of newborns with a prenatal diagnosis of CHD require a multidisciplinary team composed of fetal and pediatric cardiologists, obstetricians and maternal–fetal specialists, neonatologists, and other pediatric specialists.

CONSENT FOR PUBLICATION

Not applicable.

CONFLICT OF INTEREST

The authors confirm that the contents of this chapter have no conflict of interest.

ACKNOWLEDGEMENTS

Declare none.

REFERENCES

[1]   Hoffman JI, Kaplan S. The incidence of congenital heart disease. J Am Coll Cardiol 2002; 39(12): 1890-900.
       [http://dx.doi.org/10.1016/S0735-1097(02)01886-7] [PMID: 12084585]

[2]   Nelle M, Raio L, Pavlovic M, Carrel T, Surbek D, Meyer-Wittkopf M. Prenatal diagnosis and treatment planning of congenital heart defects-possibilities and limits. World J Pediatr 2009; 5(1): 18-22.
       [http://dx.doi.org/10.1007/s12519-009-0003-8] [PMID: 19172327]

[3]   Eurocat – European Surveillance of Congenital Anomalies. http://www.eurocat-network.eu /statisticalmonitoring-2009

[4]   Clur SA, Van Brussel PM, Mathijssen IB, Pajkrt E, Ottenkamp J, Bilardo CM. Audit of 10 years of referrals for fetal echocardiography. Prenat Diagn 2011; 31(12): 1134-40.
       [http://dx.doi.org/10.1002/pd.2847] [PMID: 21915886]

[5]   Berg KA, Clark EB, Astemborski JA, Boughman JA. Prenatal detection of cardiovascular malformations by echocardiography: an indication for cytogenetic evaluation. Am J Obstet Gynecol 1988; 159(2): 477-81.
       [http://dx.doi.org/10.1016/S0002-9378(88)80113-3] [PMID: 3407707]

[6]   Paladini D, Calabrò R, Palmieri S, D'Andrea T. Prenatal diagnosis of congenital heart disease and fetal karyotyping. Obstet Gynecol 1993; 81(5 (Pt 1)): 679-82.
       [PMID: 8469453]

[7]   Nicolaides K, Shawwa L, Brizot M, Snijders R. Ultrasonographically detectable markers of fetal chromosomal defects. Ultrasound Obstet Gynecol 1993; 3(1): 56-69.
       [http://dx.doi.org/10.1046/j.1469-0705.1993.03010056.x] [PMID: 12796906]

[8]   Słodki M. Habilitation Thesis 2012. https://www.researchgate.net/publication/2913377775_ Prenatal_and_perinatal_management_for_pregnant_women_with_fetal_cardiac_defects_based_on_ne w_prenatal_cardiac_anomalies_classification_Polish

[9]   Allan LD, Huggon IC. Counselling following a diagnosis of congenital heart disease. Prenat Diagn 2004; 24(13): 1136-42.
       [http://dx.doi.org/10.1002/pd.1071] [PMID: 15614846]

[10]   Tworetzky W, McElhinney DB, Reddy VM, Brook MM, Hanley FL, Silverman NH. Improved surgical outcome after fetal diagnosis of hypoplastic left heart syndrome. Circulation 2001; 103(9): 1269-73.
       [http://dx.doi.org/10.1161/01.CIR.103.9.1269] [PMID: 11238272]

[11]   Kipps AK, Feuille C, Azakie A, *et al.* Prenatal diagnosis of hypoplastic left heart syndrome in current era. Am J Cardiol 2011; 108(3): 421-7.
       [http://dx.doi.org/10.1016/j.amjcard.2011.03.065] [PMID: 21624547]

[12]   Colaco SM, Karande T, Bobhate PR, Jiyani R, Rao SG, Kulkarni S. Neonates with critical congenital heart defects: Impact of fetal diagnosis on immediate and short-term outcomes. Ann Pediatr Cardiol 2017; 10(2): 126-30.
       [http://dx.doi.org/10.4103/apc.APC_125_16] [PMID: 28566819]

[13]   Mahle WT, Clancy RR, McGaurn SP, Goin JE, Clark BJ. Impact of prenatal diagnosis on survival and early neurologic morbidity in neonates with the hypoplastic left heart syndrome. Pediatrics 2001; 107(6): 1277-82.
       [http://dx.doi.org/10.1542/peds.107.6.1277] [PMID: 11389243]

[14]   Donofrio MT, Moon-Grady AJ, Hornberger LK, *et al.* American Heart Association Adults With Congenital Heart Disease Joint Committee of the Council on Cardiovascular Disease in the Young and Council on Clinical Cardiology, Council on Cardiovascular Surgery and Anesthesia, and Council on Cardiovascular and Stroke Nursing. Diagnosis and treatment of fetal cardiac disease: a scientific

statement from the American Heart Association. Circulation 2014; 129(21): 2183-242.
[http://dx.doi.org/10.1161/01.cir.0000437597.44550.5d] [PMID: 24763516]

[15] Brown KL, Sullivan ID. Prenatal detection for major congenital heart disease: a key process measure for congenital heart networks. Heart 2014; 100(5): 359-60.
[http://dx.doi.org/10.1136/heartjnl-2013-305161] [PMID: 24402769]

[16] Sanapo L, Pruetz JD, Słodki M, Goens MB, Moon-Grady AJ, Donofrio MT. Fetal echocardiography for planning perinatal and delivery room care of neonates with congenital heart disease. Echocardiography 2017; 34(12): 1804-21.
[http://dx.doi.org/10.1111/echo.13672] [PMID: 29287132]

[17] Berkley EM, Goens MB, Karr S, Rappaport V. Utility of fetal echocardiography in postnatal management of infants with prenatally diagnosed congenital heart disease. Prenat Diagn 2009; 29(7): 654-8.
[http://dx.doi.org/10.1002/pd.2260] [PMID: 19340841]

[18] Clur SA, Van Brussel PM, Ottenkamp J, Bilardo CM. Prenatal diagnosis of cardiac defects: accuracy and benefit. Prenat Diagn 2012; 32(5): 450-5.
[http://dx.doi.org/10.1002/pd.3837] [PMID: 22495905]

[19] Respondek-Liberska M. Atlas of congenital heart disease.Lodz: Adi Art;. 2011.

[20] Donofrio MT, Levy RJ, Schuette JJ, et al. Specialized delivery room planning for fetuses with critical congenital heart disease. Am J Cardiol 2013; 111(5): 737-47.
[http://dx.doi.org/10.1016/j.amjcard.2012.11.029] [PMID: 23291087]

[21] Pruetz JD, Carroll C, Trento LU, et al. Outcomes of critical congenital heart disease requiring emergent neonatal cardiac intervention. Prenat Diagn 2014; 34(12): 1127-32.
[http://dx.doi.org/10.1002/pd.4438] [PMID: 24947130]

[22] Wald N, Kennard A. Routine ultrasound scanning for congenital abnormalities. Ann N Y Acad Sci 1998; 847: 173-80.
[http://dx.doi.org/10.1111/j.1749-6632.1998.tb08937.x] [PMID: 9668709]

[23] Copel JA, Pilu G, Kleinman CS. Congenital heart disease and extracardiac anomalies: associations and indications for fetal echocardiography. Am J Obstet Gynecol 1986; 154(5): 1121-32.
[http://dx.doi.org/10.1016/0002-9378(86)90773-8] [PMID: 2939723]

[24] Fogel M, Copel JA, Cullen MT, Hobbins JC, Kleinman CS. Congenital heart disease and fetal thoracoabdominal anomalies: associations *in utero* and the importance of cytogenetic analysis. Am J Perinatol 1991; 8(6): 411-6.
[http://dx.doi.org/10.1055/s-2007-999427] [PMID: 1839950]

[25] Tennstedt C, Chaoui R, Körner H, Dietel M. Spectrum of congenital heart defects and extracardiac malformations associated with chromosomal abnormalities: results of a seven year necropsy study. Heart 1999; 82(1): 34-9.
[http://dx.doi.org/10.1136/hrt.82.1.34] [PMID: 10377306]

[26] Russo MG, Paladini D, Pacileo G, et al. Changing spectrum and outcome of 705 fetal congenital heart disease cases: 12 years, experience in a third-level center. J Cardiovasc Med (Hagerstown) 2008; 9(9): 910-5.
[http://dx.doi.org/10.2459/JCM.0b013e32830212cf] [PMID: 18695428]

[27] Respondek-Liberska M, Papis A, Oszukowski P, et al. [Fetal echocardiography in 83 fetuses with omphalocele from Dept. for Diagnoses and Prevention of Fetal Malformations, Research Institute Polish Mother's Memorial Hospital, and Medical University of Lodz, (1999-2006)]. Ginekol Pol 2008; 79(9): 602-11.
[PMID: 18939510]

[28] Paladini D, Tartaglione A, Agangi A, et al. The association between congenital heart disease and Down syndrome in prenatal life. Ultrasound Obstet Gynecol 2000; 15(2): 104-8.

[http://dx.doi.org/10.1046/j.1469-0705.2000.00027.x] [PMID: 10775990]

[29] Pierpont ME, Markwald RR, Lin AE. Genetic aspects of atrioventricular septal defects. Am J Med Genet 2000; 97(4): 289-96.
[http://dx.doi.org/10.1002/1096-8628(200024)97:4<289::AID-AJMG1279>3.0.CO;2-U] [PMID: 11376440]

[30] Friedberg MK, Kim N, Silverman NH. Atrioventricular septal defect recently diagnosed by fetal echocardiography: echocardiographic features, associated anomalies, and outcomes. Congenit Heart Dis 2007; 2(2): 110-4.
[http://dx.doi.org/10.1111/j.1747-0803.2007.00082.x] [PMID: 18377486]

[31] Słodki M, Respondek-Liberska M, Pruetz JD, Donofrio MT. Fetal cardiology: changing the definition of critical heart disease in the newborn. J Perinatol 2016; 36(8): 575-80.
[http://dx.doi.org/10.1038/jp.2016.20] [PMID: 26963427]

[32] Trines J, Hornberger LK. Evolution of heart disease *in utero*. Pediatr Cardiol 2004; 25(3): 287-98.
[http://dx.doi.org/10.1007/s00246-003-0592-2] [PMID: 15360119]

[33] Lin MH, Wang NK, Hung KL, Shen CT. Spontaneous closure of ventricular septal defects in the first year of life. J Formos Med Assoc 2001; 100(8): 539-42.
[PMID: 11678004]

[34] Apitz C, Webb GD, Redington AN. Tetralogy of Fallot. Lancet 2009; 374(9699): 1462-71.
[http://dx.doi.org/10.1016/S0140-6736(09)60657-7] [PMID: 19683809]

[35] Starr JP. Tetralogy of fallot: yesterday and today. World J Surg 2010; 34(4): 658-68.
[http://dx.doi.org/10.1007/s00268-009-0296-8] [PMID: 20091166]

[36] Escribano D, Herraiz I, Granados M, Arbues J, Mendoza A, Galindo A. Tetralogy of Fallot: prediction of outcome in the mid-second trimester of pregnancy. Prenat Diagn 2011; 31(12): 1126-33.
[http://dx.doi.org/10.1002/pd.2844] [PMID: 21928295]

[37] Donofrio MT, Skurow-Todd K, Berger JT, *et al.* Risk-stratified postnatal care of newborns with congenital heart disease determined by fetal echocardiography. J Am Soc Echocardiogr 2015; 28(11): 1339-49.
[http://dx.doi.org/10.1016/j.echo.2015.07.005] [PMID: 26298099]

[38] Pepas LP, Savis A, Jones A, Sharland GK, Tulloh RM, Simpson JM. An echocardiographic study of tetralogy of Fallot in the fetus and infant. Cardiol Young 2003; 13(3): 240-7.
[http://dx.doi.org/10.1017/S1047951103000477] [PMID: 12903870]

[39] Hornberger LK, Sanders SP, Sahn DJ, *et al. In utero* pulmonary artery and aortic growth and potential for progression of pulmonary outflow tract obstruction in tetralogy of Fallot. J Am Coll Cardiol 1995; 25(3): 739-45.
[http://dx.doi.org/10.1016/0735-1097(94)00422-M] [PMID: 7860923]

[40] Simpson JM, Sharland GK. Natural history and outcome of aortic stenosis diagnosed prenatally. Heart 1997; 77(3): 205-10.
[http://dx.doi.org/10.1136/hrt.77.3.205] [PMID: 9093035]

[41] Gardiner HM. Progression of fetal heart disease and rationale for fetal intracardiac interventions. Semin Fetal Neonatal Med 2005; 10(6): 578-85.
[http://dx.doi.org/10.1016/j.siny.2005.08.001] [PMID: 16213202]

[42] Słodki M, Rychik J, Moszura T, Janiak K, Respondek-Liberska M. Measurement of the great vessels in the mediastinum could help distinguish true from false-positive coarctation of the aorta in the third trimester. J Ultrasound Med 2009; 28(10): 1313-7.
[http://dx.doi.org/10.7863/jum.2009.28.10.1313] [PMID: 19778876]

[43] Słodki M, Moszura T, Janiak K, *et al.* The three-vessel view in the fetal mediastinum in the diagnosis of interrupted aortic arch. Ultrasound Med Biol 2011; 37(11): 1808-13.
[http://dx.doi.org/10.1016/j.ultrasmedbio.2011.06.002] [PMID: 21840641]

[44]   Więckowska K, Zych-Krekora K, Słodki M, Respondek-Liberska M. Do umbilical cord wrapped around the fetal body can mimic signs of aortal coarctation? Prenat Cardiol 2016; 6: 82-6.
[http://dx.doi.org/10.1515/pcard-2016-0011]

[45]   Słodki M, Taranenko K, Zych-Krekora K, Respondek-Liberska M. New explanation of false-positive diagnosis of coarctation of the aorta during fetal life. Ultrasound Obstet Gynecol 2018; 52 (Suppl. 1): 184.
[http://dx.doi.org/10.1002/uog.19758]

[46]   Moszura T, Janiak K, Respondek-Liberska M, *et al*. Prenatal diagnosis of major aortopulmonary collateral arteries. Kardiol Pol 2011; 69(2): 146-51.
[PMID: 21332055]

[47]   Kordjalik P, Tobota Z, Respondek-Liberska M. Selected data from the Polish National Prenatal Cardiac Pathology Registry from the year 2016. Prenat Cardiol 2017; 7: 7-11.
[http://dx.doi.org/10.1515/pcard-2017-0002]

[48]   Goldberg CS, Gomez CA. Hypoplastic left heart syndrome: new developments and current controversies. Semin Neonatol 2003; 8(6): 461-8.
[http://dx.doi.org/10.1016/S1084-2756(03)00116-7] [PMID: 15001118]

[49]   Brackley KJ, Kilby MD, Wright JG, *et al*. Outcome after prenatal diagnosis of hypoplastic left-heart syndrome: a case series. Lancet 2000; 356(9236): 1143-7.
[http://dx.doi.org/10.1016/S0140-6736(00)02756-2] [PMID: 11030293]

[50]   Feinstein JA, Benson DW, Dubin AM, *et al*. Hypoplastic left heart syndrome: current considerations and expectations. J Am Coll Cardiol 2012; 59(1) (Suppl.): S1-S42.
[http://dx.doi.org/10.1016/j.jacc.2011.09.022] [PMID: 22192720]

[51]   Rychik J, Szwast A, Natarajan S, *et al*. Perinatal and early surgical outcome for the fetus with hypoplastic left heart syndrome: a 5-year single institutional experience. Ultrasound Obstet Gynecol 2010; 36(4): 465-70.
[http://dx.doi.org/10.1002/uog.7674] [PMID: 20499409]

[52]   Rychik J. Hypoplastic left heart syndrome: from *in-utero* diagnosis to school age. Semin Fetal Neonatal Med 2005; 10(6): 553-66.
[http://dx.doi.org/10.1016/j.siny.2005.08.006] [PMID: 16243013]

[53]   Michelfelder E, Gomez C, Border W, Gottliebson W, Franklin C. Predictive value of fetal pulmonary venous flow patterns in identifying the need for atrial septoplasty in the newborn with hypoplastic left ventricle. Circulation 2005; 112(19): 2974-9.
[http://dx.doi.org/10.1161/CIRCULATIONAHA.105.534180] [PMID: 16260632]

[54]   Glatz JA, Tabbutt S, Gaynor JW, *et al*. Hypoplastic left heart syndrome with atrial level restriction in the era of prenatal diagnosis. Ann Thorac Surg 2007; 84(5): 1633-8.
[http://dx.doi.org/10.1016/j.athoracsur.2007.06.061] [PMID: 17954074]

[55]   Yoo SJ, Lee YH, Kim ES, *et al*. Three-vessel view of the fetal upper mediastinum: an easy means of detecting abnormalities of the ventricular outflow tracts and great arteries during obstetric screening. Ultrasound Obstet Gynecol 1997; 9(3): 173-82.
[http://dx.doi.org/10.1046/j.1469-0705.1997.09030173.x] [PMID: 9165680]

[56]   Bonnet D, Coltri A, Butera G, *et al*. Detection of transposition of the great arteries in fetuses reduces neonatal morbidity and mortality. Circulation 1999; 99(7): 916-8.
[http://dx.doi.org/10.1161/01.CIR.99.7.916] [PMID: 10027815]

[57]   Calderon J, Angeard N, Moutier S, Plumet MH, Jambaqué I, Bonnet D. Impact of prenatal diagnosis on neurocognitive outcomes in children with transposition of the great arteries. J Pediatr 2012; 161(1): 94-8.e1.
[http://dx.doi.org/10.1016/j.jpeds.2011.12.036] [PMID: 22284567]

[58]   Maeno YV, Kamenir SA, Sinclair B, van der Velde ME, Smallhorn JF, Hornberger LK. Prenatal

features of ductus arteriosus constriction and restrictive foramen ovale in d-transposition of the great arteries. Circulation 1999; 99(9): 1209-14.
[http://dx.doi.org/10.1161/01.CIR.99.9.1209] [PMID: 10069789]

[59]   Jouannic JM, Gavard L, Fermont L, *et al*. Sensitivity and specificity of prenatal features of physiological shunts to predict neonatal clinical status in transposition of the great arteries. Circulation 2004; 110(13): 1743-6.
[http://dx.doi.org/10.1161/01.CIR.0000144141.18560.CF] [PMID: 15364811]

[60]   Punn R, Silverman NH. Fetal predictors of urgent balloon atrial septostomy in neonates with complete transposition. J Am Soc Echocardiogr 2011; 24(4): 425-30.
[http://dx.doi.org/10.1016/j.echo.2010.12.020] [PMID: 21324642]

[61]   Słodki M, Axt-Fliedner R, Zych-Krekora K, *et al*. International Prenatal Cardiology Collaboration Group. New method to predict need for Rashkind procedure in fetuses with dextro-transposition of the great arteries. Ultrasound Obstet Gynecol 2018; 51(4): 531-6.
[http://dx.doi.org/10.1002/uog.17469] [PMID: 28295809]

[62]   Atz AM, Feinstein JA, Jonas RA, Perry SB, Wessel DL. Preoperative management of pulmonary venous hypertension in hypoplastic left heart syndrome with restrictive atrial septal defect. Am J Cardiol 1999; 83(8): 1224-8.
[http://dx.doi.org/10.1016/S0002-9149(99)00087-9] [PMID: 10215289]

[63]   Rychik J, Rome JJ, Collins MH, DeCampli WM, Spray TL. The hypoplastic left heart syndrome with intact atrial septum: atrial morphology, pulmonary vascular histopathology and outcome. J Am Coll Cardiol 1999; 34(2): 554-60.
[http://dx.doi.org/10.1016/S0735-1097(99)00225-9] [PMID: 10440172]

[64]   Vlahos AP, Lock JE, McElhinney DB, van der Velde ME. Hypoplastic left heart syndrome with intact or highly restrictive atrial septum: outcome after neonatal transcatheter atrial septostomy. Circulation 2004; 109(19): 2326-30.
[http://dx.doi.org/10.1161/01.CIR.0000128690.35860.C5] [PMID: 15136496]

[65]   Better DJ, Apfel HD, Zidere V, Allan LD. Pattern of pulmonary venous blood flow in the hypoplastic left heart syndrome in the fetus. Heart 1999; 81(6): 646-9.
[http://dx.doi.org/10.1136/hrt.81.6.646] [PMID: 10336926]

[66]   Taketazu M, Barrea C, Smallhorn JF, Wilson GJ, Hornberger LK. Intrauterine pulmonary venous flow and restrictive foramen ovale in fetal hypoplastic left heart syndrome. J Am Coll Cardiol 2004; 43(10): 1902-7.
[http://dx.doi.org/10.1016/j.jacc.2004.01.033] [PMID: 15145119]

[67]   Klein AL, Hatle LK, Burstow DJ, *et al*. Comprehensive Doppler assessment of right ventricular diastolic function in cardiac amyloidosis. J Am Coll Cardiol 1990; 15(1): 99-108.
[http://dx.doi.org/10.1016/0735-1097(90)90183-P] [PMID: 2295749]

[68]   Reed KL, Appleton CP, Anderson CF, Shenker L, Sahn DJ. Doppler studies of vena cava flows in human fetuses. Insights into normal and abnormal cardiac physiology. Circulation 1990; 81(2): 498-505.
[http://dx.doi.org/10.1161/01.CIR.81.2.498] [PMID: 2404632]

[69]   Allan L. Pulmonary venous flow reversal. Ultrasound Obstet Gynecol 1996; 8(3): 212.
[http://dx.doi.org/10.1046/j.1469-0705.1996.08030210-4.x] [PMID: 8915095]

[70]   Lenz F, Machlitt A, Hartung J, Bollmann R, Chaoui R. Fetal pulmonary venous flow pattern is determined by left atrial pressure: report of two cases of left heart hypoplasia, one with patent and the other with closed interatrial communication. Ultrasound Obstet Gynecol 2002; 19(4): 392-5.
[http://dx.doi.org/10.1046/j.1469-0705.2002.00684.x] [PMID: 11952970]

[71]   Vida VL, Bacha EA, Larrazabal A, *et al*. Hypoplastic left heart syndrome with intact or highly restrictive atrial septum: surgical experience from a single center. Ann Thorac Surg 2007; 84(2): 581-5.

[http://dx.doi.org/10.1016/j.athoracsur.2007.04.017] [PMID: 17643639]

[72] Divanović A, Hor K, Cnota J, Hirsch R, Kinsel-Ziter M, Michelfelder E. Prediction and perinatal management of severely restrictive atrial septum in fetuses with critical left heart obstruction: clinical experience using pulmonary venous Doppler analysis. J Thorac Cardiovasc Surg 2011; 141(4): 988-94.
[http://dx.doi.org/10.1016/j.jtcvs.2010.09.043] [PMID: 21130471]

[73] Phillipos EZ, Robertson MA, Still DK. Prenatal detection of foramen ovale obstruction without hydrops fetalis. J Am Soc Echocardiogr 1990; 3(6): 495-8.
[http://dx.doi.org/10.1016/S0894-7317(14)80367-2] [PMID: 2278716]

[74] Hagen A, Albig M, Schmitz L, *et al.* Prenatal diagnosis of isolated foramen ovale obstruction. A report of two cases. Fetal Diagn Ther 2005; 20(1): 70-3.
[http://dx.doi.org/10.1159/000081373] [PMID: 15608464]

[75] Rasanen J, Wood DC, Weiner S, Ludomirski A, Huhta JC. Role of the pulmonary circulation in the distribution of human fetal cardiac output during the second half of pregnancy. Circulation 1996; 94(5): 1068-73.
[http://dx.doi.org/10.1161/01.CIR.94.5.1068] [PMID: 8790048]

[76] Sutton MS, Groves A, MacNeill A, Sharland G, Allan L. Assessment of changes in blood flow through the lungs and foramen ovale in the normal human fetus with gestational age: a prospective Doppler echocardiographic study. Br Heart J 1994; 71(3): 232-7.
[http://dx.doi.org/10.1136/hrt.71.3.232] [PMID: 8142191]

[77] Tworetzky W, Wilkins-Haug L, Jennings RW, *et al.* Balloon dilation of severe aortic stenosis in the fetus: potential for prevention of hypoplastic left heart syndrome: candidate selection, technique, and results of successful intervention. Circulation 2004; 110(15): 2125-31.
[http://dx.doi.org/10.1161/01.CIR.0000144357.29279.54] [PMID: 15466631]

[78] Selamet Tierney ES, Wald RM, McElhinney DB, *et al.* Changes in left heart hemodynamics after technically successful *in-utero* aortic valvuloplasty. Ultrasound Obstet Gynecol 2007; 30(5): 715-20.
[http://dx.doi.org/10.1002/uog.5132] [PMID: 17764106]

[79] Tworetzky W, McElhinney DB, Marx GR, *et al. In utero* valvuloplasty for pulmonary atresia with hypoplastic right ventricle: techniques and outcomes. Pediatrics 2009; 124(3): e510-8.
[http://dx.doi.org/10.1542/peds.2008-2014] [PMID: 19706566]

[80] Respondek M, Wilczyński J, Oszukowski P, *et al.* [Prenatal echocardiography of aortic stenosis]. Pediatr Pol 1996; 71(6): 505-10.
[PMID: 8756768]

[81] Respondek-Liberska M, Polaczek A, Słodki M, *et al.* Wybrane problemy kliniczne 56 płodów i 38 noworodków z krytyczną stenozą aortalną. ECHO Płodu 2012; 3: 10-4.

[82] Wieczorek A, Żarkowska A, Radzymińska-Chruściel B, *et al.* Krytyczna stenoza zastawki aortalnej - diagnostyka i postępowanie w ośrodku referencyjnym kardiologii prenatalnej. Polski Przegląd Kardiologiczny 2008; 10: 78-84.

[83] Dubiel M, Moszczyńska K, Dryżek P, *et al.* Prenatalna krytyczna stenoza aortalna – opis 2 przypadków z dobrym zakończeniem Echo płodu 2012; 1: 17-22.

[84] Marshall AC, Levine J, Morash D, *et al.* Results of *in utero* atrial septoplasty in fetuses with hypoplastic left heart syndrome. Prenat Diagn 2008; 28(11): 1023-8.
[http://dx.doi.org/10.1002/pd.2114] [PMID: 18925607]

CHAPTER 2

Cardiovascular Development

Maya Reddy[1,2] and **Daniel L. Rolnik**[1,*]

[1] *Department of Obstetrics and Gynaecology, Monash Womens, Monash Health, Clayton, Victoria, Australia*

[2] *Department of Obstetrics and Gynaecology, Faculty of Medicine, Nursing and Health Sciences, Monash University, Clayton, Victoria, Australia*

Abstract: An understanding of normal cardiovascular development is essential to appreciating the abnormalities seen in congenital heart disease. The cardiovascular system develops within the mesoderm and through the process of folding, and establishment of the body axis, patterning and laterality it transforms from blood islands into the primitive heart tube and then the complex cardiac structures that supply the fetus. This chapter will discuss the embryological formation of the cardiovascular system and how deviations from normal development result in common cardiac defects.

Keywords: Cardiovascular development, Cardiovascular embryology, Congenital heart defects, Embryology.

INTRODUCTION

The development of cardiovascular structures is a complex process that is crucial to the formation of the embryo, fetus and neonate. The rudimentary heart begins to beat and pump blood as early as day 22 of gestation. This is essential to meet the ongoing requirements of the embryo. Cardiovascular development not only relies on a variety of genes and transcription factors, but also on appropriate patterning and laterality of the embryo, without which various congenital heart defects can occur. In this chapter, we will explore the embryological development of the heart and vasculature, and discuss how malfunction within this process can lead to common congenital heart defects.

* **Corresponding author Daniel Rolnik:** Department of Obstetrics and Gynaecology, Monash Medical Centre, Monash Medical Centre, Level. 5, 246 Clayton Road, Clayton, VIC, Australia (3168), Tel: +61 3 9594 6666; E-mail: daniel.rolnik2@gmail.com

EARLY EMBRYOGENESIS

When fertilisation occurs, the zygote undergoes rapid cleavage and differentiation, eventually forming the blastocyst. The blastocyst is a key structure of early pregnancy and consists of an inner cell mass and an outer cell mass, which transform into the embryo proper and the placenta, respectively [1]. During the second week of development, the inner cell mass divides further, and the base layer of cells differentiate into a bilaminar disc made up of hypoblasts and epiblasts [1]. During the third week of development, the vital process of gastrulation occurs and a trilaminar disc is formed. This involves the development of the primitive streak in the epiblast layer, which signals cells within the epiblast to differentiate and then invaginate in between the epiblast and hypoblast layers of the bilaminar disc. The subsequent development of a trilaminar disc is key to all embryogenesis, as it forms the three germ layers (endoderm, mesoderm and ectoderm) from which the body structures arise. From the ectoderm arises the nervous system, epidermis, hair, and sweat glands [1]. The endoderm will form the gastrointestinal tract, lungs, liver and pancreas [1]. The mesoderm differentiates into the skeletal system, muscles, the dermis and the genitourinary tract [1]. The mesoderm layer also gives rise to the cardiovascular system [1]. During gastrulation, the primitive streak plays a vital role in establishing the cranial-caudal, medial-lateral, left-right and dorsal-ventral body axes [2]. Correct establishment of these axes is of crucial importance to normal cardiac development.

The Mesoderm Layer and the Origins of the Heart

During gastrulation, the epiblast cells that form the mesoderm migrate to specific areas and undergo differentiation into cells that serve a particular function. The cells adjacent to the neural tube form the paraxial mesoderm, which gives rise to the somites that ultimately form the axial skeleton, the voluntary muscles of the neck, body wall and limbs, and the dermis of the neck [3]. The adjacent intermediate mesoderm consists of cells that form the urogenital structures [3]. The most lateral aspect is made up of the lateral plate mesoderm, which on day 17 divides into a splanchnic and somatic layer [3]. The somatic layer fuses with the overlying ectoderm and the splanchnic layer fuses with the underlying endoderm [3]. Cardiac structures develop within the cranial portion of the splanchnic lateral plate mesoderm.

PATHOLOGY: BODY AXES, PATTERNING, AND PATHOLOGICAL LESIONS OF THE HEART

Correct development of cardiovascular structures requires appropriate patterning of cells and laterality, which occur during gastrulation. Patterning refers to the programming of cells such that cells in a particular location differentiate to form certain structures with particular functions [2]. The development of the body axes and laterality combined with patterning is essential to left-right axis formation of the heart and its relation to the abdominal viscera [3].

Normal Body Arrangement *(Situs Solitus)*

In normal development, laterality and patterning result in asymmetrical development of the left and right side of the body axes such that different structures populate these areas [4]. In the abdomen, the stomach and the spleen are located on the left, and the liver and inferior vena cava (IVC) are located on the right. The IVC drains into the right atrium which is located on the right aspect of the heart. In the thorax, the right lung is made up of three lobes and a shorter bronchus, whereas the left lung consists of two lobes only and a longer bronchus .

Complete Reversal of the Left - Right Axis *(Situs Inversus)*

Situs inversus occurs due to abnormalities in laterality and involves complete reversal of the abdominal and thoracic organs such that it is a mirror image of normal development [4]. In this scenario, the liver and IVC are located on the left, and the stomach and spleen on the right. The left sided IVC drains into the morphologically right atria and ventricle, which are now located on the left. The morphologically left atria and ventricle are now located on the right . As there is total reversal *in situs inversus*, the organs and vessels maintain concordance. Therefore, *situs inversus* is rarely problematic. However, in some cases it is associated with genetic syndromes, such as an autosomal recessive disorder causing primary ciliary dyskinesia (Kartagener's syndrome) [4]. Twenty percent of patients with *situs inversus* are known to have Kartageners syndrome [5].

Visceral Heterotaxy with Isomerism

Visceral heterotaxy with isomerism occurs when there is symmetrical development of the left and right body, rather than the asymmetrical development that normally takes place [6]. In visceral heterotaxy with right sided isomerism, both left and right sides of the abdomen and thorax reflect right sided development and structures. As such, both lungs consist of a short bronchus and three lobes; both atria contain right atrial appendages; and the liver is located in the midline, with a malrotated gut and asplenia. In visceral heterotaxy with left sided isomerism, both left and right sides resemble left sided development. As a result, there are two lobes in each lung; two left atrial appendages; a midline liver with a malrotated gut and multiple accessory spleens (polysplenia) . Isomerism is often accompanied by multiple cardiac defects including anomalous venous connections [7].

DEVELOPMENT OF THE PRIMITIVE HEART TUBE

The development of the primitive heart tube requires 1) formation of blood islands on either side of the lateral plate mesoderm, 2) coalescing of these blood islands into cardiac crescents, and 3) the fusion of these cardiac crescents with embryonic folding. This process generally occurs between day 19-21 of development. Whilst these are not distinctive or necessarily chronological stages, it is useful to view them as such in order to understand development.

Stage 1 - Progenitor Heart Cells and the Formation of Blood Islands

Progenitor heart cells migrate from the cranial end of the primitive streak to the splanchnic layer of the lateral plate mesoderm. These cells migrate to two main areas on both sides of the embryo - 1) the primary heart field and 2) the secondary heart field [3, 8]. The cells that migrate to the primary heart field will eventually form the atria, left ventricle, and part of the right ventricle [3, 8]. The cells that form the secondary heart field will form part of the right ventricle and outflow tracts, and function to lengthen the primitive heart tube [8]. The surrounding intraembryonic cavity will later develop into the pericardial cavity.

Stage 2 - Formation of the Cardiac Crescents

The underlying endoderm induces the cells within the primary heart field to differentiate into myoblasts, endothelial cells, and blood islands. These blood islands fuse to form a horseshoe shaped endocardial tube (cardiac crescent) that is lined with endothelial cells and surrounded by myoblasts.

Stage 3 - Embryonic Folding and the Formation of the Primitive Heart Tube

By the end of third week of development, as the embryo folds in the lateral-medial direction, the cardiac crescents fuse together to form the primitive heart tube. Simultaneously, rapid development of cranial structures and embryonic folding causes this primitive heart tube to migrate ventrally and caudally to lie in front of the foregut endoderm. The primitive heart tube is now surrounded by an enclosed cavity of intraembryonic coelom, which forms the pericardial cavity. Initially this tube is attached to the foregut dorsally by the dorsal mesocardium, which eventually ruptures, and leaves the heart suspended within the pericardial cavity by its vasculature. The cellular and anatomical components of the primitive heart tube are shown in Table **1**.

Table 1. Anatomical and cellular structures of the primitive heart tube [1].

Cellular Components of the Primitive Heart Tube	Anatomical Components of the Primitive Heart Tube
Endocardium - formed by the fused endocardial tubes of the cardiac crescents and is lined by endothelial cells. Cardiac jelly - a layer of extracellular matrix that is secreted by the myoblasts and functions to separate the endocardium and myocardium during development. Myocardium - an enveloping outer tube made up of the myoblasts that eventually form the contractile muscle of the heart.	*Sinus venosus* (left and right) - primary source of venous return. Primitive Atrium - divides into left and right atrium. Ventricle - forms mainly the left ventricle. *Bulbus cordis* - forms the right ventricle. Conotruncal region - made up of the *conus cordis* (the cranial end of the bulbus cordis) and *truncus arteriosus*. These form the ascending aorta and pulmonary trunk. Aortic sac and aortic roots - give rise to the aortic arches and part of the ascending aorta.

Stage 4 - Blood Flow Through the Primitive Heart Tube

By day 28, blood flows through the primitive heart tube and its various structures. Initially, blood from the embryo enters the heart *via* the paired *sinus venosus* into the atrium. It is then directed into the ventricle through the atrioventricular canal. Blood subsequently flows from the ventricle into the *bulbus cordis*, and then into the conotruncal region and aortic sac. The conotruncal region and aortic sac then attach to the dorsal aortae *via* the aortic arches.

CARDIAC LOOPING

The folding of the primitive heart tube is key to the formation of the four-chamber heart, and the correct positioning of cardiac structures to facilitate normal blood flow. During week four, the primitive heart tube lengthens as cells are added from the secondary heart field [8]. As lengthening occurs, the primitive heart tube folds such that the *bulbus cordis* and conotruncal region move ventrally, caudally and to the right; the ventricle is pushed to the left; and the atria and *sinus venosus* migrate to the left and in a dorsocranial direction. As the atria move dorsocranially they dilate [9]. This causes a relative shift of the conotruncal region in the midline direction with the bulging atria on either side, thus positioning the outflow tracts so that they communicate with the appropriate ventricles.

DEVELOPMENT OF THE ATRIA, VENTRICLES AND FOUR-CHAMBER HEART

The development of a four-chamber heart predominately occurs between days 28 and 37 of gestation. This involves several processes:

1. Development of endocardial cushions
2. Separation of the atria
3. Separation of the ventricles
4. Separation of the outflow tract

Development of Endocardial Cushions

Endocardial cushions are involved in the separation of the four heart chambers and in the division of the outflow tracts. As cardiac looping occurs, the myocardium secretes an extracellular matrix, which forms a cushion-like structure between the myocardium and endocardium [10]. This structure expands into the heart lumen in two locations, 1) at the level of the atrioventricular canal, and 2) within the conotruncal region. The extracellular matrix then transforms into mesenchymal tissue, which ultimately forms the connective tissue that separates the structures of the heart. The four endocardial cushions at the atrioventricular canal are related to the formation of 1) the atrioventricular septum, which divides the heart into left and right chambers, 2) the atrial septum which separates the right and left atria, 3) the ventricular septum that separates the ventricles and 4) the atrioventricular valves [11]. These endocardial cushions eventually fuse to close atrioventricular canal, and form the central region of the heart known as the *crux cordis*. Similarly, the endocardial cushions in the conotruncal region separate the aortic and pulmonary vasculature and also form the outflow valves.

PATHOLOGY- ATRIOVENTRICULAR CANAL DEFECTS

Atrioventricular canal defects are divided into complete and partial defects, and occur due to failure of fusion of the superior and inferior endocardial cushions. These malformations account for 3-5% of all congenital heart defects and are commonly associated with trisomy 21 (Down's syndrome) [12, 13]. Complete failure of fusion of these endocardial cushions results in a large atrial and ventricular septal defect and a common atrioventricular valve (atrioventricular septal defect - AVSD) [13]. Partial failure of fusion results in an atrial septal defect (ASD) only, and two atrioventricular valves sharing a single annulus [13].

Separation of the Atria

Division of the atria occurs through the formation of two septa, which fuse together in extrauterine life. An opening exists in both septum in order to allow for the right-left shunting of blood *in utero*. The first septum to form, the *septum primum*, grows inferiorly from the roof of the atria towards the dorsal endocardial cushion [1, 3, 11]. An opening between the growing septum and endocardial cushion is known as the *ostium primum*. As the septum fuses with the dorsal endocardial cushion, the *ostium primum* closes. Simultaneously, the superior aspect of the septum undergoes apoptosis, creating a second opening known as the *ostium secundum* [1, 3, 11]. As the right atrium enlarges, the *septum secundum*, a second more muscular septum, forms and grows towards the endocardial cushions. However, this septum falls short of fusing with the atrioventricular cushions, leaving an opening called the *foramen ovale* [3]. The adjacent septum primum forms a flap like valve over the *foramen ovale*. Thus, a passageway for blood remains from the right atrium through the *foramen ovale*, across the *ostium secundum* and into the left atrium. With the transition to extrauterine life, the change in pressures results in reversal of the right to left shunt. This causes the *septum primum* to push against the *septum secundum*, which fuse together to completely separate the atria. The *foramen ovale* closes and becomes an indentation in the right atrium known as the *fossa ovalis*.

PATHOLOGY - ATRIAL SEPTAL DEFECTS

Atrial septal defects (ASD) account for 10-15% of congenital heart disease, and are defined by their location [14]. The morbidity associated with ASD depends on its size, location and association with other anomalies.

1. Primum ASD: Primum ASDs develop when the *septum primum* fails to fuse with the endocardial cushions, resulting in a persistent *ostium primum*. These defects are most commonly seen in atrioventricular canal defects such as complete or partial AVSD and are a result of deficiencies in the endocardial cushions and atrioventricular septum [15, 16].

2. Secundum ASD: Secundum ASDs often occur due inadequate closure of the *ostium secundum*, such that when the septa fuse in extrauterine life, an opening remains in this ostium. This can occur due to inadequate growth of the *septum secundum* or excessive resorption of the *septum primum* resulting in a large *ostium secundum* [15, 16].

3. *Sinus venosus* defects: *Sinus venosus* ASDs are defects in the upper portion of the atrial septum. They occur due to malposition and incomplete resorption of the *sinus venosus* or abnormal development of the *septum secundum*. This results in malposition of the superior vena cava (SVC) or inferior vena cava (IVC) such that an interatrial communication forms between the vena cavae and pulmonary veins. These defects are almost always associated with partial anomalous pulmonary venous return [16].

4. Patent Foramen Ovale: A patent *foramen ovale* (PFO) occurs during transition to extrauterine life and results from incomplete adhesion of the septum primum to the septum secundum. Although it occurs in up to 25% of the population, this defect is not considered a true atrial septal defect and most patients with a PFO are asymptomatic [17].

STRUCTURES OF THE LEFT AND RIGHT ATRIA - THE VENOUS STRUCTURES OF THE CARDIOVASCULAR SYSTEM

Right Atrium

The right atrium is the primary chamber for venous return from the superior and inferior vena cava. Blood is then pumped from the right atrium into the right ventricle and subsequently the pulmonary circulation. In early development, the venous return to the right atrium is from the paired *sinus venosus* [1]. Venous blood from the cardinal veins enters the left and right sinus horns which then push blood into the atrium [1]. Between week 4 and week 8 there is remodelling of this venous system so that all venous flow drains into the right sinus horn *via* the superior and inferior vena cava [11]. This sinus horn then implants into the right atrium. The residual left sinus horn also drains into the right atrium, and transforms into a sac that carries the venous return from the coronary sinus [11]. Eventually, through the process of intussusception, the superior vena cava, inferior vena cava and coronary sinus directly embed into the right atrial wall, in a smooth walled area known as the *sinus venarum* [1].

Left Atrium

The majority of the left atrium is composed of the openings of the pulmonary veins, and as a result, it is largely a smooth walled structure. The left atrium continues to expand as the septa are forming in order to accommodate for the pulmonary veins. A single pulmonary vein forms as a growth from the posterior left atrial wall [1]. It then connects with the developing lung tissue distally and proximally, and bifurcates twice to produce four pulmonary veins [1]. Again, through the process of intussusception, the four pulmonary veins embed into the left atrium [1].

SEPARATION OF THE VENTRICLES

Similar to the atria, a muscular septum grows from the apex of the ventricle towards the endocardial cushions surrounding the atrioventricular canal . Simultaneously, the right endocardial cushion at the atrioventricular canal projects inferiorly towards the muscular septum. The left and right ventricle remain partially separated with an opening superior to the muscular septum to allow for communication between the left and right side. This opening is important, as it enables ongoing communication between the left ventricle and outflow tract. By the seventh to eight weeks of gestation, this opening is closed by a membranous septum, which arises from the outflow tract. This delay in closure allows time for septation and remodelling of both the left ventricle and outflow tract [3].

PATHOLOGY BOX - VENTRICULAR SEPTAL DEFECTS

Ventricular septal defects (VSD) are common heart malformations that can occur at various locations of the ventricular septum. These defects can occur in isolation or in combination with other malformations, in particular those of the atrioventricular canal or outflow tract. The type of ventricular septal defect is dependent on the location of the malformation, and the severity is often dependent on size.

1. Muscular VSD: These occur due to inadequate development of the muscular septum.
2. Perimembranous VSD: These occur due to failure of fusion of the muscular and membranous septum.
3. Conoseptal or supracristal VSD - The proximal end of the outflow tract (conotruncal region) contributes to the membranous interventricular septum. Failure of fusion or development of the proximal conotruncal ridge contributes to a conoseptal VSD.
4. Inlet/Atrioventricular canal VSD: These VSD's occur as a result of atrioventricular canal defects resulting from complete failure in fusion of the endocardial cushions.

Separation of the Outflow Tract

The outflow tracts of the heart include the pulmonary trunk and the aorta, which arise from the structures that constitute the conotruncal region (*conus cordis* and *truncus arteriosus*. These vessels have an unusual formation, and spiral around each other as they exit the heart. In order to achieve this intricate formation, in week five of development, two spiralling membranous ridges form within the conotruncal region [1, 18]. Endocardial cushions derived from both mesoderm and neural crest cells then populate these ridges. Over the next week, these ridges fuse to form the conotruncal septum, which divides the area into left and right outflow tracts. Fusion begins distally in the *truncus arteriosus* region and moves proximally to the *conus cordis* region [18]. The final area of fusion is at the proximal end of the outflow tracts, where this membranous ridge also facilitates closure of the interventricular septum [1]. Eventually, the endocardial cushions that form the conotruncal ridge are replaced by muscle in the *conus cordis* region, such that this forms the outflow portion of the left and right ventricles [1].

PATHOLOGY - MALFORMATIONS OF THE OUTFLOW TRACT

Persistent *Truncus Arteriosus*

Persistent *truncus arteriosus* occurs due to the lack of separation of the proximal outflow tract (conotruncal region) as it exits the left and right ventricle [19]. As a result, the proximal outflow tract receives blood from both left and right ventricle, causing a mixing of circulations and cyanotic heart disease [19]. It is important to note that the proximal end of the conotruncal region is also responsible for the development of the membranous portion of the interventricular septum. As such a persistent *truncus arteriosus* is often accompanied by a ventricular septal defect (VSD) [3].

Transposition of the Great Arteries (TGA)

The typical transposition of the great arteries is characterised by a reversal in the location of the outflow tracts such that the aorta empties the right ventricle and the pulmonary trunk empties the left. It is thought that this malformation arises from abnormal partitioning of the conotruncal region, and a failure of the aorticopulmonary septum to spiral in a helical formation as it separates the outflow tracts [3].

Tetralogy of Fallot

Tetralogy of Fallot is a relatively common cardiac defect characterised by pulmonary stenosis, ventricular septal defect, aorta overriding the interventricular septum, and right ventricular hypertrophy. This lesion arises due to asymmetrical division of the outflow tracts [3]. Firstly, asymmetrical fusion of the conotruncal ridges results in a larger aorta (in relation to a smaller pulmonary artery). Consequently, it is overriding in that the aortic opening extends into both left and right ventricles. Secondly, asymmetry of the conotruncal ridges contributes to malalignment during the formation of the aortic and pulmonary valves, resulting in pulmonary stenosis. Fusion of the proximal conotruncal ridges is also key to the formation of the interventricular septum. Thus, the asymmetry and abnormal fusion contributes to a ventricular septal defect. As a result of these three lesions, there is increased flow and pressure in the right ventricle, causing right ventricular hypertrophy.

DEVELOPMENT OF HEART VALVES

Formation of the Atrioventricular Valves

The mitral and tricuspid valves separate the atria from the ventricles. The mitral valve is a bicuspid valve formed by an anterior and a posterior leaflet [20]. In contrast, the tricuspid valve contains a small additional third leaflet. These valves are predominantly derived from the endocardial cushions, which project into the heart lumen [20]. Structures that support these valves include the *chordae tendinae* and papillary muscles. These structures form in the process of ventricular remodelling and play an important role in the opening and closing of the atrioventricular valves [20].

Development of the Outflow Valves

The aortic and pulmonary valves are semilunar valves that form through remodelling of the conotruncal septum. As the conotruncal septum develops, additional endocardial cushions develop on either side of the outflow tract [20]. As remodelling occurs these endocardial cushions are transformed into six semilunar sinuses. Finally, when the left and right outflow tracts divide, these semilunar sinuses form the aortic valve and pulmonary valve respectively [1].

DEVELOPMENT OF THE PERIPHERAL VASCULATURE

The peripheral vasculature also arises from the splanchnic layer of the lateral plate mesoderm. The formation of the arterial vasculature relies on vasculogenesis (formation of blood vessels) and angiogenesis (branching of vessels). To appreciate this process, one requires an understanding of the development of the dorsal aortae and aortic arches. This will be discussed briefly in this section.

Development of the Dorsal Aortae

The dorsal aortae are a pair of vessels that attach to the heart *via* the aortic arches and fuse distally to form the descending aorta. The dorsal aortae are also linked to the vitelline arteries at the level of the umbilicus [21]. Similar to the cardiac crescents, the dorsal aortae form as blood islands in the splanchnic layer of the lateral plate mesoderm, on either side of the embryo. These blood islands coalesce together to form left and right tubes. As the embryo folds, these tubes (dorsal aortae) attach to the *truncus arteriosus via* the formation of the first aortic arch. The subsequent paired aortic arches develop in a sequential fashion and connect the aortic sac and *truncus arteriosus* to the paired dorsal aortae. Some of these aortic arches regress with development, leaving residual arteries. However, given that this happens in a sequential manner, the dorsal aortae always remain connected to the *truncus arteriosus* and aortic sac.

Sequential Development of the Aortic Arches

The formation of the aortic arches follows the development of the pharyngeal arches and occurs between six to eight weeks of gestation. The first aortic arch is followed by the formation of a second aortic arch [15]. However, both of these arches regress as the third and fourth aortic arches develop. The third aortic arch branches into the left and right common carotid arteries that supply the head, brain, and neck structures. Around this time, the dorsal aortae between the third and fourth aortic arches regress, and the sixth aortic arch also forms. In humans, the fifth aortic arch either never forms or forms as a rudimentary structure that ultimately regresses. Simultaneous to the development of the sixth aortic arch is the development of the lung buds which form the respiratory system. These aortic arches thus branch into the left and right pulmonary artery, which provide the arterial supply to the respiratory system. On the left side the sixth aortic arch maintains a connection to the dorsal aorta, whilst on the right side this connection regresses. The left sided connection forms the *ductus arteriosus*, a key vessel in the fetal circulation. By the seventh week of development, the right dorsal aorta degenerates leaving a residual component that is attached to the fourth aortic arch. On the left-hand side, the fourth arch remains connected to the left dorsal aorta and forms the arch of the aorta. It also branches here to form the left subclavian artery, which supplies the left upper limb. On the right side, as the right dorsal aorta degenerates it remains connected to the fourth aortic arch, and branches into the right subclavian artery which supply the right upper limb. The remaining left dorsal aorta forms the descending aorta, which supplies the gastrointestinal system, the genitourinary structures and the lower limbs [15].

PATHOLOGY: RIGHT AORTIC ARCH AND DOUBLE AORTIC ARCH

Double Aortic Arch

A double aortic arch is a malformation that arises when the right dorsal aorta fails to regress between the seventh intersegmental artery and its connection to the left dorsal aorta [22]. As a result, both dorsal aortae remain connected to ascending and descending aorta. At the level of the ascending aorta, the left and right dorsal aortae traverse anterior to the trachea and oesophagus [22]. When the dorsal aortae reunite and form the descending aortae they travel posterior to the trachea and oesophagus. This creates a vascular ring that encircles and compresses the trachea and oesophagus causing difficulties in breathing and swallowing [22].

Right Aortic Arch

A right aortic arch is an anatomical variation such that the right dorsal aorta and right fourth aortic arch persist and the left dorsal aorta and left fourth aortic arch regress [22]. When this is a "true mirror image" of normal vascular development, there is no compression of the oesophagus or trachea [22]. However, in a small portion of the population this is not a true mirror image and there is a persistent left ductus arteriosus and aberrant left subclavian artery [22]. This creates a vascular ring that completely encircles the oesophagus and trachea, which when compressed can cause issues with breathing and swallowing [22]. An isolated right aortic arch has been associated with chromosomal abnormalities, in particular, 22q11 microdeletion [23].

FETAL CIRCULATION

The fetal circulation is a relatively hypoxic intrauterine environment that is designed to provide adequate oxygen and nutrients to the fetus, and allow for the excretion of waste products. Central to this process is the placenta and the numerous shunts within the fetal circulation that bypass the liver and lungs. Through the process of diffusion oxygenated blood is transported from the placental villi into the umbilical vein. As the umbilical vein enters the fetus, blood is directed in two pathways. A small amount of blood perfuses the liver while the rest is redirected through the ductus venosus and into the IVC. Blood from the IVC then enters the right atrium, and is combined with poorly oxygenated venous return from the head and neck *via* the SVC [24]. The majority of blood from the ductus venosus and IVC is directed through the foramen ovale, and into the left atrium, left ventricle, and then the ascending aorta. In contrast, blood from the SVC is preferentially shifted through the right ventricle into the pulmonary arteries [24].

At the level of the pulmonary arteries, 80-90% of blood bypasses the pulmonary circulation *via* the ductus arteriosus, which forms due to the persistent connection between the sixth aortic arch and the left dorsal aorta [24]. As a result, this blood directly enters the systemic circulation. The oxygenated blood from the aorta is then distributed through the fetus to supply the 1) head and neck *via* the common carotid and vertebral arteries, 2) upper limbs *via* the subclavian arteries, and the 3) abdominal structures and lower limbs *via* the descending aorta. Deoxygenated blood from the fetus is then transported back towards the placenta *via* the umbilical arteries. Here, through the process of diffusion, carbon dioxide and other waste products are excreted.

In the transition to extrauterine life, the process of labour, initial breaths, and clamping of the umbilical cord result in a decrease in pulmonary vascular resistance and an increase in systemic vascular resistance. As a result, the right-to-left shunts within the fetal circulation begin to reverse, stimulating functional closure of 1) the *foramen ovale* within minutes to hours of life, and 2) the *ductus arteriosus* at 96 hours of life [24]. Anatomical closure of these shunts occurs a later stage such that the *foramen ovale* becomes the *fossa ovalis* and the *ductus arteriosus* becomes the *ligamentum arteriosum*. With the removal of the placental circulation, the flow through the *ductus venosus* also falls significantly. By day 3 to day 10 of life the *ductus venosus* also closes, forming the *ligamentum venosum* [24].

CONSENT FOR PUBLICATION

Not applicable.

CONFLICT OF INTEREST

The authors confirm that the contents of this chapter have no conflict of interest.

ACKNOWLEDGEMENTS

Declare none.

REFERENCES

[1]   Schoenwolf G, Bleyl S, Brauer P, Francis-West P. Larsen's Human Embryology. Philadelphia, PA: Churchill Livignstone Elsevier 2009.

[2]   Hackett BP. Formation and malformation of the vertebrate left-right axis. Curr Mol Med 2002; 2(1): 39-66.
        [http://dx.doi.org/10.2174/1566524023363031] [PMID: 11898848]

[3]   Sadler TW, Sadler-Redmond SL, Tosney K, *et al.* Langmans Medical Embryology. Philadelphia, PA: Wolters Kluwer 2010.

[4]   Casey B. Two rights make a wrong: human left-right malformations. Hum Mol Genet 1998; 7(10): 1565-71.
        [http://dx.doi.org/10.1093/hmg/7.10.1565] [PMID: 9735377]

[5]   Imbrie JD. Kartagener's syndrome: a genetic defect affecting the function of cilia. Am J Otolaryngol 1981; 2(3): 215-22.
        [http://dx.doi.org/10.1016/S0196-0709(81)80018-X] [PMID: 6974512]

[6]   Applegate KE, Goske MJ, Pierce G, Murphy D. Situs revisited: imaging of the heterotaxy syndrome. Radiographics 1999; 19(4): 837-52.
        [http://dx.doi.org/10.1148/radiographics.19.4.g99jl31837] [PMID: 10464794]

[7]   Phoon CK, Neill CA. Asplenia syndrome: insight into embryology through an analysis of cardiac and extracardiac anomalies. Am J Cardiol 1994; 73(8): 581-7.
        [http://dx.doi.org/10.1016/0002-9149(94)90338-7] [PMID: 8147305]

[8]   Moorman A, Webb S, Brown NA, Lamers W, Anderson RH. Development of the heart: (1) formation of the cardiac chambers and arterial trunks. Heart 2003; 89(7): 806-14.
        [http://dx.doi.org/10.1136/heart.89.7.806] [PMID: 12807866]

[9]   Gittenberger-de Groot AC, Bartelings MM, Deruiter MC, Poelmann RE. Basics of cardiac development for the understanding of congenital heart malformations. Pediatr Res 2005; 57(2): 169-76.
        [http://dx.doi.org/10.1203/01.PDR.0000148710.69159.61] [PMID: 15611355]

[10]   Person AD, Klewer SE, Runyan RB. Cell biology of cardiac cushion development. Int Rev Cytol 2005; 243: 287-335.
        [http://dx.doi.org/10.1016/S0074-7696(05)43005-3] [PMID: 15797462]

[11]   Anderson RH, Webb S, Brown NA, Lamers W, Moorman A. Development of the heart: (2) Septation of the atriums and ventricles. Heart 2003; 89(8): 949-58.
        [http://dx.doi.org/10.1136/heart.89.8.949] [PMID: 12860885]

[12]   Craig B. Atrioventricular septal defect: from fetus to adult. Heart 2006; 92(12): 1879-85.
        [http://dx.doi.org/10.1136/hrt.2006.093344] [PMID: 17105897]

[13]   Baumgartner H, Bonhoeffer P, De Groot NM, *et al*. ESC Guidelines for the management of grown-up congenital heart disease (new version 2010). Eur Heart J 2010; 31(23): 2915-57.
        [http://dx.doi.org/10.1093/eurheartj/ehq249] [PMID: 20801927]

[14]   van der Linde D, Konings EE, Slager MA, *et al*. Birth prevalence of congenital heart disease worldwide: a systematic review and meta-analysis. J Am Coll Cardiol 2011; 58(21): 2241-7.
        [http://dx.doi.org/10.1016/j.jacc.2011.08.025] [PMID: 22078432]

[15]   Moore KLPT, Torchia M. The developing human: Clinically oriented embryology. 10ᵗʰ ed., Philadelphia: Elsevier 2016.

[16]   Rojas CA, El-Sherief A, Medina HM, *et al*. Embryology and developmental defects of the interatrial septum. AJR Am J Roentgenol 2010; 195(5): 1100-4.
        [http://dx.doi.org/10.2214/AJR.10.4277] [PMID: 20966313]

[17]   Hagen PT, Scholz DG, Edwards WD. Incidence and size of patent foramen ovale during the first 10 decades of life: an autopsy study of 965 normal hearts. Mayo Clin Proc 1984; 59(1): 17-20.
        [http://dx.doi.org/10.1016/S0025-6196(12)60336-X] [PMID: 6694427]

[18]   Anderson RH, Webb S, Brown NA, Lamers W, Moorman A. Development of the heart: (3) formation of the ventricular outflow tracts, arterial valves, and intrapericardial arterial trunks. Heart 2003; 89(9): 1110-8.
        [http://dx.doi.org/10.1136/heart.89.9.1110] [PMID: 12923046]

[19]   Volpe P, Paladini D, Marasini M, *et al*. Common arterial trunk in the fetus: characteristics, associations, and outcome in a multicentre series of 23 cases. Heart 2003; 89(12): 1437-41.
        [http://dx.doi.org/10.1136/heart.89.12.1437] [PMID: 14617557]

[20]   Combs MD, Yutzey KE. Heart valve development: regulatory networks in development and disease. Circ Res 2009; 105(5): 408-21.
        [http://dx.doi.org/10.1161/CIRCRESAHA.109.201566] [PMID: 19713546]

[21]   Sato Y. Dorsal aorta formation: separate origins, lateral-to-medial migration, and remodeling. Dev Growth Differ 2013; 55(1): 113-29.
        [http://dx.doi.org/10.1111/dgd.12010] [PMID: 23294360]

[22]   Bravo C, Gámez F, Pérez R, Álvarez T, De León-Luis J. Fetal Aortic Arch Anomalies: Key Sonographic Views for Their Differential Diagnosis and Clinical Implications Using the Cardiovascular System Sonographic Evaluation Protocol. J Ultrasound Med 2016; 35(2): 237-51.
        [http://dx.doi.org/10.7863/ultra.15.02063] [PMID: 26715656]

[23]   Vigneswaran TV, Allan L, Charakida M, *et al*. Prenatal diagnosis and clinical implications of an apparently isolated right aortic arch. Prenat Diagn 2018; 38(13): 1055-61.
        [http://dx.doi.org/10.1002/pd.5388] [PMID: 30421794]

[24]   Murphy PJ. The Fetal Circulation. Contin Educ Anaesth Crit Care Pain 2005; 5: 107-12.
        [http://dx.doi.org/10.1093/bjaceaccp/mki030]

CHAPTER 3

Utero-Placental Circulation Development

Kersti K. Linask[*]

Department of Pediatrics, USF Morsani College of Medicine, Tampa and St. Petersburg, FL, USA

Abstract: With increasing obesity and diabetes in our population, and alcohol, marijuana, and tobacco use among women of child-bearing years, there is a high probability of embryonic exposure to risk factors before pregnancy is recognized. These metabolic changes and environmental factors are known in animals to induce birth defects and specifically, congenital heart defects (CHDs). This study discusses an interrelationship between placental and heart development in which blood flow between these developing organs needs to be maintained at specific levels. When blood flow is altered in the mouse by embryonic exposure to environmental factors, dysmorphogenesis occurs. Additionally, with gene expression analysis of the embryonic heart it was demonstrated that with elevated homocysteine (HCy) a natural metabolite, and alcohol exposures, numerous Gene Ontology classifications relating to lipid metabolism were altered. As for example, relative to the female embryo, significantly more alterations occurred in the male embryonic heart transcriptome with homocysteine exposure. That lipid metabolism was altered was validated by staining for localization of neutral lipids in the embryonic mouse embryos. We demonstrated that lipid droplet amount and the localization patterning were changed with exposures in both the fetal four-chambered heart and in the placenta. More changes occurred, however, in the placental tissue. We have demonstrated that a regimen of high folic acid supplementation of the pregnant mouse diet started with the morning after conception prevented the environmentally induced alterations. The importance of lipids in trophoblast and placental development, the relationship to gender, and how folate supplementation normalizes development through epigenetic programming is reviewed.

Keywords: Alcohol, Bioinformatics, Congenital heart defects, Environmental effects, Ethanol, Gender, Heart, Homocysteine, Human embryology, Lithium, Lipid metabolism, Mouse embryo, Placenta, Trophoblasts.

---

[*] **Corresponding author Kersti K. Linask:** Department of Pediatrics, USF Morsani College of Medicine, 601- 4th Street South, St. Petersburg, FL 33701; USA; E-mail: klinask@usf.edu

Edward Araujo Júnior, Nathalie Jeanne M. Bravo-Valenzuela and Alberto Borges Peixoto (Eds.)

INTRODUCTION

Heart organogenesis begins during gastrulation, that is, within the second week after conception [1]. It is the first organ to develop in the embryo, followed closely by the brain. Because of the early timing during embryonic development, congenital heart defects (CHDs) are the most prevalent type of human birth defects, taking place approximately in one out of every 100 live births. CHDs are usually not caused by changes in single genes. Even in cases in families where a defect in a single gene has been identified, there is often variable expression or incomplete penetrance.

The majority of CHDs are believed to be multifactorial in nature occurring as sporadic, non-syndromic events. Causes for CHDs have been difficult to define. From research in my laboratory using animal models, as well as from other laboratories, embryonic exposures to even a single dose of an environmental factor during gastrulation, can induce cardiac defects and placental abnormalities [2, 3]. Environmental factors such as alcohol, cigarette smoking, marijuana-associated cannabinoids, certain prescription drugs, or even higher than normal concentrations of normal metabolites, have been shown to induce CHDs [4 - 8]. Because confirmation of human pregnancy usually occurs at 5 to 6 weeks after conception, the early gestational period of cardiogenesis that happens between the second and third week after fertilization, is a high-risk time frame for embryonic exposure to environmental factors. The mother in her second and third week of pregnancy is most likely not yet aware of being pregnant, continues with her usual lifestyle, or maybe taking prescribed medications, and is not yet taking precautions to protect her developing embryo from possible deleterious environmental factors.

In the context that 49% of pregnancies are not planned [9], it is suggested that the first four weeks of pregnancy is especially at high risk for the initiation of birth defects. Due to the potential for a high incidence of CHDs being induced by environmental exposures so early in gestation, one of the first studies we carried out in the laboratory was to define the timing during gestation when we can induce the highest percentage of heart defects. We initially used avian embryos to answer this question and then followed this up experimentally in the mouse model [2, 3]. Our experimental paradigm was to give the pregnant mouse a single exposure by intraperitoneal injection (i.p.). We then allowed the embryos to develop to mid-gestation to embryonic day (ED) 15.5, when the heart has developed four cardiac chambers and valves. The environmental factors that we focused on were (i) lithium (Li^+), a drug often prescribed for bipolar disorder, (ii) elevating the concentration of homocysteine (HCy), a natural metabolite in the embryo and a marker of folic acid deficiency, or (iii) alcohol (ethanol). All three chemical factors are known to induce a high number of CHDs in human pregnancies. In both the chick and mouse embryos, after exposure to the defined substance, we analyzed for changes in specific key genes and in protein expression during subsequent heart development. We additionally carried out cardiac function analyses in the mouse using Doppler ultrasound noninvasively [10]. The answer to our question regarding the timing of exposure using the above listed three substances and the two vertebrate models was that the highest percentage of heart defects were initiated by an acute embryonic exposure occurring during gastrulation [2, 3, 5, 6, 11]. In the avian embryonic model this timing was late stage 4/early stage 5. We defined ED 6.75 using the mouse model with exposure occurring on embryonic day (ED) 6 at 6 PM. This timing of exposure in the mouse coincides with gastrulation.

Only a single exposure during gastrulation is necessary to induce heart defects. If we exposed a half day earlier, the effect was lethal. This latter result regarding lethality seemingly relates to the finding that in approximately 13% of human miscarriages and spontaneous abortions, adverse heart development is observed in the aborted conceptuses [12]. When we exposed increasingly later, CHDs can still be induced, but the incidence, lethality, and severity of the defects decreased. Besides defining gastrulation as the period of the highest incidence of CHD induction, the other outcome of our studies in the mouse demonstrated that also placental development was negatively affected with the acute environmental exposures. During the course of this research, my laboratory was involved in collaborative studies focusing on biomechanical/biophysical parameters of heart development and the role of blood flow. Taken together, our research results led to our proposing the concept of blood flow within the heart-placenta axis being important in normal cardiac development. When changes occur either in the placenta or in the heart with environmental exposures affecting blood flow, cardiac malformations can occur [13]. This chapter is to review recent literature on heart and placental development, how they intersect, and why both are especially vulnerable to environmental exposures to result in cardiac birth defects. Lastly, the protective role of folate supplementation to prevent the adverse effects is reviewed. Although my focus is on the heart, it is noted that with our early exposures we usually also observed neural tube defects and abnormal brain development. This to us was not surprising, because it is known that in brain development many of the same genetic pathways, growth factors, and proteins are active as in heart development. For example, mothers drinking alcohol during pregnancy are known to give birth to babies with fetal alcohol spectrum disorders (FASD) characterized by neural anomalies, congenital heart defects [4], learning disabilities, craniofacial malformations, and fetal growth restriction among other abnormalities [14, 15].

EMBRYONIC YOLK SAC, TROPHOBLASTS AND CHORIOALLAN-TOIC PLACENTAL DEVELOPMENT

For survival and normal fetal growth, the development of a circulatory system in the embryo is necessary to take place early in pregnancy in order for the embryo to interact with its uterine environment for the exchange of nutrients and oxygen between the mother and the fetus. For this exchange, the vitelline and placental extraembryonic circulations develop. It has been demonstrated that blood flow forces from the extraembryonic circulations can contribute to normal embryonic heart development. Based upon investigations by others and by my laboratory, the results demonstrated that changes in blood flow in the vitelline or in placental circulations can lead to abnormal heart development to result in heart defects. In analysis of the role of hemodynamic forces in normal heart development, we used four-dimensional optical coherence tomography (OCT) to define the relationships of the endocardium, myocardium, and cardiac jelly compartments during a single cardiac cycle during the heart looping stages of development [16]. Heart looping is a process that forms the four-chambered heart from the initial single heart tube. OCT allows for dynamic and high-resolution imaging of the functioning early, beating, embryonic heart. Combining the dynamic and high-resolution imaging OCT data with immunohistohemical studies, the data demonstrated the structural form of the heart develops in such a way that it can accommodate increasing blood flow and through synthesis of mechanotransducing molecules, the cardiac cells are attuned to pressure- and stress-related changes. Immunohistochemical analysis for specific mechanotransducing extracellular matrix networks, including fibronectin, tenascin C, nonmuscle myosin-IIA and -IIB demonstrated an organization that facilitates heart looping to form the trabeculated four-chambered heart [17]. This relationship between heart development and the extraembryonic circulations that develop, we refer to as the heart-placenta axis [13, 18]. More recent treatments of this topic reviewing biomechanical considerations and hemodynamics have confirmed our initial data [19, 20]. This data indicated the importance of defining how even small changes in embryonic blood flow can result in CHDs. Analyses of studies whereby blood flow was changed in a controlled manner during chick heart development demonstrated that reproducible types of heart defects can be induced [20, 21]. As an example, the results showed that constricting the outflow tract by 10-35% led to mainly ventricular septal defects; constricting by 35-60% resulted in a double outlet right ventricle. Ligation of the vitelline vein caused mainly pharyngeal arch artery defects. Experimental manipulation of mouse embryos in culture, followed by optical projection tomography imaging and morphometric analyses showed how reducing hemodynamic loading altered mammalian heart volume, myocardial thickness, trabeculation, and looping [22]. Intermediate levels of loading were sufficient for normal myocardial growth and heart size, but not for heart looping to form a four-chambered heart or for trabeculation. Myocardial growth and heart size were negatively affected by low levels of hemodynamic loading. Both studies using either the avian or mouse models demonstrated that cardiac anomalies can be finely regulated by the specific hemodynamic environment of the embryo at a given time of pregnancy. These results also demonstrate the need to understand the development of the extraembryonic membranes and placenta that contribute to the embryos' hemodynamics and how changes extraembryonically result in embryonic malformations. It is only with this knowledge that effective future prevention and treatments can be defined for human pregnancy.

Vitelline Circulation: Initially during embryonic development, the need for nutrient and oxygen exchange is taken care of by the vitelline circulation to the yolk sac. Changes in normal yolk sac hemodynamics have been observed to result in embryonic dysmorphogenesis or lethality [23, 24].

In the mouse embryo, heart formation occurs coincidentally along with blood and vascular development in the extraembryonic yolk sac. The first blood cells and endothelial cells are known to form in yolk sac blood islands at approximately ED 7.0 in the mouse [25]. McGrath *et al.* analyzed the establishment of early circulation in mouse embryos by examining the redistribution of yolk sac-derived primitive erythroblasts and definitive hematopoietic progenitors [25]. Their studies revealed that small numbers of erythroblasts first enter the embryo proper at ED 8.25, concomitant with the onset of cardiac function. Hours later at ED 8.5, most red cells remained in the yolk sac. A steady state of approximately 40% red cells was not reached until ED 10. The erythroblasts were observed to be unevenly distributed within the embryo's vasculature during the early stages. These data suggest that a fully functional circulation is established after ED 10. This timing during gestation correlates with remodeling of the vasculature, suggesting that vessel arborization and smooth muscle recruitment, or both, are necessary. Further study was carried out relating to the localization of committed hematopoietic progenitors during early embryogenesis. Before ED 8.0, all precursors were present in the yolk sac. When normalized to circulating erythroblasts, there was a significant enrichment of precursors in the yolk sac compared within the embryo proper, even later between ED 9.5 to ED 10.5. These observations indicate that the yolk sac vascular network remains a site of progenitor cell production, even after the fetal liver is developing into a hematopoietic organ. The investigators concluded that a functional vascular system develops gradually and that specialized vascular- hematopoietic environments exist well after circulation becomes fully established. Importantly, our timing of exposure during mouse gestation of ED 6.75, a time when we administer a *single* injection of an experimental factor to the pregnant female, coincides closely with the formation of vascular - hematopoietic environments. It is currently not known how these vascular-hematopoietic environments may be altered by exposures to external factors such as alcohol or cannabinoids, and other drugs. As described in the above studies, reducing-hemodynamic loading to even slightly different levels affected differentially mouse heart volume, myocardial thickness, trabeculation, and looping, resulting in different types of cardiac malformations [22]. Thus, the hemodynamic fine-tuning of heart development is evident, but what is missing is a more detailed clarification of the hemodynamic mechanisms that underlie the adverse effects of environmental exposures to commonly used substances as alcohol, marijuana, or even specific prescription drugs that have been linked to heart birth defects.

Early studies that analyzed the impact of vitelline hemodynamics on heart development were carried out using avian embryos. It is relatively easy to experimentally manipulate early-stage chick and quail embryos and to visualize the results under the microscope. Using what is described as the venous clip model, whereby the right lateral vitelline vein is constricted, the venous return and intracardiac laminar blood flow patterns were able to be experimentally changed, with secondary effects then observed on the mechanical load of the embryonic myocardium [26]. All hemodynamic parameters that were measured were observed to decrease acutely after the constriction. The cardiac malformations that formed in these embryos were ascribed to the effects of the decreased hemodynamics. Subsequently, in a pressure-volume loop analysis of the venous clipped model, it was shown that vessel constriction also resulted in abnormal systolic and diastolic ventricular function. The ventricular functional changes were found to precede the morphological abnormalities that only became apparent in later developmental stages. In the chicken embryo, permanent obstruction of the right lateral vitelline vein by clipping, reduced the mechanical load on the embryonic myocardium and was demonstrated to induce a spectrum of outflow tract anomalies [27].

The hemodynamic changes correlate with changes of shear stress and strains that are associated with embryonic heart remodeling. Shear stress is positively correlated to blood flow. Blood flow-related shear stress and circumferential strains have been analyzed in the developing embryonic heart and are a normal aspect of the formation of the four-chambered heart structure. These blood flow forces are transduced intra-cellularly to the cardiomyocytes *via* mechano-transducing molecular complexes some of which we defined by our immunohistochemical studies [16, 17]. In addition to the molecular sensing complexes, an ultrastructural cellular mechanosensing adaptation known as the primary cilium has been shown to have an important role [28, 29]. The primary cilia are connected to the cytoskeletal microtubules and transmit information into the endothelia cells about the direction and amount of blood flow. Not only do the endothelial cells have cilia, but also my laboratory reported that primary cilia are associated with embryonic cardiomyocytes within the myocardium during heart looping, as the myocardial tube bends rightward and loops to form the four-chambered heart [16]. These myocardial microcilia we suggested recognized forces exerted by the extraembryonic chorioalllantoic membrane on the myocardial wall during the looping process. Additionally, it has been shown that during looping and heart remodeling from a C-shaped tube, the highest shear stress is experienced by the inner heart curvature. When the shear stress is experimentally changed, this inner curvature region is highly affected and is associated with the development of congenital heart defects [30]. The changes in shear stress have been shown also to change gene expression in the cells located in these regions of high shear stress [31, 32]. Thus, there is a finely tuned control and interplay of biomechanical and biochemical sensing mechanisms and their signaling pathways that ultimately control genetic responses during the formation of the heart.

Trophoblasts and Chorioallantoic Placenta: According to our experimental paradigm, we acutely exposed mouse embryos to different environmental factors by a single i.p. injection given to the pregnant female during gastrulation at ED 6.75. The exposure was followed by more than a week of continuing pregnancy and embryonic development up to ED 15.5 at which time the embryonic blood flow of the individual embryos within the uterine horns was analyzed noninvasively by Doppler ultrasound to observe cardiac and placental blood flow [10, 33]. Both cardiac and abnormal placental function were observed with environmental exposures. Upon sectioning, in comparison to normal control embryos, we found disorganized placental organization and using histochemistry, we described abnormal protein expression, as well as abnormal neutral lipid localization in the placenta with the exposures [34 - 36]. In the mouse, a fully functional placental circulation is established by approximately ED 10.0. By embryonic day ED 10.5 during mouse gestation, embryonic/fetal growth is dependent on umbilical blood flow *via* the chorioallantoic placenta. It has been ascertained that at ED 13.5 in the mouse, the placental circulation becomes most important [18].

In human pregnancy, the vitelline artery and umbilico-placental circulations are functional from the onset of the initial heartbeats that are driven by the sodium-calcium exchanger (NCX-1) until the end of the organogenetic period, approximately defined as 9 weeks post conception [37]. After organ development is completed during the first trimester, the human yolk sac regresses and vitelline blood velocities are no longer detected. Vascular remodeling during utero-placental circulation provides blood flow throughout pregnancy and is mediated by trophoblast invasion of uterine spiral arteries. Vascular remodeling is characterized by increasing shear stress, as well as by angiogenic and humoral biochemical factors [38].

What is unique to the maternal placental vasculature in both the human and mouse, is that it is lined by fetal cells of the trophoblast lineage and not by maternal endothelial cells. Based upon the trophoblast fetal lineage of the maternal vasculature, we suggest that an answer as to why our early acute exposure on E 6.75 in the mouse resulted in placental abnormalities relates to our timing of exposure to when trophoblast differentiation and migration is taking place. The primary trophoblast cells that undergo invasion of the maternal blood vessels already begin to develop from the trophectoderm layer at the blastocyst stage [39]. These primary trophoblast cells eventually contribute to the formation of the decidua and promote the formation of maternal blood vessels that deliver blood to the placenta.

In a recent study it is noteworthy that many more trophoblast subtypes exist in the placenta than were previously known and were shown to vary with gestational age [40]. After fertilization has occurred, the first cell fate decision during embryo development separates the embryonic cells into two lineages, the inner cell mass that develops into the embryo proper and the trophectoderm that eventually forms the main part of the placenta [41]. The functions of nutrient and waste exchange between the mother and the fetus, as well as prevention of rejection of the fetus by the maternal immune system are performed by the placenta *via* the multiple specialized cell types. The mature placenta is composed of three main types of trophoblasts: cytotrophoblasts (CTBs), the syncytiotrophoblast (STBs) and extravillous trophoblast (EVTs). The CTBs line the stromal core and replenish STBs and EVTs. EVTs are differentiated trophoblasts that proliferate and differentiate to form a trophoblast cell column. The extravillous trophoblasts eventually invade the maternal uterine wall to anchor the fetus and to remodel the uterine spiral artery enabling fetal-maternal nutrient transfer. The STBs cover the surface of the villous tree throughout pregnancy. During pregnancy, the STB surface sheds apoptotic nuclei and cytoplasm into the maternal circulation and there is a continuous incorporation into the STB *via* fusion of new cell components from the CTB layer. An analysis using IT single-cell RNA sequencing of first and second trimester placental STBs, EVTs, and CTBs identified fourteen subtypes of placental cells and possible functions of those cells [40]. To define the molecular characteristics of the cells, a list of the genes that were specifically expressed at high levels in each cell type was generated and a functional annotation by gene ontology (GO) analysis was performed [40]. The authors confirm that genes associated with epigenetic modification and chromatin modification that are involved with cell differentiation and reprogramming are expressed by the different subtypes. For example, the DNMT1 (DNA methyltransferase-1) gene that maintains DNA methylation patterns during replication are highly expressed in all CTB_8W subtypes. Seemingly, in relation to my lab's analyses of mechanisms involved in mouse pregnancy, the importance of the maintenance of specific methylation patterns may be a reason why the maternal dietary folic acid supplementation protects normal mouse placental development [34 - 36]: Folic acid *via*the folate- homocysteine pathway synthesizes the primary methyl donor S-adenosylmethionine (SAM) in cells. Additionally, we demonstrated using *in vitro* culture studies that folic acid normalized trophoblast HTR8/SVneo cell line motility with environmental exposures [35, 41 - 43].

Recent studies are providing more information on trophoblast stem cells and differentiation and sex-related differences. The results of many studies have chiefly relied on the use of two different trophoblast cell lines, HTR8/SVneo or BeWo cell lines, to study placental function [44]. A recent proteomic analysis using comparative gene ontology of unique and up-regulated proteins revealed that the principal differences between these above-cited trophoblast cell lines are in proteins associated with cell junction/adhesion, the catenin complex, the spindle and microtubule associated complex, as well as in cell differentiation. The data indicated that BeWo cells express an epithelial proteome more characteristic of villous trophoblasts; whereas the HTR8/SVneo cells were a mesenchymal phenotype, more characteristic of extravillous trophoblasts. The HTR8/SVneo cells are considered in general to have more trophoblast progenitor cell-like characteristics indicative of self-renewal, repopulation activity, and expression of stem cell associated transcription factors [45]. In our study analyzing effects of environmental factors on early trophoblasts, we thus used the more precursor cell-like HTR8/SVneo human cell line and demonstrated that in our acute environmental exposure studies, a negative effect was observed on trophoblast cell migration *in vitro* and the non-muscle myosin-heavy chain-II (NMMHC -II) expression that is associated with cell motility [43]. Similar changes in NMMHC-II were observed in the *in vivo* mouse placenta and in the same mouse embryos displaying altered cardiac function [44]. In summary, with the timing of our exposures to gastrulation, the migration of trophoblasts and subtypes can be inhibited and thus would affect negatively downstream vascular remodeling during placentation.

That placental defects correlate strongly with abnormal heart, vascular, and brain development has been substantiated by a large-scale phenotyping study analyzing 103 embryonic lethal and sub-viable mouse knockout lines within the Mechanisms of Developmental Disorders program [46]. It was reported in this analysis that 68% of knockout lines that are lethal at or after mid-gestation, exhibited placental abnormalities. Early lethality between ED 9.5-14.5 was almost always associated with severe placental malformations. Furthermore, analysis of mutant trophoblast stem cells and conditional knockouts suggested that a significant number of factors that cause embryonic lethality, when ablated displayed their primary gene function in trophoblast cells [46]. Despite our studies reporting an association with placental and heart development, as well as studies from other investigators that we have reviewed [13, 18], the mechanisms underlying placental defects and their contribution to abnormal embryonic development, remains, unfortunately, a relatively under-studied area of research on effects of environmental factors. When considering that early maternal dietary folate supplementation may help to prevent these types of environmentally induced changes in the embryo and placenta, it seems necessary to have more research focused on these areas and clinical studies carried out to define an optimal dose for folate protection of heart and placental development.

BIOINFORMATICS OF EXPOSURES: ASSOCIATION WITH LIPID METABOLISM AND EMBRYO GENDER

In our research an aim was to define what common process(es) in the developing mouse heart may be changed by maternal lithium, elevated homocysteine, or alcohol exposure and whether the adverse effects can be prevented by folic acid dietary supplementation. Microarrays were carried out on embryonic mouse hearts, with and without exposures and with and without maternal folate dietary supplementation. Bioinformatic analysis of the data was validated by biochemical and genetic analyses in the mouse heart and placenta [34, 36]. The methodology that we used for our bioinformatics analyses was recently reviewed [47]. Using these approaches, lipid metabolism in the embryonic heart and in the placenta were found to be predominantly altered in comparison to control embryos. Interestingly, the lipid-related variation demonstrated a gender preference with male embryos being more adversely affected. Male embryos had greater numbers of genes changed in the lipid-related Gene Ontology biological processes than in female embryos [34]. The perturbations resulting from the environmental exposures, besides negatively affecting embryonic heart function, resulted in smaller placentas with disorganized cell and placental organization and reduced cellular neutral lipid droplet distribution. High folate supplementation of the maternal diet during early gestation protected normal mouse heart and placental function, resulted in normal gene expression, and normal neutral lipid localization [34]. A differential role for gender during early embryogenesis, as well as in lipid metabolism are aspects of development that have received little study, but are increasingly of more recent focus, as analyses have spread into the fields of diabetes, as well as obesity [48 - 52].

Lipids and Development

Lipids are essential in cellular energy production, in components of cell membranes, and in cell signaling by growth factors. We previously reported that the growth factor Wnt signaling is an important pathway in cardiogenesis [2, 3]. Wnt signaling is greatly dependent upon lipids. Active Wnt signaling and its secretion is dependent upon modification by two fatty acids [53 - 55]. Many of these cell-signaling proteins as Wnts are incorporated into lipid rafts that are dynamic regions of the plasma membrane. These lipid rafts contain high concentrations of cholesterol and glycosphingolipids [56 - 58]. Cholesterol within lipid rafts were reported to affect gene expression during skeletal muscle differentiation [59], as well as has the ability to modulate other growth factor signaling besides that of Wnt, *e.g.*, EGF receptor-mediated, signaling [60]. Interestingly, the possibility exists that the folate pathway intersects with the lipid signaling function in membranes, because an elevation of HCy, an important metabolite of our experimental paradigm, was reported to significantly increase glomerular endothelial cell permeability by stimulating lipid raft clustering to form redox signaling platforms [61]. Whether similar lipid raft clustering occurs in the embryo in response to HCy elevation, and possibly modulating Wnt signaling, is currently not known.

Lipid Metabolism

The bioinformatics analysis of our microarray data indicated that folic acid deficiency alters expression of proteins involved in fatty acid β-oxidation and lipid metabolism. The validation of the effects of HCy and Li^+ exposures on lipids was determined by Oil Red O (ORO) staining, a methodology to ascertain the presence of neutral lipid droplets. Cells can convert lipids into neutral lipids and store them as intracellular organelles that are defined as lipid droplets or adiposomes. These droplets help to maintain cell homeostasis. Droplet increase in cells, however, is linked in common disease states associated with obesity and diabetes [62].

Deficiency of *methyltetrahydrofolate reductase* (*Mthfr*; important enzyme in the folate pathway) and low dietary folic acid in the transgenic *Mthfr* model is associated with heart defects, fetal loss, intrauterine growth restriction (IUGR) and placental abnormalities [63, 64]. Because the embryos that we exposed to the environmental factors presented with abnormal heart physiology, were smaller in size with smaller placentas, and displayed changed umbilical artery blood flow, we included analysis of the placentas in our exposure studies of the animals that received and those that did not receive folate supplementation. After the earlier ED 6.75 single exposure by injection and more than a week later at mid-gestation in the ED 15.5 mouse fetus, both neutral lipid synthesis and localization were changed in the fetal heart and in the placenta. The most abnormal neutral lipid localization was seen in the placental tissue [34]. The Li^+ and HCy acute exposures on ED 6.75 resulted not only in disorganized villi in comparison to unexposed, control placentas, but also in changes in normal placental lipid localization patterns in the labyrinth and maternal decidual layers. Large areas of these placental compartments were often completely lacking in neutral lipids. The control placenta with a normal nutrient supply displayed a high number of lipid droplets in placental cells. Seemingly, with folic acid deficiency a characteristic of nutrient deprivation, the placenta degrades lipids to assist in their transfer to the embryo to facilitate embryonic growth and development. Decreased fatty acid transfer during development would change the fatty acid composition of tissue lipids resulting in both short- and long- term effects on cell structure and function, including on cell signaling. These effects would eventually contribute to cardiac pathology. A divergence in fatty acid uptake or utilization in the adult heart, for example, has been shown to lead to an increase in lipids that becomes toxic to cardiomyocytes leading to ventricular dysfunction and premature death. In the embryo, such a divergence may result in less than optimal oxygenation, nutrition, and in altered cellular bioenergetics leading to decreased embryonic myocardial function [5, 35, 65-67].

The development of cellular bioenergetics has been found to be an important part of normal cardiac cell differentiation [66]. As the embryonic heart increasingly depends upon oxidative metabolism, and as the blood vessels bring blood to the heart from the placenta, there is an increasing need for energy for maintenance of heartbeats. The energy source is primarily dependent on mitochondrial ß-oxidation of fatty acids. Myocardial fatty acid metabolism in disease has been reviewed [67]. Recent results demonstrate that cytoplasmic lipases remove fatty acids from lipid droplets when cells are starved and enable their transfer into mitochondria [68]. Although the early embryonic vertebrate heart and placenta develop in a low oxygen environment [69, 70], by ED 14 mouse cardiac mitochondria are involved in oxidative phosphorylation and fatty acid oxidation [68]. In general, underscoring the physiological importance of fatty acids for cellular energy production, in human studies genetic alterations in mitochondrial fatty acid oxidation are recognized as important causes of disease and death.

In our studies we specifically analyzed the expression of specific genes associated with lipid metabolism and also expressed in the embryonic heart. Two genes involved in fatty acid oxidation were studied, *Acyl CoA dehydrogenase medium chain* (*Acadm*) and *Acyl CoA dehydrogenase long* chain (*Acadl*). Both genes appeared several times in the lists of lipid-related Gene Ontology (GO) categories that we had identified from the embryonic mouse heart microarray analysis. These genes were deemed to be of importance because both genes are expressed within the heart and have been associated with disease states. For example, *Acadm* is associated with cardiomyocyte differentiation and cold tolerance in mice [71]. *Acadl* is linked with sudden death occurring closely after birth, as well as possibly before birth because decreased litter sizes were noted, as well as a link with cardiomyopathy [72]. A gender difference was also noted in our studies: The male placental tissue displayed a highly significant difference in *Acadm* expression level in response to an elevation of HCy than the placenta of female embryos. Similarly, in the human population genetic mutations of fatty acid oxidation-related genes are known to be present and are identified as being involved in certain disease states and in death [73]. Human ACADM (*MCAD*) deficiency is a most frequently cited disorder of the fatty acid oxidation pathway and in general is one of the most recognizable inborn error of metabolism [73].

Another area of increasing attention on lipids during pregnancy is the study of what effect maternal obesity has on embryonic development. Rate of maternal obesity has increased over a number of years in the United States with close to 60% of pregnant women being overweight and 25% being obese, the latter class defined by a body mass index – BMI >30kg/m^2) [74]. Maternal obesity during pregnancy is associated with various conditions, such as IUGR, as well as miscarriage. On the mother's side, obesity is associated with gestational hypertension, gestational diabetes, premature labor, as well as preeclampsia. Dysregulated serum fatty acids are linked to a creation of a lipotoxic environment within the placenta that then contributes to the pregnancy complications, seemingly by decreasing human extravillous trophoblast invasion by extending the exposure of the embryo to saturated fatty acids [75]. Hirschmugl *et al.* [52] demonstrated that the expression of placental genes related to transport and storage of neutral lipids was significantly changed by pre-gravid obesity. High maternal adiposity was associated also with a high level of reactive oxygen species (ROS) and decreased placental ATP levels in both male and female fetuses [74]. To define how maternal obesity affected cellular bioenergetics of the placenta, the expression of genes encoding the complexes of the mitochondrial electron transport chain was measured. All five mitochondrial complexes displayed a trend to decrease with increasing adiposity. To analyze the effect of maternal obesity on placental trophoblast respiration, an *in vitro* syncytiotrophoblast culture model was used. The investigators observed a decrease in mitochondrial respiration with increasing adiposity. The reduction in maximum respiration and spare respiratory capability suggested that syncytiotrophoblasts from placentae of overweight and obese women have a decreased ability to meet cellular bioenergetic needs.

Gender Association

At the time we were analyzing a possible gender bias in relation to lipid related genes that were changed and defects that arise during mouse heart development, similar gender relationships based on outcome studies of human pregnancy had been published in association with severity of congenital heart defects (CHDs) present in newborns.

Two studies [76, 77] analyzing the prevalence of CHDs at live births used Doppler ultrasound screening, as we had with our mouse screening studies. The Shanghai study screened 5,190 babies [77], and a second earlier study with similar echo screening, was carried out in Germany [76]. Both studies arrived at a similar conclusion that there was a male preponderance noted where severe CHDs existed (*e.g.*, hypoplastic left heart syndrome; interruption of the aortic arch, single ventricle, double outlet right ventricle, tetralogy of Fallot, among others). A female preponderance was found in cases of mild CHDs (*e.g.* small ventricular septal defect, mild pulmonary stenosis). A large US population study of sex differences in mortality in children undergoing congenital heart disease surgery, similarly concluded that more male children had CHD surgery and more had higher-risk procedures than the female children [78]. Mechanisms for these gender-based differences in the human population are not understood, but may relate to dyslipidemia as based on our mouse studies where heart defects were noted and an association with embryonic gender. Severe CHD is usually associated with prematurity and low birth weight. The fetus is dependent on the placenta for supplying long chain polyunsaturated fatty acids that are essential in growth of the fetus and development. When the fatty acid supply is reduced, low birth weight can result. Other studies have demonstrated that maternal dyslipidemia during human pregnancy increases the risk of adverse pregnancy outcomes and congenital heart defects [79, 80]. Arriving at similar results in other vertebrate models, a baboon model of moderate maternal nutrient deprivation resulted in growth restriction in the offspring. Furthermore, the investigators found that the IUGR was related to a gender -dependent abnormal regulation of cardiac structure, miRNA expression, and also abnormal cardiac lipid metabolism [81]. Analyzing a swine model of IUGR, the female offspring in general appeared to show better adaptive responses to maternal malnutrition than the male offspring [82, 83].

Our studies of mouse pregnancy were extended to alcohol exposure and to an analysis of neutral lipid modulation in the placentas of those same embryos displaying cardiac defects. Using biochemical and molecular assays, similar results in response to alcohol on lipid modulation were obtained, as had been observed with an elevation of HCys and that were prevented by folic acid [34].

Because the timing of the single exposure by i.p. injection during mouse gastrulation, *i.e.*, before organ formation at ED 7.5 and before the formation of the gonads at ED 10.5, the results indicate that the gender effect may be explained by a role for genes on the X/Y sex chromosomes during early embryogenesis. The Y-chromosome contains the male sex determination gene *SRY* and about 70 additional genes important for spermatogenesis. The Y-linked genes are known to function also beyond reproduction, because they are amply expressed in multiple adult tissues and during development [84]. Importantly, in relation to our research on the placenta, it has been demonstrated that sex-specific gene expression differences exist in trophoblastic progenitor cells, as well as in human embryonic stem cells, indicating that sex-biased gene expression is inherently present in early human placental progenitor cells [85]. The authors observed significant sex differences in transcriptomic profiles of human embryonic stem cells (hESCs) and trophoblastic progenitors, and also with the trophoblast differentiation process itself between the genders [85].

EPIGENETCS

A large number of genes expressed differentially between the sexes are suggested to be under the control of sex-specific epigenetic marks [86]. Epigenetic marks relate to heritable changes that are not part of the DNA sequence and form key modifications of the DNA or chromatin. Key epigenetic regulation of gene expression involves DNA methylation of CpG islands or sequences in the promoter regions of the DNA, as well as in histone methylation, acetylation or phosphorylation in chromatin remodeling complexes. As described earlier, the folic acid cycle by leading to the synthesis of the primary methyl donor S-adenosylmethionine (SAM), specifically contributes to the cells' epigenetic methylation capabilities. Dietary nutrient deficiency that results in an elevation of HCy levels within the folic acid cycle, decreases SAM production and thus reduces methylation capability. This decrease has the potential to critically inhibit normal epigenetic regulation and gene expression programming during specific phases of development and to do so in a sex-biased manner. There is evidence to indicate that sexual dimorphism underlies major aspects of imprinted gene regulation as well [87]. The physiological and molecular biological basis for the observed sexual bias in fetal programming is not well understood.

FOLATE PROTECTION OF NORMAL EMBRYOGENESIS

There is general agreement that folate supplementation during pregnancy has helped in the prevention of neural tube defects. There is increasing evidence that folate supplementation can prevent or reduce the risk and severity of CHD in human pregnancy as well. Prenatal supplementation with folate in clinical studies has been shown to protect the embryo from developing neural tube defects, to reduce preterm birth, and the severity of heart defects [88 - 93]. In our animal studies using the chick and mouse vertebrate models, folate supplementation or supplementation with both folate and myo-inositol were shown to prevent the teratogenic effects of a number of environmental molecules that affect human pregnancy, including of alcohol exposure [5, 36]. In human epidemiological studies, relatively high doses of folate of 10 mg/kg were shown effective in preventing cardiovascular defects [89]. In our mouse studies, a metabolic weight dose equivalent of 10.5 mg/kg maternal weight completely prevented cardiac defects from being induced during gastrulation. A more moderate dose of 6.2 mg/kg, however, provided only partial protection. No deleterious effects of folate at these doses were noted on normal development in the control animals receiving only physiological saline injections. These results indicate that a slightly higher dose of folate may be necessary for the prevention of cardiac birth defects than for neural tube defects where 1 mg/kg folate acid (FA) are given for high risk pregnancies. A mouse study using a folate dose 4 times higher than ours, that is, 40mg /kg, showed that such a high dose was deleterious to normal embryonic development [94]. These latter investigators administered a dose within a toxic range. If an equivalency of 10 mg/kg dose is already effective in preventing defects, it is not apparent why one would go to a higher range of concentration that has the potential to be toxic. To use a minimal effective dose is always optimal.

Another methyl donor in addition to the B vitamins folate and choline is betaine. All three participate in HCy metabolism and are known to exist in a delicate balance [95]. When folate levels are low, an elevation of HCy occurs. Remethylation of the HCy to form methionine in the folic acid cycle is catalyzed by methionine synthase with cobalamin used as a cofactor and 5-methyltetrahydrofolate as the methyl donor for this reaction. With low folate, HCy remethylation can be carried out by betaine HCy methyltransferase. Dimethylglycine is the other product of this reaction. Choline oxidation leads to the formation of betaine. Choline is also known to be an essential nutrient that functions in cell structure and signaling, lipid transport and neurotransmission. Choline is either supplied by the diet or is synthesized *de novo* from phosphatidylethanolamine. Choline cannot, however, be synthesized at necessary amounts, if both choline and folate levels are low. Evidence exists to show that the amount of folate one takes in, dictates how much choline is necessary [96]. Similarly, folate status affects plasma betaine and dimethylglycine concentrations in the cell and the association between betaine and total HCy during pregnancy [97, 98]. All of the above results indicate optimal cell folate concentrations will be the important factor in determining concentrations of the various methyl donors that will be available for methylation reactions in the embryo. Any of the methyl donors, as folate, betaine and choline, most likely will be helpful to prevent birth defects, as long as plasma folate concentrations are at a certain high enough level within the cell. Previously we reviewed the use of folate clinically to prevent CHDs [99]. Further clinical studies are necessary to define an optimal minimal FA dose for the prevention of congenital heart defects in human pregnancy.

CONCLUSION

In the 1990s the theory of the developmental origins of health and adult disease led to increasing studies and experimentation on this topic due to the pioneering work of Barker [100 - 103]. Epidemiological, clinical, and animal investigations demonstrate that the intrauterine environment will affect the growth and development of the embryo and fetus. My results from experimental studies using the mammalian mouse model, when extrapolated to human pregnancy, show that already between 16 to 19 days after fertilization of the egg by the sperm, the human embryo is highly at risk to exposure to environmental factors encountered by the pregnant female or ingested. As late as 5 weeks after conception, a woman usually is unaware of her pregnancy. Thus, during the first month of pregnancy, the mother most likely is not yet taking precautions to protect a developing embryo. The critical window of gastrulation that we targeted with our single injection coincides with a developmental period of cell specification and differentiation of cardiomyocytes and trophoblast cells, as well as of neural development. Thus, an early intrauterine exposure, even a single exposure, as we demonstrated may have long-lasting deleterious effects on tissue and organ formation and function during early pregnancy, postnatally, and well into adulthood. Counseling of couples of child-bearing age and planning pregnancy would be advisable along with dietary folate supplementation to protect the early embryo from developing birth defects of the heart and brain.

CONSENT FOR PUBLICATION

Not applicable.

CONFLICT OF INTEREST

The authors confirm that the contents of this chapter have no conflict of interest.

ACKNOWLEDGEMENTS

The author acknowledges NHLBI, American Heart Association, Suncoast Cardiovascular Research and Education Foundation founded by Helen Harper Brown and the David and Janice Mason Foundation of the USF Morsani College of Medicine for support of the research reviewed in this chapter.

REFERENCES

[1]   Linask KK. Regulation of heart morphology: current molecular and cellular perspectives on the coordinated emergence of cardiac form and function. Birth Defects Res C Embryo Today 2003; 69(1): 14-24.
[http://dx.doi.org/10.1002/bdrc.10004] [PMID: 12768654]

[2]   Chen J, Han M, Manisastry SM, *et al.* Molecular effects of lithium exposure during mouse and chick gastrulation and subsequent valve dysmorphogenesis. Birth Defects Res A Clin Mol Teratol 2008; 82(7): 508-18.
[http://dx.doi.org/10.1002/bdra.20448] [PMID: 18418887]

[3]   Manisastry SM, Han M, Linask KK. Early temporal-specific responses and differential sensitivity to lithium and Wnt-3A exposure during heart development. Dev Dyn 2006; 235(8): 2160-74.
[http://dx.doi.org/10.1002/dvdy.20878] [PMID: 16804895]

[4]   Grewal J, Carmichael SL, Ma C, Lammer EJ, Shaw GM. Maternal periconceptional smoking and alcohol consumption and risk for select congenital anomalies. Birth Defects Res A Clin Mol Teratol 2008; 82(7): 519-26.
[http://dx.doi.org/10.1002/bdra.20461] [PMID: 18481814]

[5]   Serrano M, Han M, Brinez P, Linask KK. Fetal alcohol syndrome: cardiac birth defects in mice and prevention with folate. Am J Obstet Gynecol. 2010; 203(1): e7- e15.
[http://dx.doi.org/10.1016/j.ajog.2010.03.017]

[6]   Serrano MC, Linask KK, Acharya G, Chen J, Han M, Huhta JC. Folate rescues lithium-, homocysteine- and Wnt3A-induced vertebrate cardiac anomalies. Dis Model Mech 2009; 2(9-10): 467-78.
[http://dx.doi.org/10.1242/dmm.001438]

[7]   Rosenquist TH, Ratashak SA, Selhub J. Homocysteine induces congenital defects of the heart and neural tube: effect of folic acid. Proc Natl Acad Sci USA 1996; 93(26): 15227-32.
[http://dx.doi.org/10.1073/pnas.93.26.15227] [PMID: 8986792]

[8]   Kenney SP, Kekuda R, Prasad PD, Leibach FH, Devoe LD, Ganapathy V. Cannabinoid receptors and their role in the regulation of the serotonin transporter in human placenta. Am J Obstet Gynecol 1999; 181(2): 491-7.
[http://dx.doi.org/10.1016/S0002-9378(99)70583-1] [PMID: 10454705]

[9]   Walker DS, Fisher CS, Sherman A, Wybrecht B, Kyndely K. Fetal alcohol spectrum disorders prevention: an exploratory study of women's use of, attitudes toward, and knowledge about alcohol. J Am Acad Nurse Pract 2005; 17(5): 187-93.
[http://dx.doi.org/10.1111/j.1745-7599.2005.0031.x] [PMID: 15854108]

[10]   Gui YH, Linask KK, Khowsathit P, Huhta JC. Doppler echocardiography of normal and abnormal embryonic mouse heart. Pediatr Res 1996; 40(4): 633-42.
[http://dx.doi.org/10.1203/00006450-199610000-00020] [PMID: 8888295]

[11]   Manisastry SM, Han M, Linask K. Anterior to posterior progression of heart development: Clinical implications of lithium exposure. Microsc Microanal 2004; 10 (Suppl. 2): 196-7.
[http://dx.doi.org/10.1017/S1431927604884800]

[12]   Chinn A, Fitzsimmons J, Shepard TH, Fantel AG. Congenital heart disease among spontaneous abortuses and stillborn fetuses: prevalence and associations. Teratology 1989; 40(5): 475-82.
[http://dx.doi.org/10.1002/tera.1420400510] [PMID: 2623637]

[13]   Linask KK. The heart-placenta axis in the first month of pregnancy: induction and prevention of cardiovascular birth defects. J Pregnancy 2013; 2013: 320413.
[http://dx.doi.org/10.1155/2013/320413] [PMID: 23691322]

[14]   Burd L, Deal E, Rios R, Adickes E, Wynne J, Klug MG. Congenital heart defects and fetal alcohol spectrum disorders. Congenit Heart Dis 2007; 2(4): 250-5.

[http://dx.doi.org/10.1111/j.1747-0803.2007.00105.x] [PMID: 18377476]

[15] Burd L, Klug MG, Bueling R, Martsolf J, Olson M, Kerbeshian J. Mortality rates in subjects with fetal alcohol spectrum disorders and their siblings. Birth Defects Res A Clin Mol Teratol 2008; 82(4): 217-23.
[http://dx.doi.org/10.1002/bdra.20445] [PMID: 18338392]

[16] Garita B, Jenkins MW, Han M, *et al.* Blood flow dynamics of one cardiac cycle and relationship to mechanotransduction and trabeculation during heart looping. Am J Physiol Heart Circ Physiol 2011; 300(3): H879-91.
[http://dx.doi.org/10.1152/ajpheart.00433.2010] [PMID: 21239637]

[17] Linask KK, Vanauker M. A role for the cytoskeleton in heart looping. ScientificWorldJournal 2007; 7: 280-98.
[http://dx.doi.org/10.1100/tsw.2007.87] [PMID: 17334619]

[18] Linask KK, Han M, Bravo-Valenzuela NJ. Changes in vitelline and utero-placental hemodynamics: implications for cardiovascular development. Front Physiol. 2014; 5: 390.
[http://dx.doi.org/10.3389/fphys.2014.00390]

[19] Maslen CL. Recent Advances in Placenta-Heart Interactions. Front Physiol 2018; 9: 735.
[http://dx.doi.org/10.3389/fphys.2018.00735] [PMID: 29962966]

[20] Midgett M, Thornburg K, Rugonyi S. Blood flow patterns underlie developmental heart defects. Am J Physiol Heart Circ Physiol 2017; 312(3): H632-42.
[http://dx.doi.org/10.1152/ajpheart.00641.2016] [PMID: 28062416]

[21] Midgett M, Rugonyi S. Congenital heart malformations induced by hemodynamic altering surgical interventions. Front Physiol. 2014; 5: 287. eCollection 2014.
[http://dx.doi.org/10.3389/fphys.2014.00287]

[22] Hoog TG, Fredrickson SJ, Hsu CW, Senger SM, Dickinson ME, Udan RS. The effects of reduced hemodynamic loading on morphogenesis of the mouse embryonic heart. Dev Biol 2018; 442(1): 127-37.
[http://dx.doi.org/10.1016/j.ydbio.2018.07.007] [PMID: 30012423]

[23] Hogers B, DeRuiter MC, Baasten AMJ, Gittenberger-de Groot AC, Poelmann RE. Intracardiac blood flow patterns related to the yolk sac circulation of the chick embryo. Circ Res 1995; 76(5): 871-7.
[http://dx.doi.org/10.1161/01.RES.76.5.871] [PMID: 7729004]

[24] Hogers B, DeRuiter MC, Gittenberger-de Groot AC, Poelmann RE. Extraembryonic venous obstructions lead to cardiovascular malformations and can be embryolethal. Cardiovasc Res 1999; 41(1): 87-99.
[http://dx.doi.org/10.1016/S0008-6363(98)00218-1] [PMID: 10325956]

[25] McGrath KE, Koniski AD, Malik J, Palis J. Circulation is established in a stepwise pattern in the mammalian embryo. Blood 2003; 101(5): 1669-76.
[http://dx.doi.org/10.1182/blood-2002-08-2531] [PMID: 12406884]

[26] Stekelenburg-de Vos S, Ursem NT, Hop WC, Wladimiroff JW, Gittenberger-de Groot AC, Poelmann RE. Acutely altered hemodynamics following venous obstruction in the early chick embryo. J Exp Biol 2003; 206(Pt 6): 1051-7.
[http://dx.doi.org/10.1242/jeb.00216] [PMID: 12582147]

[27] Stekelenburg-de Vos S, Steendijk P, Ursem NT, Wladimiroff JW, Poelmann RE. Systolic and diastolic ventricular function in the normal and extra-embryonic venous clipped chicken embryo of stage 24: a pressure-volume loop assessment. Ultrasound Obstet Gynecol 2007; 30(3): 325-31.
[http://dx.doi.org/10.1002/uog.5137] [PMID: 17721868]

[28] Clement CA, Kristensen SG, Møllgård K, *et al.* The primary cilium coordinates early cardiogenesis and hedgehog signaling in cardiomyocyte differentiation. J Cell Sci 2009; 122(Pt 17): 3070-82.
[http://dx.doi.org/10.1242/jcs.049676] [PMID: 19654211]

[29]   Van der Heiden K, Egorova AD, Poelmann RE, Wentzel JJ, Hierck BP. Role for primary cilia as flow detectors in the cardiovascular system. Int Rev Cell Mol Biol. 2011; 290: 87-119.
[http://dx.doi.org/10.1016/B978-0-12-386037-8.00004-1]

[30]   Hierck BP, Van der Heiden K, Poelma C, Westerweel J, Poelmann RE. Fluid shear stress and inner curvature remodeling of the embryonic heart. Choosing the right lane! Sci World J 2008; 8: 212-22.
[http://dx.doi.org/10.1100/tsw.2008.42]

[31]   Groenendijk BC, Hierck BP, Vrolijk J, *et al.* Changes in shear stress-related gene expression after experimentally altered venous return in the chicken embryo. Circ Res 2005; 96(12): 1291-8.
[http://dx.doi.org/10.1161/01.RES.0000171901.40952.0d] [PMID: 15920020]

[32]   Groenendijk BC, Van der Heiden K, Hierck BP, Poelmann RE. The role of shear stress on ET-1, KLF2, and NOS-3 expression in the developing cardiovascular system of chicken embryos in a venous ligation model. Physiology (Bethesda) 2007; 22: 380-9.
[http://dx.doi.org/10.1152/physiol.00023.2007] [PMID: 18073411]

[33]   Linask KK, Huhta JC. Use of Doppler echocardiography to monitor embryonic mouse heart function. Methods Mol Biol 2000; 135: 245-52.
[PMID: 10791321]

[34]   Han M, Evsikov AV, Zhang L, Lastra-Vicente R, Linask KK. Embryonic Exposures of Lithium and Homocysteine and Folate Protection Affect Lipid Metabolism during Mouse Cardiogenesis and Placentation. Reprod Toxicol. 2016: 61: 82-96.
[http://dx.doi.org/10.1016/j.reprotox.2016.03.039]

[35]   Han M, Serrano MC, Lastra-Vicente R, *et al.* Folate rescues lithium-, homocysteine- and Wnt3A-induced vertebrate cardiac anomalies. Dis Model Mech 2009; 2(9-10): 467-78.
[http://dx.doi.org/10.1242/dmm.001438] [PMID: 19638421]

[36]   Linask KK, Han M. Acute alcohol exposure during mouse gastrulation alters lipid metabolism in placental and heart development: Folate prevention. Birth Defects Res A Clin Mol Teratol 2016; 106(9): 749-60.
[http://dx.doi.org/10.1002/bdra.23526] [PMID: 27296863]

[37]   Linask KK, Han MD, Artman M, Ludwig CA. Sodium-calcium exchanger (NCX-1) and calcium modulation: NCX protein expression patterns and regulation of early heart development. Dev Dyn 2001; 221(3): 249-64.
[http://dx.doi.org/10.1002/dvdy.1131] [PMID: 11458386]

[38]   Osol G, Mandala M. Maternal uterine vascular remodeling during pregnancy. Physiology (Bethesda) 2009; 24: 58-71.
[http://dx.doi.org/10.1152/physiol.00033.2008] [PMID: 19196652]

[39]   Rai A, Cross JC. Development of the hemochorial maternal vascular spaces in the placenta through endothelial and vasculogenic mimicry. Dev Biol. 2014; 387(2):131-41.
[http://dx.doi.org/10.1016/j.ydbio.2014.01.015]

[40]   Liu Y, Fan X, Wang R, *et al.* Single-cell RNA-seq reveals the diversity of trophoblast subtypes and patterns of differentiation in the human placenta. Cell Res 2018; 28(8): 819-32.
[http://dx.doi.org/10.1038/s41422-018-0066-y] [PMID: 30042384]

[41]   Nelson DM. How the placenta affects your life, from womb to tomb. Am J Obstet Gynecol 2015; 213(4) (Suppl.): S12-3.
[http://dx.doi.org/10.1016/j.ajog.2015.08.015] [PMID: 26428490]

[42]   Linask KK, Huhta J. Folate protection from congenital heart defects linked with canonical Wnt signaling and epigenetics. Curr Opin Pediatr 2010; 22(5): 561-6.
[http://dx.doi.org/10.1097/MOP.0b013e32833e2723] [PMID: 20844350]

[43]   Han M, Neves AL, Serrano M, *et al.* Effects of alcohol, lithium, and homocysteine on nonmuscle myosin-II in the mouse placenta and human trophoblasts. Am J Obstet Gynecol. 2012; 207(2):140 e7-

19.
[http://dx.doi.org/10.1016/j.ajog.2012.05.007]

[44] Szklanna PB, Wynne K, Nolan M, Egan K, Áinle FN, Maguire PB. Comparative proteomic analysis of trophoblast cell models reveals their differential phenotypes, potential uses, and limitations. Proteomics 2017; 17(10): e1700037.
[http://dx.doi.org/10.1002/pmic.201700037] [PMID: 28317260]

[45] Weber M, Knoefler I, Schleussner E, Markert UR, Fitzgerald JS. HTR8/SVneo cells display trophoblast progenitor cell-like characteristics indicative of self-renewal, repopulation activity, and expression of "stemness-" associated transcription factors. BioMed Res Int 2013; 2013: 243649.
[http://dx.doi.org/10.1155/2013/243649] [PMID: 23586024]

[46] Perez-Garcia V, Fineberg E, Wilson R, *et al.* Placentation defects are highly prevalent in embryonic lethal mouse mutants. Nature 2018; 555(7697): 463-8.
[http://dx.doi.org/10.1038/nature26002] [PMID: 29539633]

[47] Linask KK. Bioinformatics of Embryonic Exposures: Lipid metabolism and gender as biomedical variables. In: al. X.Wang *et al* (eds), Lipidomics in Health & Disease, Translational Bioinformatics 14, Springer Nature Singapore Pte Ltd. 2018.
[http://dx.doi.org/10.1007/978-981-13-0620-4_3]

[48] Altmäe S, Segura MT, Esteban FJ, *et al.* Maternal pre-Pregnancy obesity associated with altered placental transcriptome. PLoS One 2017; 12(1): e0169223.
[http://dx.doi.org/10.1371/journal.pone.0169223] [PMID: 28125591]

[49] Calabuig-Navarro V, Haghiac M, Minium J, *et al.* Effect of maternal obesity on placental lipid metabolism. Endocrinology 2017; 158(8): 2543-55.
[http://dx.doi.org/10.1210/en.2017-00152] [PMID: 28541534]

[50] Duan Y, Sun F, Que S, Li Y, Yang S, Liu G. Prepregnancy maternal diabetes combined with obesity impairs placental mitochondrial function involving Nrf2/ARE pathway and detrimentally alters metabolism of offspring. Obes Res Clin Pract. 2018; 12(Suppl 2): 90-100.
[http://dx.doi.org/10.1016/j.orcp.2017.01.002]

[51] Ruiz-Palacios M, Ruiz-Alcaraz AJ, Sanchez-Campillo M, Larqué E. Role of Insulin in Placental Transport of Nutrients in Gestational Diabetes Mellitus. Ann Nutr Metab 2017; 70(1): 16-25.
[http://dx.doi.org/10.1159/000455904] [PMID: 28110332]

[52] Hirschmugl B, Desoye G, Catalano P, Klymiuk I, Scharnagl H, Payr S, *et al.* Maternal obesity modulates intracellular lipid turnover in the human term placenta. Int J Obes 2017; 41(2):317-23.
[http://dx.doi.org/10.1038/ijo.2016.188]

[53] Steinhauer J, Treisman JE. Lipid-modified morphogens: functions of fats. Curr Opin Genet Dev 2009; 19(4): 308-14.
[http://dx.doi.org/10.1016/j.gde.2009.04.006] [PMID: 19442512]

[54] Takada R, Satomi Y, Kurata T, *et al.* Monounsaturated fatty acid modification of Wnt protein: its role in Wnt secretion. Dev Cell 2006; 11(6): 791-801.
[http://dx.doi.org/10.1016/j.devcel.2006.10.003] [PMID: 17141155]

[55] Vrablik TL, Watts JL. Emerging roles for specific fatty acids in developmental processes. Genes Dev 2012; 26(7): 631-7.
[http://dx.doi.org/10.1101/gad.190777.112] [PMID: 22474257]

[56] Zhai L, Chaturvedi D, Cumberledge S. Drosophila wnt-1 undergoes a hydrophobic modification and is targeted to lipid rafts, a process that requires porcupine. J Biol Chem 2004; 279(32): 33220-7.
[http://dx.doi.org/10.1074/jbc.M403407200] [PMID: 15166250]

[57] Pike LJ. Lipid rafts: bringing order to chaos. J Lipid Res 2003; 44(4): 655-67.
[http://dx.doi.org/10.1194/jlr.R200021-JLR200] [PMID: 12562849]

[58] Simons K, Toomre D. Lipid rafts and signal transduction. Nat Rev Mol Cell Biol 2000; 1(1): 31-9.

[http://dx.doi.org/10.1038/35036052] [PMID: 11413487]

[59]   Possidonio AC, Miranda M, Gregoracci GB, Thompson FL, Costa ML, Mermelstein C. Cholesterol depletion induces transcriptional changes during skeletal muscle differentiation. BMC Genomics. 2014; 15: 544.
[http://dx.doi.org/10.1186/1471-2164-15-544]

[60]   Pike LJ, Casey L. Cholesterol levels modulate EGF receptor-mediated signaling by altering receptor function and trafficking. Biochemistry 2002; 41(32): 10315-22.
[http://dx.doi.org/10.1021/bi025943i] [PMID: 12162747]

[61]   Yi F, Jin S, Zhang F, *et al.* Formation of lipid raft redox signalling platforms in glomerular endothelial cells: an early event of homocysteine-induced glomerular injury. J Cell Mol Med 2009; 13(9B): 3303-14.
[http://dx.doi.org/10.1111/j.1582-4934.2009.00743.x] [PMID: 20196779]

[62]   Thiam AR, Farese RV Jr, Walther TC. The biophysics and cell biology of lipid droplets. Nat Rev Mol Cell Biol 2013; 14(12): 775-86.
[http://dx.doi.org/10.1038/nrm3699] [PMID: 24220094]

[63]   Li D, Pickell L, Liu Y, Wu Q, Cohn JS, Rozen R. Maternal methylenetetrahydrofolate reductase deficiency and low dietary folate lead to adverse reproductive outcomes and congenital heart defects in mice. Am J Clin Nutr 2005; 82(1): 188-95.
[http://dx.doi.org/10.1093/ajcn/82.1.188] [PMID: 16002818]

[64]   Pickell L, Li D, Brown K, *et al.* Methylenetetrahydrofolate reductase deficiency and low dietary folate increase embryonic delay and placental abnormalities in mice. Birth Defects Res A Clin Mol Teratol 2009; 85(6): 531-41.
[http://dx.doi.org/10.1002/bdra.20575] [PMID: 19215022]

[65]   Adams RH, Porras A, Alonso G, *et al.* Essential role of p38alpha MAP kinase in placental but not embryonic cardiovascular development. Mol Cell 2000; 6(1): 109-16.
[http://dx.doi.org/10.1016/S1097-2765(05)00014-6] [PMID: 10949032]

[66]   Hom JR, Quintanilla RA, Hoffman DL, *et al.* The permeability transition pore controls cardiac mitochondrial maturation and myocyte differentiation. Dev Cell 2011; 21(3): 469-78.
[http://dx.doi.org/10.1016/j.devcel.2011.08.008] [PMID: 21920313]

[67]   Lopaschuk GD, Ussher JR, Folmes CDL, Jaswal JS, Stanley WC. Myocardial fatty acid metabolism in health and disease. Physiol Rev 2010; 90(1): 207-58.
[http://dx.doi.org/10.1152/physrev.00015.2009] [PMID: 20086077]

[68]   Rambold AS, Cohen S, Lippincott-Schwartz J. Fatty Acid trafficking in starved cells: regulation by lipid droplet lipolysis, autophagy, and mitochondrial fusion dynamics. Dev Cell. 2015; 32(6): 678-92.
[http://dx.doi.org/10.1016/j.devcel.2015.01.029]

[69]   Han M, Trotta P, Coleman C, Linask KK. MCT-4, A511/Basigin and EF5 expression patterns during early chick cardiomyogenesis indicate cardiac cell differentiation occurs in a hypoxic environment. Dev Dyn 2006; 235(1): 124-31.
[http://dx.doi.org/10.1002/dvdy.20531] [PMID: 16110503]

[70]   Chang CW, Wakeland AK, Parast MM. Trophoblast lineage specification, differentiation and their regulation by oxygen tension. J Endocrinol 2018; 236(1): R43-56.
[http://dx.doi.org/10.1530/JOE-17-0402] [PMID: 29259074]

[71]   Tolwani RJ, Hamm DA, Tian L, *et al.* Medium-chain acyl-CoA dehydrogenase deficiency in gene-targeted mice. PLoS Genet 2005; 1(2): se23.
[http://dx.doi.org/10.1371/journal.pgen.0010023] [PMID: 16121256]

[72]   Spiekerkoetter U, Wood PA. Mitochondrial fatty acid oxidation disorders: pathophysiological studies in mouse models. J Inherit Metab Dis 2010; 33(5): 539-46.
[http://dx.doi.org/10.1007/s10545-010-9121-7] [PMID: 20532823]

[73]   Rinaldo P, Matern D, Bennett MJ. Fatty acid oxidation disorders. Annu Rev Physiol 2002; 64: 477-502.
[http://dx.doi.org/10.1146/annurev.physiol.64.082201.154705] [PMID: 11826276]

[74]   Fisher SC, Kim SY, Sharma AJ, Rochat R, Morrow B. Is obesity still increasing among pregnant women? Prepregnancy obesity trends in 20 states, 2003-2009. Prev Med 2013; 56(6): 372-8.
[http://dx.doi.org/10.1016/j.ypmed.2013.02.015] [PMID: 23454595]

[75]   Hong YJ, Ahn HJ, Shin J, *et al.* Unsaturated fatty acids protect trophoblast cells from saturated fatty acid-induced autophagy defects. J Reprod Immunol 2018; 125: 56-63.
[http://dx.doi.org/10.1016/j.jri.2017.12.001] [PMID: 29253794]

[76]   Lindinger A, Schwedler G, Hense HW. Prevalence of congenital heart defects in newborns in Germany: Results of the first registration year of the PAN Study (July 2006 to June 2007). Klin Padiatr 2010; 222(5): 321-6.
[http://dx.doi.org/10.1055/s-0030-1254155] [PMID: 20665366]

[77]   Zhao QM, Ma XJ, Jia B, Huang GY. Prevalence of congenital heart disease at live birth: an accurate assessment by echocardiographic screening. Acta paediatrica. 2013; 102(4): 397-402.
[http://dx.doi.org/10.1111/apa.12170]

[78]   Marelli A, Gauvreau K, Landzberg M, Jenkins K. Sex differences in mortality in children undergoing congenital heart disease surgery: a United States population-based study. Circulation 2010; 122(11) (Suppl.): S234-40.
[http://dx.doi.org/10.1161/CIRCULATIONAHA.109.928325] [PMID: 20837919]

[79]   Smedts HP, van Uitert EM, Valkenburg O, *et al.* A derangement of the maternal lipid profile is associated with an elevated risk of congenital heart disease in the offspring. Nutr Metab Cardiovasc Dis 2012; 22(6): 477-85.
[http://dx.doi.org/10.1016/j.numecd.2010.07.016] [PMID: 21186113]

[80]   Vrijkotte TG, Krukziener N, Hutten BA, Vollebregt KC, van Eijsden M, Twickler MB. Maternal lipid profile during early pregnancy and pregnancy complications and outcomes: the ABCD study. J Clin Endocrinol Metab 2012; 97(11): 3917-25.
[http://dx.doi.org/10.1210/jc.2012-1295] [PMID: 22933545]

[81]   Muralimanoharan S, Li C, Nakayasu ES, *et al.* Sexual dimorphism in the fetal cardiac response to maternal nutrient restriction. J Mol Cell Cardiol 2017; 108: 181-93.
[http://dx.doi.org/10.1016/j.yjmcc.2017.06.006] [PMID: 28641979]

[82]   Cogollos L, Garcia-Contreras C, Vazquez-Gomez M, *et al.* Effects of fetal genotype and sex on developmental response to maternal malnutrition. Reprod Fertil Dev 2017; 29(6): 1155-68.
[http://dx.doi.org/10.1071/RD15385] [PMID: 27184893]

[83]   Garcia-Contreras C, Vazquez-Gomez M, Astiz S, *et al.* Ontogeny of Sex-Related Differences in Foetal Developmental Features, Lipid Availability and Fatty Acid Composition. Int J Mol Sci 2017; 18(6): E1171.
[http://dx.doi.org/10.3390/ijms18061171] [PMID: 28561768]

[84]   Hughes JF, Page DC. The biology and evolution of mammalian Y chromosomes. Annu Rev Genet 2015; 49: 507-27.
[http://dx.doi.org/10.1146/annurev-genet-112414-055311] [PMID: 26442847]

[85]   Syrett CM, Sierra I, Berry CL, Beiting D, Anguera MC. Sex-specific gene expression differences are evident in human embryonic stem cells and during *in vitro* differentiation of human placental progenitor cells. Stem Cells Dev 2018; 27(19): 1360-75.
[http://dx.doi.org/10.1089/scd.2018.0081] [PMID: 29993333]

[86]   Gabory A, Attig L, Junien C. Sexual dimorphism in environmental epigenetic programming. Mol Cell Endocrinol 2009; 304(1-2): 8-18.
[http://dx.doi.org/10.1016/j.mce.2009.02.015] [PMID: 19433243]

[87]   Bourc'his D, Proudhon C. Sexual dimorphism in parental imprint ontogeny and contribution to embryonic development. Mol Cell Endocrinol 2008; 282(1-2): 87-94.
[http://dx.doi.org/10.1016/j.mce.2007.11.025] [PMID: 18178305]

[88]   Cains S, Shepherd A, Nabiuni M, Owen-Lynch PJ, Miyan J. Addressing a folate imbalance in fetal cerebrospinal fluid can decrease the incidence of congenital hydrocephalus. J Neuropathol Exp Neurol 2009; 68(4): 404-16.
[http://dx.doi.org/10.1097/NEN.0b013e31819e64a7] [PMID: 19287311]

[89]   Czeizel AE. Reduction of urinary tract and cardiovascular defects by periconceptional multivitamin supplementation. Am J Med Genet 1996; 62(2): 179-83.
[http://dx.doi.org/10.1002/(SICI)1096-8628(19960315)62:2<179::AID-AJMG12>3.0.CO;2-L] [PMID: 8882400]

[80]   Czeizel AE, Dudás I, Vereczkey A, Bánhidy F. Folate deficiency and folic acid supplementation: the prevention of neural-tube defects and congenital heart defects. Nutrients 2013; 5(11): 4760-75.
[http://dx.doi.org/10.3390/nu5114760] [PMID: 24284617]

[91]   Czeizel AE, Puhó EH, Langmar Z, Acs N, Bánhidy F. Possible association of folic acid supplementation during pregnancy with reduction of preterm birth: a population-based study. Eur J Obstet Gynecol Reprod Biol 2010; 148(2): 135-40.
[http://dx.doi.org/10.1016/j.ejogrb.2009.10.016] [PMID: 19926391]

[92]   Ionescu-Ittu R, Marelli AJ, Mackie AS, Pilote L. Prevalence of severe congenital heart disease after folic acid fortification of grain products: time trend analysis in Quebec, Canada. BMJ 2009; 338: b1673.
[http://dx.doi.org/10.1136/bmj.b1673] [PMID: 19436079]

[93]   Thompson S, Torres M, Stevenson R, Dean J, Best R. Periconceptional vitamin use, dietary folate and occurrent neural tube defected pregnancies in a high risk population. Ann Epidemiol 2000; 10(7): 476.
[http://dx.doi.org/10.1016/S1047-2797(00)00107-1] [PMID: 11018417]

[94]   Pickell L, Brown K, Li D, *et al.* High intake of folic acid disrupts embryonic development in mice. Birth Defects Res A Clin Mol Teratol 2011; 91(1): 8-19.
[http://dx.doi.org/10.1002/bdra.20754] [PMID: 21254354]

[95]   Ueland PM, Holm PI, Hustad S. Betaine: a key modulator of one-carbon metabolism and homocysteine status. Clin Chem Lab Med 2005; 43(10): 1069-75.
[http://dx.doi.org/10.1515/CCLM.2005.187] [PMID: 16197300]

[96]   Jacob RA, Jenden DJ, Allman-Farinelli MA, Swendseid ME. Folate nutriture alters choline status of women and men fed low choline diets. J Nutr 1999; 129(3): 712-7.
[http://dx.doi.org/10.1093/jn/129.3.712] [PMID: 10082779]

[97]   Chiuve SE, Giovannucci EL, Hankinson SE, *et al.* The association between betaine and choline intakes and the plasma concentrations of homocysteine in women. Am J Clin Nutr 2007; 86(4): 1073-81.
[http://dx.doi.org/10.1093/ajcn/86.4.1073] [PMID: 17921386]

[98]   Fernàndez-Roig S, Cavallé-Busquets P, Fernandez-Ballart JD, *et al.* Low folate status enhances pregnancy changes in plasma betaine and dimethylglycine concentrations and the association between betaine and homocysteine. Am J Clin Nutr 2013; 97(6): 1252-9.
[http://dx.doi.org/10.3945/ajcn.112.054189] [PMID: 23595875]

[99]   Huhta JC, Linask K. When should we prescribe high-dose folic acid to prevent congenital heart defects? Curr Opin Cardiol 2015; 30(1): 125-31.
[http://dx.doi.org/10.1097/HCO.0000000000000124] [PMID: 25389654]

[100] Barker DJ. The origins of the developmental origins theory. J Intern Med 2007; 261(5): 412-7.
[http://dx.doi.org/10.1111/j.1365-2796.2007.01809.x] [PMID: 17444880]

[101] Barker DJ. Human growth and cardiovascular disease. Nestle Nutr Workshop Ser Pediatr Program

2008; 61: 21-38.
[PMID: 18196942]

[102]   Barker DJ, Bagby SP, Hanson MA. Mechanisms of disease: *in utero* programming in the pathogenesis
        of hypertension. Nat Clin Pract Nephrol 2006; 2(12): 700-7.
        [http://dx.doi.org/10.1038/ncpneph0344] [PMID: 17124527]

[103]   Barker DJ, Bergmann RL, Ogra PL. Concluding remarks. The Window of Opportunity: Pre-Pregnancy
        to 24 Months of Age. Nestle Nutr Workshop Ser Pediatr Program 2008; 61: 255-60.
        [PMID: 18360965]

CHAPTER 4

Placenta Circulation

Leonor Ferreira and **Jader Cruz**[*]

Fetal Medicine Unit, Centro Hospitalar Universitário de Lisboa Central, Lisboa, Portugal

Abstract: The placenta is a complex organ with a distinct characteristic, it receives blood supplies from maternal and fetal circulation, forming two distinct, yet connected, systems: the maternal-placental (uteroplacental) blood circulation and the fetal-placental (fetoplacental) blood circulation. In the past decades, there have been considerable advances in the understanding of human placental circulatory physiology. Placental circulation is established early in pregnancy and adequate placental circulation and perfusion ensure that the fetus obtains an adequate supply of oxygen and nutrients. Placental vascularization involves the interaction of several regulatory pathways. Pregnancy-associated uterine vascular adaptions are the basis of the regulation of the maternal placental flow rate. Hemodynamic and structural changes ensure a low placental vascular resistance and normal umbilical blood flow which is suitable to supply oxygen and substrates needed to the fetus. This chapter reviews the structure of the human placental circulation and its development.

Keywords: Fetal-maternal circulation, Placenta, Placentation, Vascular growth factors.

INTRODUCTION

The placenta is a complex organ with an important vascular structure that receives blood from the mother (utero-placental circulation) and from the fetus (feto-placental circulation). Its implantation process establishes an interface between maternal and fetal vascular systems. An adequate placenta formation with appropriate circulation and perfusion ensure that the fetus obtains an adequate supply of oxygen and nutrients [1, 2].

Placenta vasculogenesis involves the interaction of several regulatory pathways. Vascular endothelial growth factor (VEGF) is required for all steps of placenta vascular formation and development. Inactivation of a single VEGF allele or abnormalities in genes encoding VEGF receptor can lead to severe vascular abnormalities in the placenta. VEGF (including placental growth factor) and its

---

[*] **Corresponding author Dr. Jader Cruz:** Centro Hospitalar Universitário Lisboa Central, Rua Viriato, 1069-089, Lisboa, Portugal; E-mail: jaderjcruz@gmail.com

Edward Araujo Júnior, Nathalie Jeanne M. Bravo-Valenzuela and Alberto Borges Peixoto (Eds.)

receptors have been localized in placenta tissue, in the maternal decidual cells, and in cytotrophoblasts. In normal pregnancies, VEGF expression increases with gestational age. This pattern suggests that VEGF is involved in regulating trophoblast invasion and in trophoblast differentiation and migration [3, 4].

Extensive neovascularization in the placenta is accompanied with periodic increases in uterine and placental blood flows during gestation. Blood flows to the maternal, fetal, and placental units are established when the maternal-fetal circulations connect within the placenta. It gradually increases until mid-gestation, then substantially increases at the last third trimester of gestation, keeping pace with the rate of fetus growth. Animal studies have shown that angiogenesis and vasodilatation of the uterine and placental vessels are important mechanisms to increase placental blood flow during late gestation, which is imperative for normal fetal growth and survival and is also directly linked to the well-beings of the fetus and the mother during pregnancy [4].

Placental angiogenesis is an important process that creates feto-maternal circulation, plays a key role in the elaboration of the placental villous tree and ensures efficient exchanges between the mother and the fetus. Failure in these processes is highly linked to the development of placental pathologies such as preeclampsia and fetal growth restriction [4].

UTEROPLACENTAL BLOOD CIRCULATION

The uterine artery is a branch of the internal iliac artery, and divides into four arcuate arteries, which in time, divide into more than 25 spiral arteries each. Pregnancy-associated uterine vascular adaptations, especially in the spiral arteries, are the key regulation of the materno-placental flow rate. Maternal vessels must be remodeled to achieve a successful uteroplacental circulation. Trophoblast invasion is an important event in placentation. Prior to trophoblast invasion, the walls of spiral arteries undergo a variety of reorganization processes. During the invasion period, cytotrophoblastic cells migrate out from the anchoring villi, invade the spiral arteries and remodels them. As a result, the spiral arteries obtain the physiologic properties that are required to perfuse the placenta (Fig. **1**).

Trophoblasts also penetrate the endothelium and reach the lumen of the vessel where they accumulate and form trophoblast plugs (Fig. **2**). These plugs block the blood flow from the mother towards the placenta during the first trimester allowing only plasma to pass through [2]. The maternal plasma that reaches the trophoblast has low oxygen levels. The low oxygen environment present in early placenta helps to promote angiogenesis throw the secretion of vascular endothelial growth factor [5]. The presence of intervillous blood flow on the sixth week has been associated to miscarriages or later gestational complications [6]. Invasion of the venous side of the uterine circulation is minimal, sufficient to enable venous return [7]. These plugs finally disintegrate at the end of the first trimester, allowing maternal blood to flow towards the intervillous space of the placenta. The maternal blood leaves the spiral arteries, circulates throughout the intervillous spaces and the surfaces of the villi and is then collected by the uterine veins.

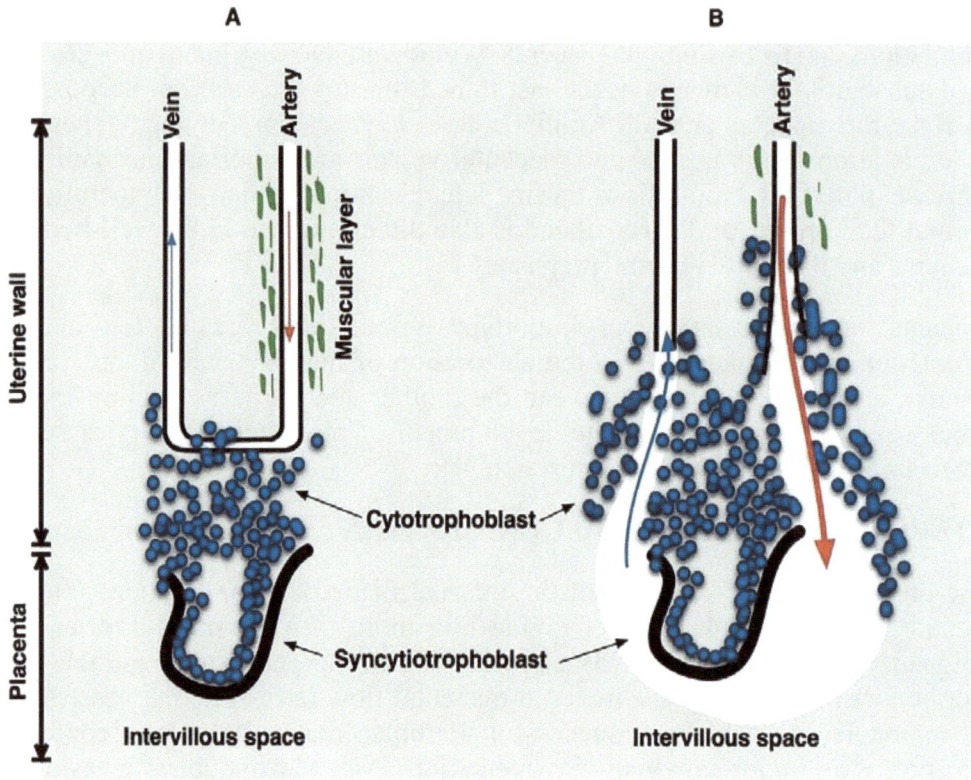

Fig. (1). Schematic drawing of placenta invasion of spiral arteries. A) early gestational age, B) after first trimester of pregnancy.

These modifications determine the quality of uteroplacental circulation and normal fetal growth. They are only fully established at the end of the first trimester [8]. When this process is successful, a low resistance, high capacitance placental compartment is established [9, 10]. The low-resistance of uteroplacental vessels and the contrast of blood pressure between uterine arteries and placental intervillous space allow the maternal blood to perfuse the intervillous space and the blood in the intervillous space to exchange two to three times per minute [9]. The progressive thinning of the villous trophoblast down to 4 μm by around 16th week and the prompt increased placental exchange area to reach a surface area of up to 12 m² at term, results in low placental blood flow resistance with a pressure around 10 mmHg in the intervillous space [10, 11]. The volume of placental blood increases throughout pregnancy, reaching about 600–700 ml/minute (80% of the uterine perfusion) at term [11, 12].

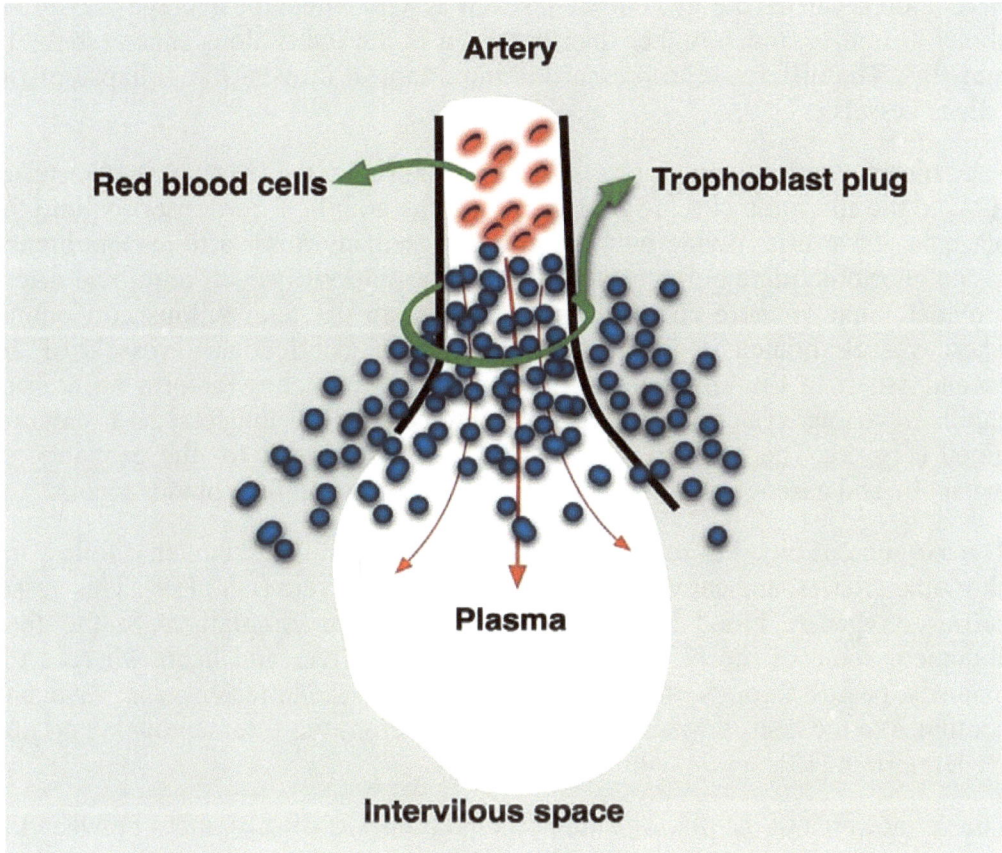

Fig. (2). Schematic drawing of placenta invasion of spiral arteries demonstrating the trophoblast plug.

Uterine vasculature has strict regulation and remains dilated under normal pregnancy conditions. Variations in maternal blood pressure and umbilical artery resistance play a role in regulating the blood flow to the utero-placenta circulation [13]. Placenta flow is additionally regulated by local paracrine factors such as nitric oxide, endothelin red blood cell adenosine and fetal atrial natriuretic peptide [14, 15]. The sum of these changes increases nutrient carrying capacity in maternal and fetal vascular beds and improves the efficiency of active and passive transplacental exchange [15].

THE FETOPLACENTAL CIRCULATION

The fetoplacental circulation can be divided into two broad categories the macrovascular, involving the umbilical and chorionic plate vessels, and the microvasculature, including intravillous vessels and capillaries [16]. The fetal circulation is carried out in a closed vascular system where the average pressure is about 30 mmHg, much higher than that seen in the intervillous space (about 10 mm Hg). The difference in pressure is important to prevent the collapse of the villous vessels [17].

Fetal blood with low oxigen levels leaves the aorta by the two umbilical arteries (UA) to the chorionic villi [18]. At the site of the umbilical cord insertion into the placenta, the arteries divide into, radially disposed, chorionic arteries that branch in the chorionic plate before entering the chorionic villi. Each umbilical artery provides eight or more chorionic plate arteries to the fetal villous cotyledons. These vessels branch in four to eight horizontal cotyledonary vessels of the second order. In the villi, the third order villous branches to form an arterio-capillary venous system that allows contiguity between the fetal and maternal blood (Fig. **3**). This system provides a large surface area for the exchange of metabolic and gaseous products between the maternal and fetal bloodstreams.

The oxygenated blood in the fetal capillaries passes into the veins that follow the chorionic arteries, and converge to form the umbilical vein (UV) [19]. This vessel carries oxygenate blood back to the fetal systemic circulation. In the fetal abdomen, some of the blood is distributed to the liver and heart whereas the majority passes through the ductus venosus into the inferior vena cava and continues to the heart through the right atrium across the foramen ovale and into the left atrium [13].

The surface area of the placenta supports the transport of substances between the placenta and the maternal blood. Some areas of the placenta, approximately 5-10%, are extremely thin allowing a flowing diffusion of substances between the fetal and maternal circulation. The transfer of substances occurs both ways across the placenta. The most common substances transferred from mother to fetus are oxygen and nutrients. The transfer of gases, oxygen and carbon dioxide, happens by diffusion and is mainly dependent on blood flow. As for water and electrolytes, these are easily transferred across the placenta through osmotic pressure and function ion channels. At 12 weeks, IgG antibodies begin to move through the placenta with a peak of transfer rate after 34 weeks. For this reason, prematurely born infants do not obtain complete levels of maternal antibodies.

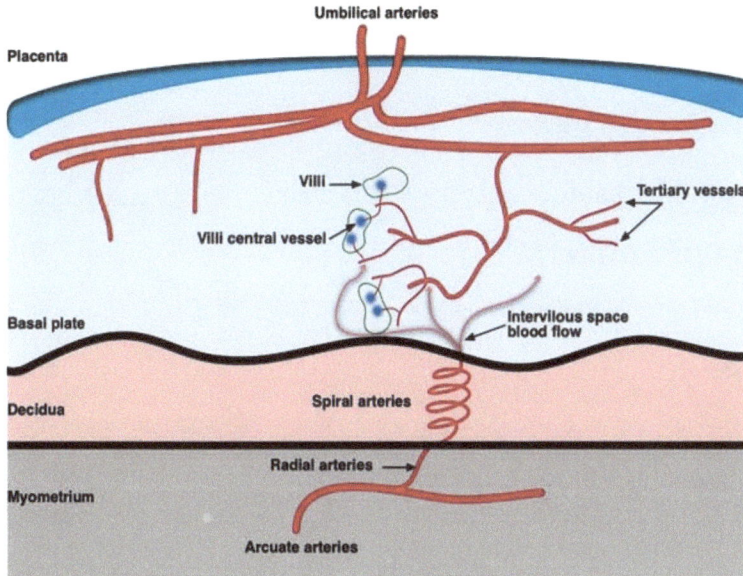

Fig. (3). Schematic drawing of feto-placenta circulation.

Umbilical blood flow is influenced by the placental resistance and gradient pressure between the descending aorta and inferior vena cava. Fetal movement and gestational age also determine the blood flow in this vessel. The umbilical artery waveforms alter during fetal breathing [20 - 22] and the UV blood flow is markedly affected by fetal respiratory movements due to changes in intrathoracic pressure in the fetus [23, 24].

In the past decades, there have been considerable advances in the understanding of human placental circulatory physiology. Placental circulation is established early in pregnancy to adapt to the necessities of the growing fetus. Hemodynamic and structural changes ensure a low placental vascular resistance and normal umbilical blood flow which is suitable to supply oxygen and substrates to the fetus. Although exact noninvasive measurement of all hemodynamic parameters of placental circulation still remains a challenge, technological developments have provided us with the tools to evaluate the umbilical and uterine circulation in order to confirm normality and diagnose fetoplacental circulatory compromise [25].

Nonetheless, with colour Doppler, it is still a challenge to noninvasively assess placental perfusion specially the visualization of small placental vessels as intra-placental villous artery that might be useful in the identification of pregnancies at risk of preeclampsia and placental insufficiency [26, 27].

CONSENT FOR PUBLICATION

Not applicable.

CONFLICT OF INTEREST

The authors confirm that the contents of this chapter have no conflict of interest.

ACKNOWLEDGEMENTS

Declare none.

REFERENCES

[1]   Acharya G, Sonesson SE, Flo K, Räsänen J, Odibo A. Hemodynamic aspects of normal human feto-placental (umbilical) circulation. Acta Obstet Gynecol Scand 2016; 95(6): 672-82.
       [http://dx.doi.org/10.1111/aogs.12919] [PMID: 27130575]

[2]   Wang Y, Zhao S. Vascular Biology of the Placenta. San Rafael, CA: Morgan & Claypool Life Sciences 2010; pp. 3-7.

[3]   Dvorak HF. Vascular permeability factor/vascular endothelial growth factor: a critical cytokine in tumor angiogenesis and a potential target for diagnosis and therapy. J Clin Oncol 2002; 20(21): 4368-80.
       [http://dx.doi.org/10.1200/JCO.2002.10.088] [PMID: 12409337]

[4]   Shibuya M. Structure and function of VEGF/VEGF-receptor system involved in angiogenesis. Cell Struct Funct 2001; 26(1): 25-35.
       [http://dx.doi.org/10.1247/csf.26.25] [PMID: 11345501]

[5]   Bruce M. Human Embryology and Developmental Biology. Philadelphia, PA: WB Saunders Company 2019; pp. 110-27.

[6]   Jaffe R, Dorgan A, Abramowicz JS. Color Doppler imaging of the uteroplacental circulation in the first trimester: value in predicting pregnancy failure or complication. AJR Am J Roentgenol 1995; 164(5): 1255-8.
       [http://dx.doi.org/10.2214/ajr.164.5.7717242] [PMID: 7717242]

[7]   Fisher SJ. Why is placentation abnormal in preeclampsia? Am J Obstet Gynecol 2015; 213(4) (Suppl.): S115-22.
       [http://dx.doi.org/10.1016/j.ajog.2015.08.042] [PMID: 26428489]

[8]   Persico MG, Vincenti V, DiPalma T. Structure, expression and receptor-binding properties of placenta growth factor (PlGF). Curr Top Microbiol Immunol 1999; 237: 31-40.
       [http://dx.doi.org/10.1007/978-3-642-59953-8_2] [PMID: 9893344]

[9]   Carbillon L, Challier JC, Alouini S, Uzan M, Uzan S. Uteroplacental circulation development: Doppler assessment and clinical importance. Placenta 2001; 22(10): 795-9.
       [http://dx.doi.org/10.1053/plac.2001.0732] [PMID: 11718565]

[10]   Junaid TO, Brownbill P, Chalmers N, Johnstone ED, Aplin JD. Fetoplacental vascular alterations associated with fetal growth restriction. Placenta 2014; 35(10): 808-15.
       [http://dx.doi.org/10.1016/j.placenta.2014.07.013] [PMID: 25145956]

[11]   Maini CL, Rosati P, Galli G, Bellati U, Bonetti MG, Moneta E. Non-invasive radioisotopic evaluation of placental blood flow. Gynecol Obstet Invest 1985; 19(4): 196-206.
       [http://dx.doi.org/10.1159/000299034] [PMID: 3928457]

[12]   Luckhardt M, Leiser R, Kingdom J, *et al.* Effect of physiologic perfusion-fixation on the

morphometrically evaluated dimensions of the term placental cotyledon. J Soc Gynecol Investig 1996; 3(4): 166-71.
[http://dx.doi.org/10.1177/107155769600300402] [PMID: 8796826]

[13]   Pardo M, Miller R. Basics of Anesthesia. Philadelphia, PA: WB Saunders Company 2018; pp. 553-8.

[14]   Kingdom JC, Burrell SJ, Kaufmann P. Pathology and clinical implications of abnormal umbilical artery Doppler waveforms. Ultrasound Obstet Gynecol 1997; 9(4): 271-86.
[http://dx.doi.org/10.1046/j.1469-0705.1997.09040271.x] [PMID: 9168580]

[15]   Kiserud T. The ductus venosus. Semin Perinatol 2001; 25(1): 11-20.
[http://dx.doi.org/10.1053/sper.2001.22896] [PMID: 11254155]

[16]   Boron W, Boulpaep E. Medical physiology. Philadelphia, PA: WB Saunders Company 2017; pp. 1151-68.

[17]   Castellucci M, Kosanke G, Verdenelli F, Huppertz B, Kaufmann P. Villous sprouting: fundamental mechanisms of human placental development. Hum Reprod Update 2000; 6(5): 485-94.
[http://dx.doi.org/10.1093/humupd/6.5.485] [PMID: 11045879]

[18]   Baschat AA. Fetal responses to placental insufficiency: an update. BJOG 2004; 111(10): 1031-41.
[http://dx.doi.org/10.1111/j.1471-0528.2004.00273.x] [PMID: 15383103]

[19]   Moore K, Persaud T, Torchia M. Before We Are Born: Essentials Of Embryology And Birth Defects. Philadelphia, PA: WB Saunders Company 2016; pp. 71-89.

[20]   Pozniak M, Allan P. Clinical Doppler Ultrasound: Expert Consult. Philadelphia, PA: Elsevier 2014; pp. 315-32.

[21]   Mulders LG, Muijsers GJ, Jongsma HW, Nijhuis JG, Hein PR. The umbilical artery blood flow velocity waveform in relation to fetal breathing movements, fetal heart rate and fetal behavioural states in normal pregnancy at 37 to 39 weeks. Early Hum Dev 1986; 14(3-4): 283-93.
[http://dx.doi.org/10.1016/0378-3782(86)90191-X] [PMID: 3803274]

[22]   Nyberg MK, Johnsen SL, Rasmussen S, Kiserud T. Fetal breathing is associated with increased umbilical blood flow. Ultrasound Obstet Gynecol 2010; 36(6): 718-23.
[http://dx.doi.org/10.1002/uog.7701] [PMID: 20521237]

[23]   Koppelaar I, Wladimiroff JW. Quantitation of breathing-related modulation of umbilical arterial and venous flow velocity waveforms in the normal term fetus. Eur J Obstet Gynecol Reprod Biol 1992; 45(3): 177-80.
[http://dx.doi.org/10.1016/0028-2243(92)90080-I] [PMID: 1511763]

[24]   Trudinger BJ, Cook CM. The fetal breath cycle. Early Hum Dev 1990; 21(3): 181-91.
[http://dx.doi.org/10.1016/0378-3782(90)90117-2] [PMID: 2178919]

[25]   Indik JH, Reed KL. Variation and correlation in human fetal umbilical Doppler velocities with fetal breathing: evidence of the cardiac-placental connection. Am J Obstet Gynecol 1990; 163(6 Pt 1): 1792-6.
[http://dx.doi.org/10.1016/0002-9378(90)90751-R] [PMID: 2256484]

[26]   Noguchi J, Hata K, Tanaka H, Hata T. Placental vascular sonobiopsy using three-dimensional power Doppler ultrasound in normal and growth restricted fetuses. Placenta 2009; 30(5): 391-7.
[http://dx.doi.org/10.1016/j.placenta.2009.02.010] [PMID: 19327824]

[27]   Babic I, Ferraro ZM, Garbedian K, *et al.* Intraplacental villous artery resistance indices and identification of placenta-mediated diseases. J Perinatol 2015; 35(10): 793-8.
[http://dx.doi.org/10.1038/jp.2015.85] [PMID: 26226247]

CHAPTER 5

Fetal Echocardiographic Evaluation

Luciane Alves da Rocha[1,*] and **Edward Araujo Júnior**[2,3]

[1] *Postgraduate Program in Health Sciences, Medical School, Federal University of Amazonas (PPHS-UFAM), Manaus-AM, Brazil*

[2] *Department of Obstetrics, Discipline of Fetal Medicine, Federal University of São Paulo (EPM-UNIFESP), São Paulo-SP, Brazil*

[3] *Medical Course, Municipal University of São Caetano do Sul (USCS), Bela Vista Campus, São Paulo-SP, Brazil*

Abstract: Congenital heart diseases are more common than chromosomal abnormalities or neural tube defects. Although been one of the cause of mortality in infants, early diagnosis of heart defects increases survival. It is of utmost importance to perform adequate cardiac screening. The International Society of Ultrasound in Obstetrics and Gynecology standardized the basic echocardiographic planes, in order to facilitate its use, increasing diagnosis. Therefore, in this chapter, we will discuss the anatomy and a systematized technical description of the fetal heart by two-dimensional (2D) echocardiography, emphasizing its indications, essential points for a good cardiac evaluation, and notions about some heart defects.

Keywords: Congenital heart disease, Echocardiography, Screening.

INTRODUCTION

The incidence of fetus cardiac defects is six times greater than chromosomal abnormalities and four times greater than neural tube defects [1 - 3]. According to data from the World Health Organization [4 - 6], infant mortality rate attributed to cardiac malformations was 42% between the years 1950 and 1994. Early diagnosis is essential for the treatment of several diseases and represents a better chance for surviving. In relation to congenital heart diseases, it is not different. With the early detection of congenital heart disease, we may: advise relatives about the nature and severity of the disease; allow intrauterine intervention when it is necessary and to allow family members and multidisciplinary staff to adequately plan childbirth, always with the aim of improving the prognosis of this child, thus reducing the rate of infant mortality and morbidity [7 - 10].

* **Corresponding author Luciane Alves da Rocha:** Postgraduate Program in Health Sciences, Medical School, Federal University of Amazonas (UFAM), 1100 Nilton Lins Teacher ave, n. 01, Flores, Zip Code: 69058-030, Manaus-AM, Brazil; Tel: +55-92-994038600; E-mail: lucianerocha.amorim@gmail.com

With cardiac screening performed during morphological ultrasonography, it was noticed an increase of suspicion of cardiac abnormalities is observed and, consequently, a higher rate of detection of cardiac diseases in the fetus by more experienced professionals in the diagnosis of these diseases is noticed. The rate of detection of cardiac defects has increased since the introduction of the concept of cardiac screening, especially after the standardization of basic echocardiographic planes by the International Society of Ultrasound in Obstetrics and Gynecology [8, 9].

The second trimester is considered the best time to perform echocardiography [9, 10]. During this period, the fetal heart is better visualized because of the relatively large fetus size and because there are very few calcified structures that can block the image (acoustic shadowing). A complete fetal echocardiographic examination includes structural and functional heart evaluation. In this chapter, we will discuss a systematized technical description and practice of the fetal heart anatomy, emphasizing the essential points for a good cardiac evaluation of the fetus, the indications of the fetal echocardiogram and notions about some heart defects.

HOW IS THE SCREENING FOR CONGENITAL HEART DISEASES PERFORMED?

Examination of the fetal heart should ideally be performed with a good ultrasound machine using the two-dimensional (2D) tools with colored and pulsed Doppler. Cardiac evaluation begins with the fetal positioning, in order to identify what is left and right, anterior and posterior, upper and lower [7].

In the transverse plane of the fetal abdomen, we can identify the stomach on the left and the liver on the right; as we directed the transducer lightly to the thoracic portion of the fetus, we are able to better register the abdominal aorta positioned posteriorly (near the vertebral body) and the left of the fetus, in addition to the inferior vena cava located to the right and anteriorly [7, 10] (Fig. **1**).

In the transverse plane of the fetus, in the thoracic region, we visualize the heart occupying a third of the thoracic area, presenting an axis around 45° (+/- 20°) when we draw two imaginary lines: a line between the vertebral body and the sternum of the fetus and another line tangentiating the interventricular septum of the fetal heart [10] (Fig. **2**).

Up to this point, we have already characterized the situs, the position and the cardiac apex that are part of the cardiac evaluation. Continuing in the transverse plane of the fetal thorax, we visualize the heart of the fetus with its four chambers. In this plane, several structures can be analyzed: the cardiac cavities, the pulmonary venous return, the atria, the ventricles and the atrioventricular valves

[7, 10] (Fig. **3**).

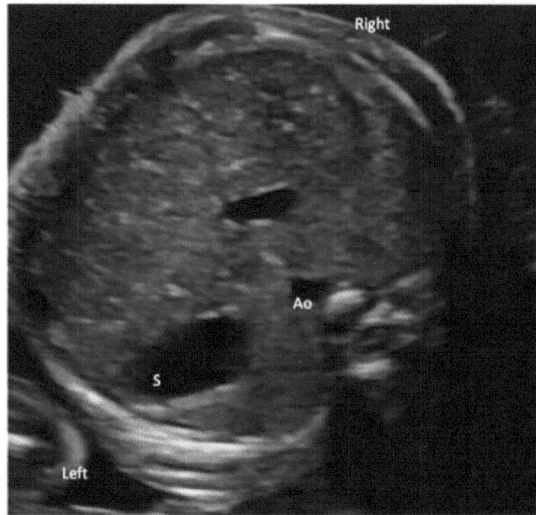

Fig. (1). Transverse plane of the fetal abdomen. Situs abdominal solitus. Fetal positioning: cephalic with posterior dorsum. S: stomach. Ao: aorta.

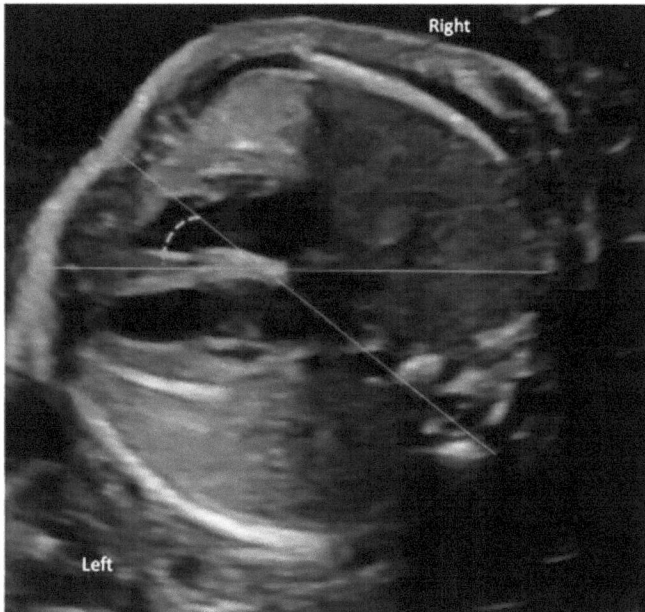

Fig. (2). Transverse plane of the fetal thorax. Cardiac axis around 45°. We draw two imaginary lines: one line between the vertebral body and the sternum of the fetus and another line tangentiating the interventricular septum of the fetal heart.

- Evaluation of the cardiac chambers: we can observe the proportional dimensions of the cardiac chambers in a more global way and then we can detail their internal characteristics in a sequential and segmental way (Fig. **3**).

- Pulmonary venous return: assessment of pulmonary veins draining into the left atrium. These structures can be visually displayed with relative ease when using color Doppler with lower velocity (between 30 and 40 cm/sec) (Fig. **4**).

- Visualization of the atria - the size of the atria and the interatrial septum are evaluated. The morphologically left atrium, located on the left side of the fetus, has visible drainage of at least two pulmonary veins and presence of the foramen ovale with good mobility for its interior. The morphologically right atrium located on the right side of the fetus has blood flow directed to both the right ventricle by tricuspid valve and the left atrium through the foramen ovale, visible with the aid of color Doppler (Fig. **3**).

- Atrioventricular valves (mitral and tricuspid valves): the mitral valve is related to the left heart cavities and the tricuspid valve, with the right cardiac cavities. The tricuspid valve is located slightly more apical than the mitral valve (Fig. **3**). We must observe the valve mobility and valve insufficiency with the help of color and pulsed Doppler.

- Visualization of the ventricles: the size and proportion of the ventricles are evaluated, besides the ventricular septum that must be intact. In the right ventricle we observe the presence of the typical moderating band of this cavity (Fig. **3**).

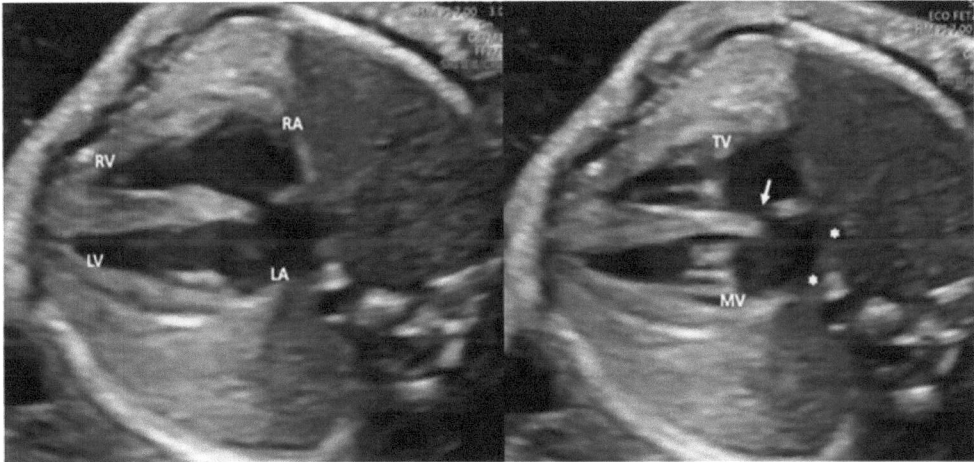

Fig. (3). Transverse plane of the fetal thorax. Four-chamber view. RA: right atrium, LA: left atrium, RV: right ventricle, LV: left ventricle, TV: tricuspid valve; MV: mitral valve. Arrow: blade of the foramen ovale. * pulmonary veins.

Following the transverse plane of the fetal thorax, the examiner should gently move the transducer toward the cranial portion of the fetus. With this slight movement, we can see the vessels that leave the heart (aorta and pulmonary arteries), a portion of the superior vena cava and the trachea. At this angle, we visualize the plane called "three vessels and trachea". With a slight movement, the examiner should observe: the left ventricular outflow tract, the right ventricular outflow tract and the plane of the three vessels and trachea (Figs. **5** to **7**). In this movement of the scale, performed with the help of color Doppler, the examiner clearly observes the crossing of the great vessels characteristic of a normal heart [7].

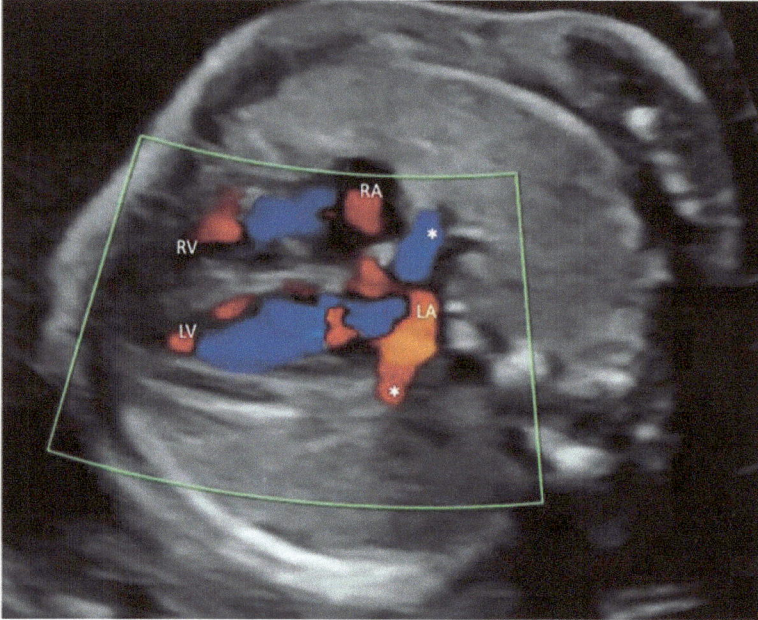

Fig. (4). Transverse plane of the fetal thorax showing the four-chamber view. Enlargement of the image to evidence the presence of the pulmonary vein arriving in the left atrium with the help of color Doppler. RA: right atrium. LA: left atrium. RV: right ventricle. LV: left ventricle. * pulmonary veins.

- The left ventricular outflow tract: is the connection of the left ventricle to the aortic artery. At this point, the integrity of the interventricular septum, the thickness of the ventricle wall, the mobility of the aortic valve and the ascending aorta should be assessed (Fig. **5**).
- The right ventricular outflow tract: the right ventricle connection to the pulmonary artery. The relation between the pulmonary artery and the right ventricle, the wall of the ventricle and the mobility of the pulmonary valve is observed. It is possible to observe the division of the pulmonary artery with its right and left pulmonary branches, different from what is observed in the aorta artery that normally emits the brachiocephalic trunk, the left carotid artery and the left subclavian artery, giving continuity as a descending aorta artery (Fig. **6**).
- Finally, the plane of the "three vessels and trachea": where the examiner

evaluates from left to right and anterior-posterior direction of the fetus, pulmonary artery, aorta, superior vena cava and trachea (Fig. **7**). The size of the pulmonary artery is larger than the aorta, and this is larger than the superior vena cava. Using color Doppler, the same direction of blood flow should be observed in the pulmonary artery and aorta, otherwise obstruction is suspected in some region of the vessel pathway that has retrograde flow. The trachea can be difficult to perceive because its reduced size can be mistaken for some vascular structure. The color Doppler tool is usually used for differentiation. The pulmonary artery emits the right and left branches, and the ductus arteriosus that communicates with the most distal aortic arch. This junction is to the left of the trachea. This anatomical description becomes important for the diagnosis of the right aortic arch, when the trachea is positioned between the pulmonary artery and the aorta. It should also be noted that there is the possibility of a fourth vessel in this plane of the three vessels and trachea, this situation is due to the existence of a persistent left superior vena cava that may be related to some obstruction of the aortic arch.

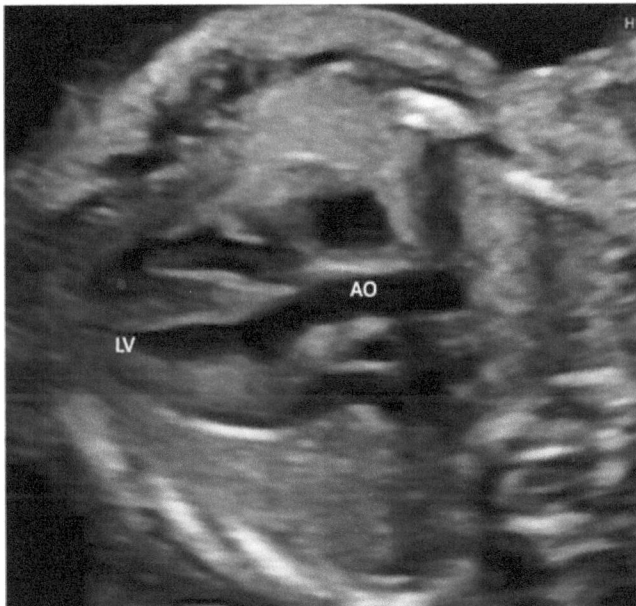

Fig. (5). Longitudinal plane of the fetal heart. The left ventricular outflow tract is observed, assessing the integrity of the interventricular septum, left ventricular wall thickness, aortic valve, and ascending aorta. LV: left ventricle. AO: ascending aorta.

Several studies have shown that the fetal heart evaluation by performing the four chamber and the three vessel and tracheal views are capable of detecting the vast majority of congenital heart defects in the fetus [11 - 15]. In 2009, Xu *et al.* [16] performed a prospective study in 5.5% of the fetuses had congenital heart disease, of which 31.5% were detected only with the four-chamber view, while 69% were detected by combining the four-chamber and the three-vessel and tracheal views.

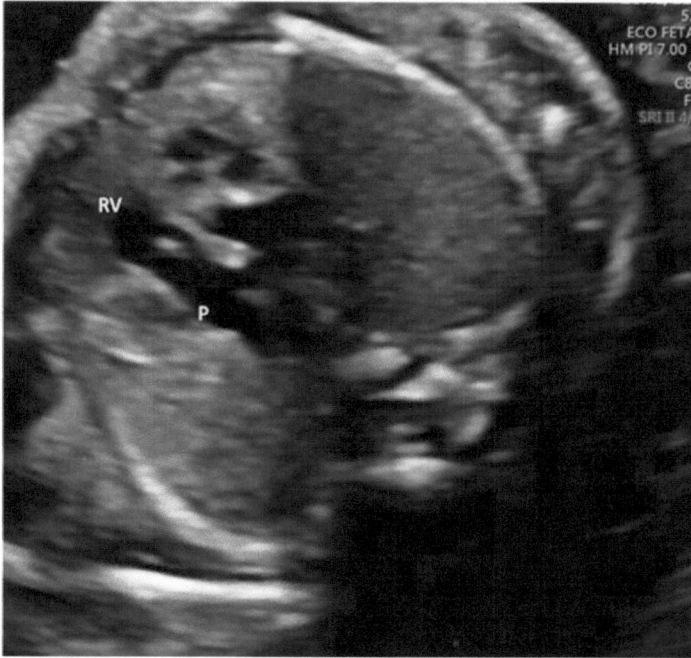

Fig. (6). Connection of the right ventricle to the pulmonary artery. The relation between the pulmonary artery and the right ventricle, the ventricle wall, the pulmonary valve, and the pulmonary trunk are observed. RV: right ventricle. P: pulmonary trunk.

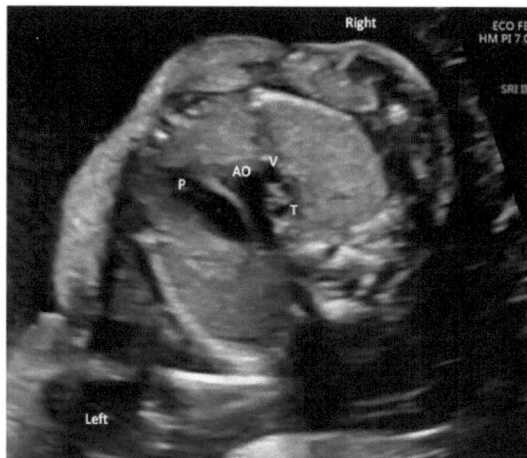

Fig. (7). Transverse plane of the fetal thorax. From the four-chamber view, the examiner performs a discrete movement directed to fetal head and obtains the image of the three vessels and trachea. P: pulmonary trunk. AO: ascending aorta. V: superior vena cava. T: trachea.

The arches of the heart are assessed through the sagittal plane of the fetus (Figs. **8** and **9**). Normally, the transducer is positioned in the sagittal plane in the opposite direction of the fetal spine, in order to minimize the imaging artifacts caused by the vertebral body and the intercostal arches of the fetus [7, 10].

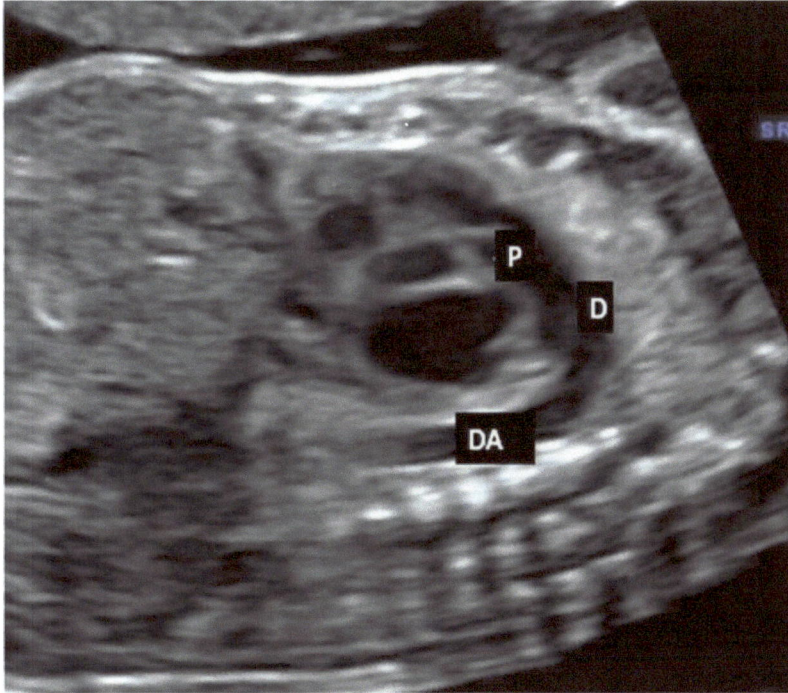

Fig. (8). Sagittal plane of the fetus. Ductal arch showing pulmonary artery, ductus arteriosus and descending aorta. P: pulmonary artery. D: ductus arteriosus. DA: descending aorta.

In the plane of the ductal arch, the right atrium is observed communicating with the right ventricle and, this, with the pulmonary artery, which divides into the pulmonary branches (right and left) and emits the ductus arteriosus (ductus arteriosus) communicating with the descending aorta (Fig. **8**).

In the plane of the aortic arch, the examiner should visualize the ascending aorta, which continues with the transverse arch that gives rise to the vessels of the neck - brachiocephalic trunk, left carotid artery and left subclavian artery - and follows the descending aorta (Fig. **9**).

One of the major advantages of fetal echocardiography is that it is a non-invasive diagnostic method and does not cause any danger to the pregnant woman or to the fetus. Therefore, it should be performed in all pregnant women as a complementary part of the second trimester scan. However, a limiting factor is the fact that many details should be evaluated, in order to avoid misdiagnosis of potential life threatening diseases. Unfortunately, there are not enough professionals able to perform the whole examination. This limitation reinforces the idea that an adequate screening, with subsequent referral to a trained professional, may increase the early diagnosis of congenital heart diseases [7, 8].

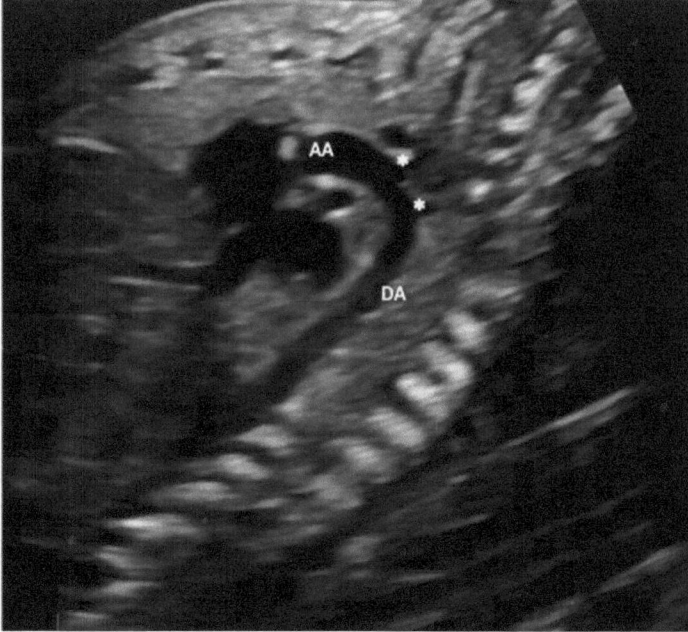

Fig. (9). Sagittal plane of the fetus. Aortic arch showing the ascending portion, the transverse arch (with the vessels of the neck) and the descending portion of the aorta. AA: ascending aorta. DA: descending aorta. *vessels of the neck.

Fetal echocardiography is a diagnostic method that is operator-dependent. The greater the experience and the knowledge of the examiner, combined with a good ultrasound equipment, the better the images obtained and the more correct the conclusions of the examinations will be. Except when the pregnant woman presents some peculiarities that hinder the proper performance of the exam, for example: obesity, scars in the abdomen, pregnancy, amniotic fluid greatly increased or decreased and advanced gestational age, which may attenuate the quality of the ultrasound images [10]. Another limiting factor of this diagnostic method is that there are some congenital heart diseases that can not be diagnosed in the intrauterine period [10]. Among them, we can mention the interatrial communications, small interventricular communications, mild valve alterations, persistent ductus arteriosus and some cases of aortic coarctation. In the case of atrial septal defect and persistent ductus arteriosus, the diagnosis cannot be made in the intrauterine period because they are structures that are patent in fetal life.

The other related heart diseases can be unnoticed in the intrauterine period due to its very discrete alterations, with diagnosis being performed in the neonatal period and, in most cases, without risk for the newborn.

INDICATIONS OF FETAL ECHOCARDIOGRAPHY

According to the guidelines of the International Society of Ultrasound in Obstetrics and Gynecology, all high-risk pregnant women should undergo more detailed fetal echocardiography, and those with a lower risk should at least receive cardiac screening [8].

Risk factors for cardiac anomaly are classified as maternal, familial and fetal factors [8]. Some indications are listed in the Table 1.

Table 1. Common indications for fetal echocardiography.

Maternal Indications Examples	
Family history	First-degree relative of proband
Pre-existing metabolic disease	Diabetes, phenylketonuria
Maternal infections	Parvovirus B19, rubella, coxsackie virus
Cardiac teratogen exposure	Retinoids, phenytoin, carbamazepine, lithium carbonate, valproic acid
Maternal antibodies	Anti-Ro (SSA), anti-La (SSB)
Fetal Indications Examples	
Suspected fetal heart anomaly	
Abnormal fetal karyotype	
Major extracardiac anomaly	
Abnormal nuchal translucency	> 3.5 mm before 14 weeks gestation
Fetal cardiac rate or rhythm disturbances	Persistent bradycardia, persistent tachycardia, persistent irregular heart rhythm

Recent research reports that low-risk pregnant women have more cases of children with congenital heart disease than pregnant women in the high-risk group. According to a retrospective study of 1395 fetuses in Turkey, 19% of female fetuses in low-risk groups were diagnosed with congenital heart disease, as opposed to 7% of female fetuses in high-risk groups [11]. Thus, reinforcing the idea that all pregnant women should undergo cardiac triage.

The early diagnosis of fetal heart disease associated with technological advances made possible some intrauterine interventions [17-19]. Pulmonary valvuloplasty, aortic valvuloplasty and atrio-septoplasty (in cases of critical pulmonary valve stenosis, aortic valve stenosis with evolution to hypoplastic left heart and hypoplastic left heart syndrome with restricted foramen ovale, respectively) are the most performed intrauterine cardiac interventions. There are few cardiac congenital anomalies that are amenable to intrauterine intervention and the number of centers of reference are also restricted. A high success rate is observed in the initial techniques of intervention with low maternal risk, however, a considerable risk of fetal morbidity and mortality [17]. However, the technological improvement and the intervention team, coupled with the exchange of experiences among the world's reference hospitals, will be fundamental for an increasingly favorable outcome of these cases.

ASSOCIATING CONGENITAL HEART DISEASES WITH CARDIAC PLANES

We can suspect some heart diseases according to the changes found in each echocardiographic plane.

In the four-chamber view may be seen the following:

- Cardiac situs: situs inversus and *situs ambiguous* (heterotaxy syndrome). In situs inversus were found to have a mirror image of the situs solitus pattern, with the aorta to the right and the inferior vena cava to the left, both vessels again being symmetrically disposed with respect to the spine [10, 20]. The term isomerism refers to the symmetrical development of normally asymmetrical organs or organ systems, which is the main feature of heterotaxy syndromes. A combination of cardiac, vascular and visceral abnormalities make up these syndromes. There are many correlates to predict the atrial situs: splenic status, lung lobation, position of abdominal viscera, bronchial morphology, pulmonary venous connection, presence or absence of coronary sinus, pulmonary artery morphology, systemic venous connection, hepatic atrial connection, position of the inferior cava and aorta. The position of the inferior vena cava and aorta alone has been shown reliably to separate those patients with situs solitus from the others situs [20]. The echocardiographic finding of left isomerism is the identification of the aorta centrally located and the presence of a vessel between the aorta and the spine: the interruption of the inferior vena cava with azygous continuation or hemiazygos vein into the superior vena cava is almost universal. In the axial plane of the fetus with left isomerism, we can see a vena (azygos vena) between the aorta and the spine [10, 20]. Many times, these characteristics are very difficult to identify, however we can differentiate them through the color Doppler: the direction of the flow in these two vessels is different, then, the colors are different, because the flow of azygos vena is going to the heart and the flow of aorta is going out of the heart [10]. Complete heart block is also found in some patients with left isomerism. In such condition, the pregnancy is often referred for fetal echocardiography because of the detection of bradycardia [10]. The echocardiographic finding of right isomerism is the identification of the inferior vena cava and aorta together on one or other side of the spine, with the aorta posterior [10, 20]. The pulmonary venous connection should be carefully examined, as by definition it is always anomalous, although the most common connection is for a venous confluence to drain directly to the center of the atrial mass [10].

- The position and the axis of the heart: dextroposition/mesoposition (heart is positioned in the right/midline hemithorax) and dextrocardia/mesocardia (heart apex is positioned to the right side of chest or midline). There are some cases where we can see dextroposition with apex still oriented to the left (levocardia). Positional abnormalities can be secondary to left diaphragmatic hernia or presence of space-occupying lesions, such as cystic adenomatoid malformation, fetal lung hypoplasia, or agenesis.

- Size of the heart: cardiomegaly or pericardial effusion.

- Pulmonary venous return: should be seen draining to the left atrium at least one left and one right pulmonary vein. In cases of abnormal venous return, the clinician can suspect of partial or total anomalous pulmonary venous drainage by seeing the collector draining in a systemic vein or in the right atrium.

- Observation of the atria: atrial dilatation in cases of atresia, stenosis, or atrioventricular valve regurgitation (as seen in Ebstein's anomaly).

- Atrial septal tissue: the clinician must use care while moving the lamina of the foramen ovale in cases of restrictive flow and if there is septum primum.

- Atrioventricular valves: significant regurgitation may be observed, as in cases of valvular dysplasia or as seen in Ebstein's anomaly. The sonographer can note valvular atresia, which is usually seen with hypoplastic ventricle (hypoplasia of the ventricle corresponding to valve atresia). At this plane, it is important when we just see a common atrioventricular valve anatomy (absent of cross of the heart due to an ostium primum atrial septal defect and an inlet ventricular septal defect), because these cases are dealing with atrioventricular canal defect (AVCD) (69% of all patients with AVCD have Down syndrome) [21].

- Anatomy of the ventricles: right ventricular hypoplasia, as seen in some cases of pulmonary or tricuspid atresia, or hypoplasia of the left ventricle, as seen in cases of mitral or aortic atresia, may be observed. The sonographer may see the right ventricle located to the left and the left ventricle located to the right, which is indicative of L loop. It is also known as ventricular inversion or congenitally corrected transposition of the great vessels. As the name suggests, there are discordant connections at both the atrioventricular and ventriculoarterial junctions.

In the images of the outflow tract of the heart and the 3 vessels and trachea axis, the clinician may observe the following:

- Left ventricular outflow tract (LVOT): in this view, stenosis or aortic atresia, ventricular septal defect or 2 vessels leaving the left ventricle featuring a double outlet left ventricle may be observed.

- Right ventricular outflow tract (RVOT): pulmonary stenosis or pulmonary atresia or 2 vessels leaving the right ventricle featuring double outlet right ventricle may be observed.

- Three vessels and trachea (3VT) axis: the clinician should suspect transposition of the great vessels when he observes only 2 vessels in this view - superior vena cava and some undefined vessel [22], beyond to be impossible to obtain the short axis view of fetal heart. When the pulmonary artery shows dimension smaller than normal, stenosis or pulmonary atresia should be suspected. A smaller than normal aorta may indicate or aortic stenosis or atresia [22]. When the trachea is seen entrapped between the aortic arch and pulmonary trunk, and the arterial ductus is seen to the right of the trachea, we should think in right-sided aortic arch [22].

The cardiac arches are observed in the sagittal plane of fetal to check for coarctation of the aorta and aortic arch interruption. These analyses are very difficult because the ductus arteriosus may hide the aortic arch and mask cardiac abnormalities [23 - 27]. Clinicians should suspect this anomaly if they observe dilatation of the right heart chambers.

CONCLUSION

In the evaluation of the cardiac structures, we must consider the segmental analysis of the heart, because in this way, we can see all the components of the heart, bringing a sequential script for the investigation of abnormalities [7, 10]. The International Society of Ultrasound in Obstetrics and Gynecology uses 2D grayscale imaging to track heart disease [8, 9]. However, we advocate the use of a very simple tool, color Doppler, which increases our accuracy in the analysis of cardiac structures. A recent study evaluated the additional use of color Doppler in grayscale imaging in a low-risk population. The authors showed that color Doppler use increased the percentage of diagnosed cases from 49% to 67% of the study population [28]. Thus, we support the idea that the addition of color

Doppler in the analysis of the structures is an important tool for the fetal cardiac tracing [7, 28]. With the technological advances and technical difficulties encountered in performing the tracking of heart disease, new tools such as STIC (spatio-temporal image correlation), which uses three-dimensional (3D) and four-dimensional (4D) to increase the morphofunctional information of the fetal heart [7, 29, 30]. There are several studies describing the advantages and disadvantages of this new tool, in order to bring improvements to its applicability [29, 30]. Fetal echocardiography is essential for the diagnosis of early congenital heart disease [7, 8, 10]. Many serious congenital heart diseases, in need of emergency clinical and surgical care soon after birth, may have their diagnosis still known in intrauterine life, leading to the early planning of the actions to be adopted by the medical team in the immediate postpartum or even during life fetal. We expect the rate of intrauterine diagnosis of congenital heart disease to increase to provide better delivery planning, thereby reducing the rate of infant mortality and morbidity due to cardiac abnormalities.

CONSENT FOR PUBLICATION

Not applicable.

CONFLICT OF INTEREST

The authors confirm that the contents of this chapter have no conflict of interest.

ACKNOWLEDGEMENTS

Declare none.

REFERENCES

[1]   Viñals F, Poblete P, Giuliano A. Spatio-temporal image correlation (STIC): a new tool for the prenatal screening of congenital heart defects. Ultrasound Obstet Gynecol 2003; 22(4): 388-94.
      [http://dx.doi.org/10.1002/uog.883] [PMID: 14528475]

[2]   Allan L. Prenatal diagnosis of structural cardiac defects. Am J Med Genet C Semin Med Genet 2007; 145C(1): 73-6.
      [http://dx.doi.org/10.1002/ajmg.c.30123] [PMID: 17304544]

[3]   Carvalho JS, Mavrides E, Shinebourne EA, Campbell S, Thilaganathan B. Improving the effectiveness of routine prenatal screening for major congenital heart defects. Heart 2002; 88(4): 387-91.
      [http://dx.doi.org/10.1136/heart.88.4.387] [PMID: 12231598]

[4]   Ferencz C, Rubin JD, McCarter RJ, *et al.* Congenital heart disease: prevalence at livebirth. The Baltimore-Washington Infant Study. Am J Epidemiol 1985; 121(1): 31-6.
      [http://dx.doi.org/10.1093/oxfordjournals.aje.a113979] [PMID: 3964990]

[5]   Cuneo BF, Curran LF, Davis N, Elrad H. Trends in prenatal diagnosis of critical cardiac defects in an integrated obstetric and pediatric cardiac imaging center. J Perinatol 2004; 24(11): 674-8.
      [http://dx.doi.org/10.1038/sj.jp.7211168] [PMID: 15284832]

[6]   Rosano A, Botto LD, Botting B, Mastroiacovo P. Infant mortality and congenital anomalies from 1950

to 1994: an international perspective. J Epidemiol Community Health 2000; 54(9): 660-6.
[http://dx.doi.org/10.1136/jech.54.9.660] [PMID: 10942444]

[7] Alves Rocha L, Araujo Júnior E, Rolo LC, *et al.* Screening of congenital heart disease in the second trimester of pregnancy: current knowledge and new perspectives to the clinical practice. Cardiol Young 2014; 24(3): 388-96.
[http://dx.doi.org/10.1017/S1047951113001558] [PMID: 24229491]

[8] International Society of Ultrasound in Obstetrics & Gynecology. Cardiac screening examination of the fetus: guidelines for performing the 'basic' and 'extended basic' cardiac scan. Ultrasound Obstet Gynecol 2006; 27(1): 107-13.
[PMID: 16374757]

[9] Lee W, Allan L, Carvalho JS, *et al.* ISUOG consensus statement: what constitutes a fetal echocardiogram? Ultrasound Obstet Gynecol 2008; 32(2): 239-42.
[http://dx.doi.org/10.1002/uog.6115] [PMID: 18663769]

[10] Allan L, Hornberger L, Sharland G. Textbook of Fetal Cardiology. London: Greenwich Medical Media 2000; pp. 3-13.

[11] Ozkutlu S, Akça T, Kafali G, Beksaç S. The results of fetal echocardiography in a tertiary center and comparison of low- and high-risk pregnancies for fetal congenital heart defects. Anadolu Kardiyol Derg 2010; 10(3): 263-9.
[http://dx.doi.org/10.5152/akd.2010.068] [PMID: 20538563]

[12] Kirk JS, Riggs TW, Comstock CH, Lee W, Yang SS, Weinhouse E. Prenatal screening for cardiac anomalies: the value of routine addition of the aortic root to the four-chamber view. Obstet Gynecol 1994; 84(3): 427-31.
[PMID: 8058243]

[13] Viñals F, Heredia F, Giuliano A. The role of the three vessels and trachea view (3VT) in the diagnosis of congenital heart defects. Ultrasound Obstet Gynecol 2003; 22(4): 358-67.
[http://dx.doi.org/10.1002/uog.882] [PMID: 14528470]

[14] Yagel S, Arbel R, Anteby EY, Raveh D, Achiron R. The three vessels and trachea view (3VT) in fetal cardiac scanning. Ultrasound Obstet Gynecol 2002; 20(4): 340-5.
[http://dx.doi.org/10.1046/j.1469-0705.2002.00801.x] [PMID: 12383314]

[15] Vettraino IM, Lee W, Bronsteen RA, Comstock CH. Sonographic evaluation of the ventricular cardiac outflow tracts. J Ultrasound Med 2005; 24(4): 566.
[http://dx.doi.org/10.7863/jum.2005.24.4.566] [PMID: 15784777]

[16] Xu Y, Hu YL, Ru T, Gu Y, Yang Y, Dai CY. [Importance of "Guidelines for performing fetal cardiac scan" in prenatal screening for fetal congenital heart disease]. Zhonghua Fu Chan Ke Za Zhi 2009; 44(2): 103-7.
[PMID: 19570419]

[17] Pedra SR, Peralta CF, Crema L, Jatene IB, da Costa RN, Pedra CA. Fetal interventions for congenital heart disease in Brazil. Pediatr Cardiol 2014; 35(3): 399-405.
[http://dx.doi.org/10.1007/s00246-013-0792-3] [PMID: 24030590]

[18] Moon-Grady AJ, Morris SA, Belfort M, *et al.* International Fetal Cardiac Intervention Registry: A Worldwide Collaborative Description and Preliminary Outcomes. J Am Coll Cardiol 2015; 66(4): 388-99.
[http://dx.doi.org/10.1016/j.jacc.2015.05.037] [PMID: 26205597]

[19] Jantzen DW, Moon-Grady AJ, Morris SA, *et al.* Hypoplastic left heart syndrome with intact or restrictive atrial septum: a report from the international fetal cardiac intervention registry. Circulation 2017; 136(14): 1346-9.
[http://dx.doi.org/10.1161/CIRCULATIONAHA.116.025873] [PMID: 28864444]

[20] Huhta JC, Smallhorn JF, Macartney FJ. Two dimensional echocardiographic diagnosis of situs. Br

Heart J 1982; 48(2): 97-108.
[http://dx.doi.org/10.1136/hrt.48.2.97] [PMID: 7093090]

[21]   Koenig P, Hijazi ZM, Zimmerman F. Essential Pediatric Cardiology. New York, NY: McGraw-Hill Medical Publishing Division 2004; pp. 131-6.

[22]   Chaoui R, McEwing R. Three cross-sectional planes for fetal color Doppler echocardiography. Ultrasound Obstet Gynecol 2003; 21(1): 81-93.
[http://dx.doi.org/10.1002/uog.5] [PMID: 12528169]

[23]   Head CE, Jowett VC, Sharland GK, Simpson JM. Timing of presentation and postnatal outcome of infants suspected of having coarctation of the aorta during fetal life. Heart 2005; 91(8): 1070-4.
[http://dx.doi.org/10.1136/hrt.2003.033027] [PMID: 16020599]

[24]   Vergani P, Mariani S, Ghidini A, *et al.* Screening for congenital heart disease with the four-chamber view of the fetal heart. Am J Obstet Gynecol 1992; 167(4 Pt 1): 1000-3.
[http://dx.doi.org/10.1016/S0002-9378(12)80027-5] [PMID: 1415383]

[25]   Hornberger LK, Sahn DJ, Kleinman CS, Copel J, Silverman NH. Antenatal diagnosis of coarctation of the aorta: a multicenter experience. J Am Coll Cardiol 1994; 23(2): 417-23.
[http://dx.doi.org/10.1016/0735-1097(94)90429-4] [PMID: 8294696]

[26]   Allan LD, Chita SK, Anderson RH, Fagg N, Crawford DC, Tynan MJ. Coarctation of the aorta in prenatal life: an echocardiographic, anatomical, and functional study. Br Heart J 1988; 59(3): 356-60.
[http://dx.doi.org/10.1136/hrt.59.3.356] [PMID: 3355726]

[27]   Sharland GK, Chan KY, Allan LD. Coarctation of the aorta: difficulties in prenatal diagnosis. Br Heart J 1994; 71(1): 70-5.
[http://dx.doi.org/10.1136/hrt.71.1.70] [PMID: 8297700]

[28]   Eggebø TM, Heien C, Berget M, Ellingsen CL. Routine use of color Doppler in fetal heart scanning in a low-risk population. ISRN Obstet Gynecol 2012; 2012496935
[http://dx.doi.org/10.5402/2012/496935] [PMID: 22685669]

[29]   Rocha LA, Rolo LC, Barros FS, Nardozza LM, Moron AF, Araujo Júnior E. Assessment of quality of fetal heart views by 3d/4d ultrasonography using spatio-temporal image correlation in the second and third trimesters of pregnancy. Echocardiography 2015; 32(6): 1015-21.
[http://dx.doi.org/10.1111/echo.12743] [PMID: 25231765]

[30]   Araujo Júnior E, Rolo LC, Rocha LA, Nardozza LM, Moron AF. The value of 3D and 4D assessments of the fetal heart. Int J Womens Health 2014; 6: 501-7.
[http://dx.doi.org/10.2147/IJWH.S47074] [PMID: 24868174]

CHAPTER 6

Early Fetal Echocardiography

Ritu Mogra[1,2] and **Jon A. Hyett**[1,2,*]

[1] *RPA Women and Babies, Royal Prince Alfred Hospital, Sydney Institute for Women, Children and their Families, Sydney, Australia*

[2] *Discipline of Obstetrics, Gynaecology and Neonatology, Central Clinical School, Faculty of Medicine, University of Sydney, Sydney, Australia*

Abstract: The role of first-trimester ultrasound has evolved from the measurement of crown-rump length (CRL), nuchal translucency (NT) and nasal bone to involve more detailed assessment of fetal anatomy. The majority of cardiac malformations are properly defined and potentially detectable by the time of the 11-13[+6] week ultrasound examination. The sensitivity of ultrasound screening for cardiac abnormalities varies according to the marker being assessed (increased NT, tricuspid regurgitation, abnormal ductus venous flow), operator experience and the extent of a protocol for formal sequential structural assessment of the heart. All cardiac structures can be visualised from 13 weeks onwards. Early fetal echocardiography has been shown to be feasible and highly sensitive and specific in experienced hands. Early identification of cardiac abnormalities allows the assessment of chromosomal abnormalities/genetic syndrome at an early stage, giving parents more reproductive autonomy. Operators should be aware of the limitations of an early cardiac examination: Some lesions progress as pregnancy advances and there is still a need for a follow up ultrasound at 20 weeks' gestation.

Keywords: Cardiac abnormalities, Early fetal echo, Prenatal screening.

INTRODUCTION

Congenital heart diseases (CHD) are the most common structural malformations resulting in stillbirth, neonatal and childhood death and are a major cause of childhood morbidity [1 - 5]. The purpose of prenatal screening to identify CHD is to allow parents to collect more information about underlying chromosomal and genetic conditions, to discuss likely prognosis and enable decisions about termination of pregnancy (where this is an option). For parents who chose to continue the pregnancy, prenatal diagnosis allows clinicians to optimise perinatal management by planning mode, time and place of delivery; delivering a stable

* **Corresponding author Jon Hyett:** RPA Women and Babies, Royal Prince Alfred Hospital, Missenden Road, Camperdown NSW 2050, Sydney, Australia; Tel: +61 2 9515 7153, Fax: +61 2 9515 3811, E-mail: jon.hyett@health.nsw.gov.au

Edward Araujo Júnior, Nathalie Jeanne M. Bravo-Valenzuela and Alberto Borges Peixoto (Eds.)

neonate in the best possible hemodynamic condition. Prenatal diagnosis has had a significant impact on morbidity and mortality associated with congenital heart defects resulting in more favourable long-term outcomes [6 - 9].

This chapter reviews the detection of major cardiac defects in early pregnancy including a description of markers defining high-risk cases, the technique of early fetal echocardiography and the sensitivity, specificity, and accuracy of screening in low- and high- risk populations.

ADJUNCTIVE PRENATAL DIAGNOSIS

Early diagnosis of structural heart defects allows earlier assessment of associated chromosomal and genetic conditions [10, 11]. The test of choice is either chorionic villous sampling (CVS) (typically offered at 11-14 weeks' gestation) or amniocentesis (from 15/16 weeks' gestation) as these tests allow assessment of the whole genome using aCGH analysis. Non-invasive prenatal testing (NIPT) - which has recently emerged as a screening tool for aneuploidy - is not normally the best tool for diagnostic assessment. A proportion of fetuses that have a chromosomal abnormality underlying the structural cardiac abnormality will have an 'atypical' chromosomal abnormality that is not normally identified through NIPT [12 - 14]. Cell free fetal DNA testing can be extended to include anomalies such as del22q11, which is commonly associated with certain cardiac abnormalities, but the sensitivity is not 100% and it is therefore difficult to advocate this as a replacement for a diagnostic test [15]. Although del22q11 is responsible for a very significant proportion of microdeletions that can be characterised, it is more appropriate to use a genome wide approach to testing rather than a targeted approach.

A number of genetic syndromes are also known to be associated with cardiac abnormalities. It may also be possible to test for specific genetic syndromes prenatally, but this is normally dependent on being able to identify other, extracardiac features on ultrasound and on having an understanding of the likely gene mutation associated with the condition [16 - 18]. In the best hands, ultrasound will identify 50% of syndromic fetuses and most genetic syndromes involve multiple potential sites of genetic variation; so establishing a firm genetic diagnosis is a complex task. A number of lab groups now produce 'panels' that can be used to assess a range of genetic conditions associated with cardiac disease either through invasive testing (CVS or amniocentesis) or a non-invasive cell free DNA based approach.

Early identification of a cardiac defect establishes the risk of a chromosomal abnormality or genetic syndrome at an early stage. If this is followed by early prenatal testing, then this gives parents time to make decisions about the ongoing pregnancy. The decision to terminate pregnancy will be influenced by the nature of the chromosomal abnormality, the severity of the cardiac condition and any extracardiac malformations. More than 90% of women that have a fetus affected by chromosomal abnormality and 45% of women that have a fetus affected by a cardiac defect opt to terminate the pregnancy [19, 20]. Early prenatal diagnosis allows safer options for termination of pregnancy [21 - 23]. Routine screening for both chromosomal abnormality and CHD has a significant impact on the prevalence of live born CHD [24].

EARLY ULTRASOUND ASSESSMENT OF THE FETAL HEART

Ultrasound screening for CHD traditionally involved the assessment of the fetal heart during the routine morphology scan that is performed at 18-23 weeks [25 - 27]. An improved understanding of the structures of the fetal heart and of patterns of malformation together with improved resolution of ultrasound machines allows earlier prenatal diagnosis. It is now appropriate to contemplate routine screening for cardiac abnormalities at the $11\text{-}13^{+6}$ week scan and to consider a window for early diagnostic echocardiography at 14-16 weeks.

The objective of screening is to identify a sub-population defined as being at 'high-risk' of a condition which can be selected for additional diagnostic testing. Identification of cardiac abnormalities differs in the detection of aneuploidy in so far as both the screening test and the diagnostic test are ultrasound based. The diagnostic assessment does, however, require a higher sonographer skill set that is unlikely to be readily available in all screening clinics.

It is possible to screen for cardiac abnormalities using ultrasound markers that have been shown to be associated with aneuploidy and that are commonly used to screen for chromosomal abnormalities during the $11\text{-}13^{+6}$ week scan. There are two markers that can be used that do not involve direct assessment of the fetal heart (nuchal translucency, abnormal ductus venosus waveform) and three markers (the axis of the four-chamber view and demonstration of tricuspid incompetence (regurgitation) and assessment of right subclavian artery that involve cardiac assessment.

i. Fetal Nuchal Translucency Thickness

Assessment of nuchal translucency thickness forms the basis of population-based screening programs for Down syndrome in many countries [28]. The test is based on early observations that fetuses with common chromosomal abnormalities (trisomies 21, 18 and 13 and 45X) often have excess fluid in the nape of the neck. The absolute risk of chromosomal abnormality depends on the amount of excess fluid - represented by measuring its thickness. This risk can be calculated for individual fetuses using a background (*a priori*) risk associated with maternal age and a likelihood ratio derived through nuchal translucency measurement that characterises how likely it is that a fetus lies in a chromosomally normal or abnormal population [29]. If ascribed risks are going to be accurate then nuchal translucency has to be measured in a standardised manner - and sonographers have to be trained and commit to an ongoing quality assurance program for best practice [30].

The observation that the prevalence of aneuploidy increases with nuchal translucency thickness holds for structural cardiac abnormalities as well. It is therefore possible to ascribe an individual risk for cardiac defects based on a likelihood ratio for nuchal translucency thickness in the same way as risks for aneuploidy are described. Once again, the risk will only be accurate if nuchal translucency is measured in a standardise manner (Fig. **1**). One important feature of this process, which also applies to aneuploidy screening, is that small nuchal translucency measures are associated with a decrease in risk of cardiac abnormality - so this screening tool can be used to reduce risk and reduce patient anxiety in women who would be deemed high-risk (perhaps because they have a previous child affected by cardiac disease) through other screening processes.

Normal NT   Thick NT

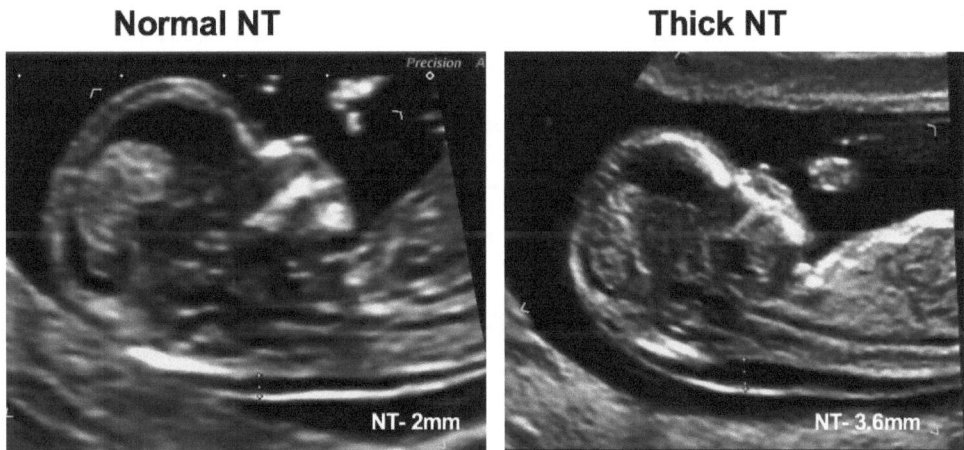

Fig. (1). (a) Ultrasound image of normal nuchal translucency (NT); (b) Ultrasound image of thick NT.

A high-risk of a cardiac abnormality was traditionally determined purely on the basis of maternal history. A woman who has a cardiac abnormality herself or who has had a previous affected pregnancy or a woman who has diabetes or who takes drugs such as lithium or sodium valproate is at higher risk of having a fetus affected by cardiac disease [31 - 33]. Using traditional maternal based screening, only 5% of cases will be referred and approximately 10% women deemed high risk would have a fetus affected by structural cardiac disease. Studies have shown that use of the routine 18-23 week scan improves detection to 40-60% depending on the extent of examination views with a positive predictive value of 1 in 9 women identified as being at risk [34]. Retrospective review of a series of 29,154 pregnancies primarily screened for chromosomal abnormality at 11-14 weeks of pregnancy identified 56% (95% CI 42-70%) of fetuses later found to have a cardiac defect (by postmortem, fetal echocardiography, or postnatal examination) with increased nuchal translucency (NT) [35]. This original series is further supported by seven other studies including a total of 88,380 pregnancies with 211 cardiac defects that show that increased first trimester NT thickness will identify 30% of fetuses that have a major cardiac defect (Table **1**) [35 - 42]. The prevalence of cardiac defects varied from 0.2% (NT <2.5mm) to 0.7% (NT 2.5-3.4mm) and 5.9% (NT ≥3.5mm). A normal NT is associated with a reduction in risk of a major cardiac abnormality (negative likelihood ratio = 6.5). An NT between 95-99th centile is associated with a modest increase in risk (positive likelihood ratio = 3.4) whilst an NT >99th centile is associated with a positive likelihood ratio of 23. One series reported a positive predictive value of 1 in 5 in cases referred for a fetal echo as they were deemed to be high risk due to increased NT [34].

Table 1. Studies reporting the effectiveness of nuchal translucency as a screening tool for major cardiac defects in chromosomally normal fetuses.

Author	n	Major Cardiac Defects (prevalence)			
		NT <2.5mm	NT 2.5-3.4mm	NT ≥3.5mm	All cases
*Hyett *et al.* 1999 [35]	29,154	22/ 27,332 (0.8 per 1000)	8/1507 (5.3 per 1000)	20/315 (63.5 per 1000)	50/291,54 (1.7 per 1000)
Mavrides *et al.* 2001 [36]	7,339	22/7,081 (3.1 per 1000)	1/198 (5.1 per 1000)	3/60 (50.0 per 1000)	26/7,339 (3.5 per 1000)
Michailidis *et al.* 2001 [37]	6,606	8/6,371 (1.2 per 1000)	1/162 (6.2 per 1000)	3/73 (41.1 per 1000)	11/6,606 (1.7 per 1000)
*□Hafner *et al.* 2003 [38]	12,978	20/12,329 (1.6 per 1000)	7/649 (10.7 per 1000)		27/12,978 (2.1 per 1000)
Bahado-Singh *et al.* 2005 [39]	8,167	18/7,789 (2.3 per 1000)	2/335 (6.0 per 1000)	1/43 (23.3 per 1000)	21/8,167 (2.6 per 1000)
Bruns *et al.* 2006 [40]	3,664	7/35,06 (4.6 per 1000)	0/127 (none reported)	3/31 (96.8 per 1000)	10/3,664 (2.7 per 1000)
*Westin *et al.* 2006 [41]	16,328	44/15,894 (2.8 per 1000)	5/382 (13.1 per 1000)	3/52 (57.7 per 1000)	55/16,328 (3.4 per 1000)

(Table 1) cont.....

Muller *et al.* 2007 [42]	4,144	11/40,44 (2.7 per 1000)	0/79 (none reported)	2/21 (95.2 per 1000)	13/4,144 (3.1 per 1000)
Total	**88380**	**152/84,346 (1.8 per 1000)**	**24/3,439 (7.0 per 1000)**	**35/595 (58.8 per 1000)**	**211/88,380 (2.4 per 1000)**

NT: nuchal translucency
*Studies using NT >95th centile rather than 2.5mm as a cut-off
□Data cannot be separated into two groups, so included as NT >95th centile

Nuchal translucency (NT) is therefore a very useful marker for structural cardiac disease although it does not have high enough sensitivity to be used as the sole screening tool for these anomalies. As a screening tool, different NT cut-offs can be set to determine the number of women referred for a more detailed fetal echo depending on local availability of resources.

ii. Blood Flow Through the Ductus Venosus

Matias *et al.* assessed fetal cardiac function by Doppler based measurement of venous return to the right atrium through the ductus venosus (DV) in a series of 143 women who had already been screened for aneuploidy and were attending for diagnostic chorion villus sampling [44]. They found that abnormality of the DV waveform - identified as absence or reversal of flow during the 'A' wave was associated with chromosome abnormality. They also noted that 7 of 11 (63%) fetuses that had increased nuchal translucency and an abnormal DV 'a' wave but had a normal karyotype were subsequently shown to have major structural heart defects.

The process of first trimester assessment of the DV differs from that used in the second and third trimester (during assessment of intrauterine growth restriction - IUGR) as the vessel is best identified in a right parasagittal rather than an axial section (Fig. **2**). The DV streams blood back to the left side of the heart at high velocity and is therefore readily identified using colour Doppler. Once the vessel has been identified, pulse wave Doppler (using a 2 mm gate) can be used to interrogate the waveform. It is important to make sure that the vessel is not confused with other vessels such as the hepatic vein or the inferior vena cava; sometimes two waveforms will overlap making it difficult to assess the 'a' wave component of the ductus (Fig. **2**).

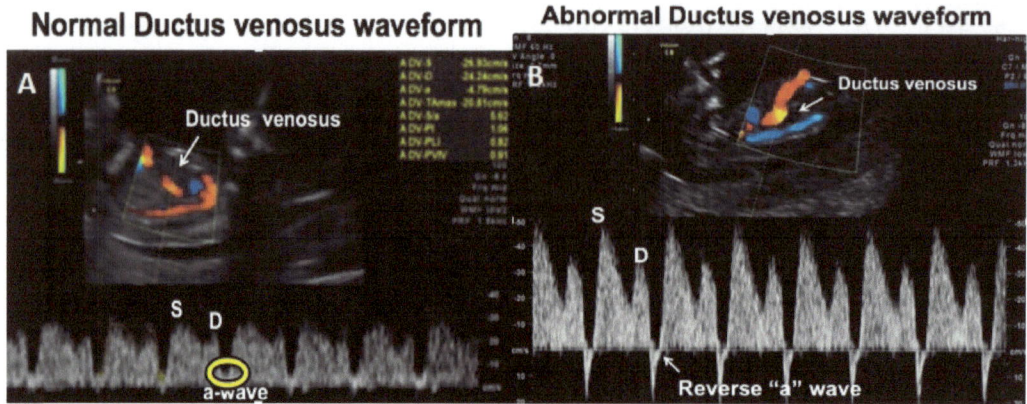

Fig. (2). (**A**) Normal ductus venosus waveform; (**B**) Abnormal Ductus venosus waveform.

A series of studies have supported the original findings of Matias *et al.* demonstrating that a significant proportion of fetuses with major cardiac defect have abnormal DV flow in the first trimester (Table **2**) [44 - 53]. An abnormal DV waveform was found in 4% of a normal population. Sensitivity and specificity of an abnormal ductus venosus in screening for cardiac defects were 50% and 93% respectively in circumstances where NT was normal and 73% and 79% respectively for increased NT.

Table 2. Studies reporting detection of major cardiac defects in chromosomally normal fetuses that had increased nuchal translucency (>95th centile) and an abnormal ductus venosus.

Author	Total (n)	Cardiac Defects (n; % total)	Abnormal Ductus Flow (n/total)	
			No Cardiac Defect	Cardiac Defect
(1) Matias *et al.* 1999 [44]	142	7 (4.9%)	4/135 (3.0%)	7/7 (100%)
(2) Bilardo *et al.* 2001 [45]	69	4 (5.8%)	19/65 (29.2%)	4/4 (100%)
(3) Murta *et al.* 2002 [46]	16	1 (6.3%)	0/15 (0%)	1/1 (100%)
(4) Zoppi *et al.* 2002 [47]	115	2 (1.7%)	30/113 (26.5%)	2/2 (100%)
(5) Favre *et al.* 2003 [48]	95	9 (9.5%)	20/86 (23.3%)	9/9 (100%)
(6) Haak *et al.* 2003 [49]	22	2 (9.1%)	8/20 (40.0%)	2/2 (100%)
(7) Toyama *et al.* 2004 [50]	141	4 (2.8%)	23/137 (16.8%)	3/4 (75%)
(8) Maiz *et al.* 2008 [51]	191	16 (8.4%)	40/175 (22.9%)	11/16 (68.8%)
(9) Timmerman *et al.* 2010 [52]	318	33 (10.4%)	74/285 (26.0%)	18/33 (55.0%)
(10) Martinez *et al.* 2010 [53]	55	11 (20.0%)	-	6/11 (54.5%)
Total	**1164**	**89 (7.6%)**	**218/1031 (21.1%)**	**63/89 (73.3%)**

Nuchal translucency and DV results are synergistic and combining of these two screening tools improves sensitivity and specificity of screening. Maiz *et al.* showed that positive and negative likelihood ratios, generated on the basis of DV findings, can be applied to a risk based on maternal history and NT thickness to effectively screen for cardiac disease [51]. Abnormal DV flow was associated with a positive likelihood ratio of 3; normal ductus venosus flow with a negative likelihood ratio of 0.5. More recent studies have measured flow through the 'S', 'D' and 'a' wave phases of the DV waveform expressing them as a pulsatility index. These studies show that flow through the DV has a similar bimodal distribution in chromosomally normal and abnormal populations as NT. The two markers appear to have some independence and the combination therefore improve screening efficacy. A similar observation has been made with cardiac defects [43, 54].

iii. The Aberrant Right Subclavian Artery

Under normal circumstances three vessels arises from the aortic arch, the first brachiocephalic artery which subdivides into right common carotid and right subclavian artery, second common left common carotid artery and third left subclavian artery. The aberrant right subclavian artery (ARSA) arises as a fourth separate branch from the aortic arch and crosses to the right side behind the trachea and oesophagus (Fig. **3**) [55]. Large autopsy and catheterization studies in adult have shown that an ARSA is the most common aortic arch anomaly and occurs in 0.5-1% of the general population [53]. Although an ARSA is often an incidental finding in asymptomatic individuals, several studies have reported that an ARSA is more prevalent in fetuses with Down syndrome (25-36%) and that a significant portion (15-20%) of cases have an associated cardiac abnormality [56 - 64]. The assessment of the right subclavian artery in the first trimester requires a skilled operator. Rembouskos *et al.* described a protocol for assessment in a prospective series of 6617 fetuses and found that through optimisation of technique it was feasible to assess this in 85% of cases [64]. Recognition of an ARSA should lead to consideration and counselling about the risk for Down syndrome or other chromosomal abnormality, taking the other findings of first trimester screening into account. If aneuploidy is excluded, then the finding of an ARSA should also initiate a referral for a detailed fetal echocardiography examination. Common associated cardiac anomalies include tetralogy of Fallot, hypoplastic left heart syndrome, aortic coarctation and AVSD.

Normal right subclavian artery- NRSA   **Aberrant right subclavian artery- ARSA**

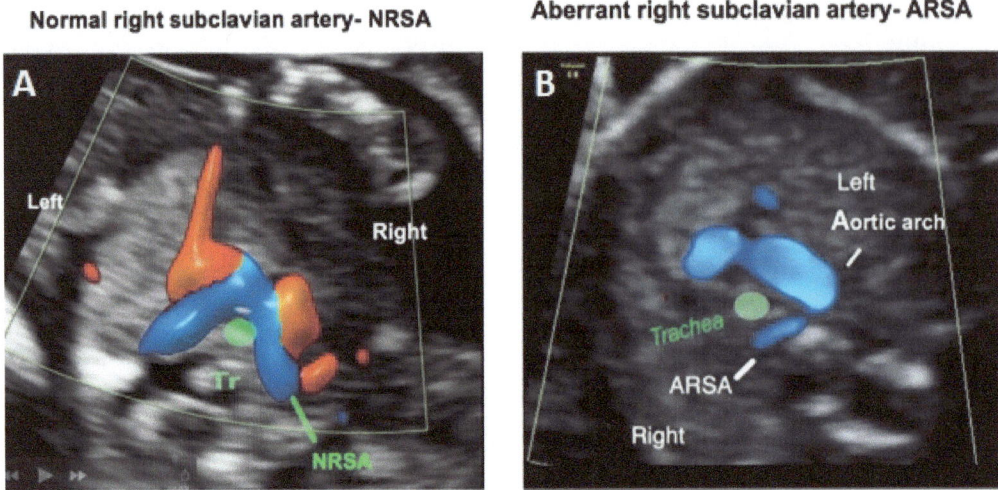

Fig. (3). (A) Ultrasound image of normal right subclavian artery (NRSA); (B) Ultrasound image of an aberrant right subclavian artery (ARSA). Tr: Trachea.

iv. Cardiac Axis in the First Trimester

As the resolution of ultrasound equipment has improved and experience with first trimester screening has increased some experts in fetal echocardiography have advocated screening based on assessment of the heart rather than on the basis of extracardiac markers. Whilst a formal cardiac echo may be technically challenging for many sonographers at 12 weeks', there are some basic parts of cardiac assessment that could easily be adapted into a routine screening program.

The first of these is assessment of cardiac axis; establishing an axial view of the thorax that shows the four-chamber view of the heart, dissecting the chest in AP diameter and establishing the angle described by this line and the interventricular septum of the heart (Fig. 4). Normal values for cardiac axis have been defined in a cohort of 100 fetus at 11-13^{+6} weeks gestation, ranging from 34.5° to 56.8° (mean (SD) 47.6° ± 5.6°) [65]. Cardiac axis could be assessed in almost all cases and excellent inter- and intra- observer variation in measurement has also been reported [66]. Cardiac axis is also recognised to change during the first trimester - as the heart starts as a relatively midline structure and levo-rotates with advancing gestation to a fixed axis by 14 weeks' gestation [67]. In this study the axis was reported to be 25° at 8 weeks and 50° at 13^{+6} weeks' gestation.

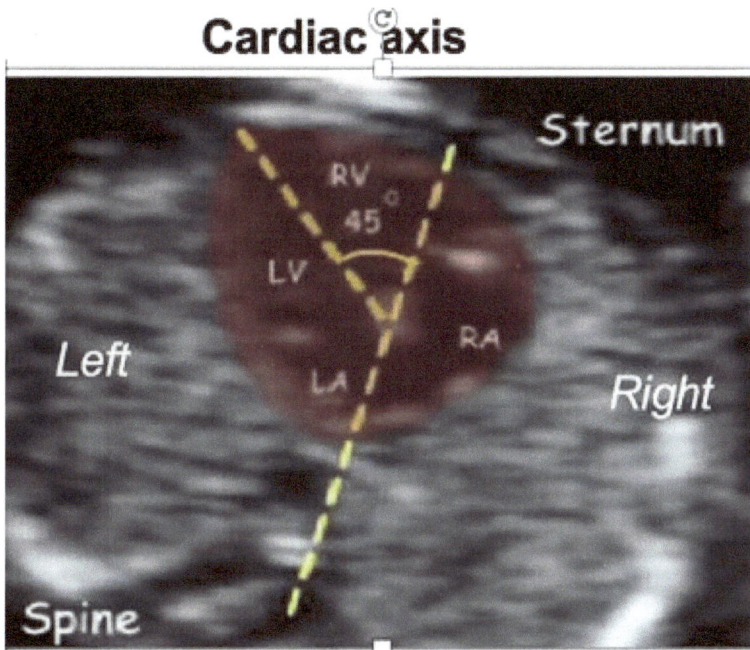

Fig. (4). Normal cardiac axis. LV: left ventricle; LA: left atrium; RV: right ventricle; RA: right atrium.

A retrospective case control study of 197 fetuses collected in three tertiary centres reported that the cardiac axis was abnormal in 74.1% of cases assessed at 11^{+0} - 14^{+6} weeks gestation and that this screening tool performed better than NT, DV or tricuspid regurgitation alone or in combination. The likelihood that a defect will be detected does, in part, depend on the nature of the structural anomaly and is more likely in fetuses that have some types of conotruncal defects or complex cardiac malformations such as a univentricular heart [68].

Use of cardiac axis was tested in a recently published prospective series of 1,568 fetuses undergoing first trimester screening, including 30 fetuses with a major structural cardiac defect [69]. The efficacy of cardiac axis was compared to that of nuchal translucency and both screening tools were found to detect 63.3% of cases - although the specificity of cardiac axis was better as false positive rates were 2.0% and 4.6% respectively. The authors assessed an additional cardiac marker - identification of the 'V' arrow head of the great arteries using colour Doppler - and found it had similar screening efficacy (66.7% sensitivity at 5.6% false positive rate). Interesting the combination of cardiac axis and the 'V' sign had a sensitivity of 93.3% for a 7.5% false positive rate.

v. Tricuspid Regurgitation

One of the original observations associated with NT was that the anomaly was more prevalent in chromosomally abnormal fetuses at 11-13^{+6} weeks' gestation than at 18-20 weeks' gestation. It was hypothesized that the dependent oedema resolved as the heart matured and cardiac function improved. Another measure of this is to assess the competence of the atrioventricular valves - most specifically the tricuspid valve. Interesting, a similar phenomenon is seen with high prevalence of tricuspid regurgitation in chromosomally abnormal infants at 11-13^{+6} weeks' gestation and lower prevalence at the 18-20-week scan.

At 11-13^{+6} weeks' gestation, flow across the tricuspid valve is assessed using an axial section of the chest that demonstrates a four-chamber view of the heart. The probe should be rotated so the apex of the heart lies at either 12 o'clock or 6 o'clock on the image, making placement of the pulse wave gate across the anterior atrioventricular (tricuspid) valve easier. A sample gate of 3mm is positioned across the tricuspid valve once the angle of insonation is <20° (Fig. **5**) and, in the original studies, valvular flow was assessed three times. Tricuspid regurgitation was defined as flow toward the atrium for at least half of systole with velocity ≥60cm/s [69].

In a population of fetuses referred for detailed echocardiography at 11-14 weeks, after the identification of increased NT (defined as ≥4mm), tricuspid regurgitation was seen in 27% of cases and 83% of these were subsequently found to have a chromosomal abnormality; most commonly trisomy 21. A second larger, prospective, study found tricuspid regurgitation in 4.4% of chromosomally normal fetuses, 67.5% of fetuses affected by trisomy 21, and 33% of fetuses affected by trisomy 18 [70]. A third study performed by the same group, again involving a selected population with a high prevalence of increased NT, chromosomal abnormalities and cardiac defects, defined tricuspid regurgitation more stringently, with flow ≥80cm/s. In this study, tricuspid flow was successfully examined in 96.8% cases and tricuspid regurgitation was found in 8.5% of chromosomally normal fetuses and 65.1% of those with trisomy 21 [71]. Further analysis of the euploid population found that tricuspid regurgitation was present in 46.9% of those cases that had a structural cardiac defect and in only 5.6% of euploid fetuses with no cardiac defect. Positive likelihood ratios describing the associations between tricuspid regurgitation and trisomy 21 or isolated cardiac defects were calculated; being 7.7 and 8.4, respectively. The authors noted an association with crown-rump length and NT thickness, and more precise likelihood ratios can be generated based on these parameters.

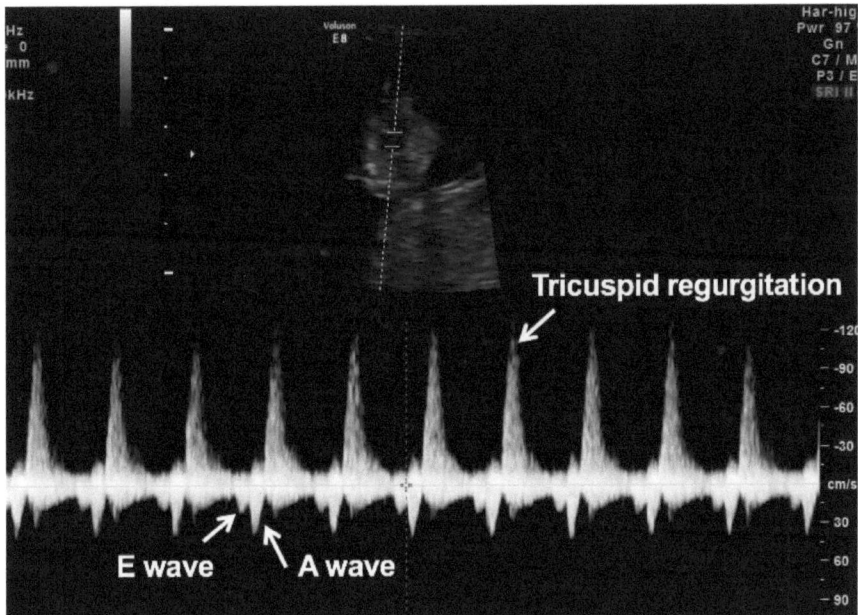

Fig. (5). Tricuspid valve regurgitation.

The combination of NT thickness, assessment of the DV 'a' wave and of tricuspid regurgitation were assessed in a large unselected population of 40,000 pregnancies that included 85 fetuses with major cardiac defects [72]. Increased fetal NT (>95th centile), reversed 'a' wave in the DV and tricuspid regurgitation were reported in 35.3%, 32.9% and 28.2% of cases respectively. If any one of these markers were considered to place the pregnancy in a high-risk group, then 57.6% of cardiac defects would have been detected for a false positive rate of 8.0%.

There are, to our knowledge, no prospective studies that have assessed the combination of all five of these sonographic markers. It is likely that using such a combination of screening tools would give high sensitivity for major cardiac defects - but the use of multiple markers also tends to be associated with an increasing false positive rate and it may be better to combine these into a multivariate algorithm using likelihood ratios (setting a risk threshold to define screen positive cases) rather than using an 'any one marker positive' approach. Finally, it is important to recognise that the discovery of extracardiac anomalies at 11-13^{+6} weeks also increases the risk that there may be a structural cardiac defect and these patients should also be referred for more targeted assessment. Left sided obstructive lesions are particularly associated with extracardiac abnormalities.

FORMAL FETAL ECHOCARDIOGRAPHY BEFORE 18 WEEKS' GESTATION

Gembruch *et al*. first demonstrated successful diagnosis of a cardiac abnormality at 11 weeks' gestation by reporting a case where fetal heart block was identified, followed by an atrioventricular septal defect (AVSD), with a diagnosis of atrial isomerism confirmed at autopsy [73]. The scan was performed transvaginally - similarly to the early reports of Bronstein *et al*. who identified a case of tetralogy of Fallot at 14 weeks' and then published a case series of 10 cases of structural heart defects diagnosed at 12-16 weeks' gestation [74]. Bronstein continued to report the screening efficacy of transvaginal ultrasonography at 14-16 weeks' gestation - being able to visualise both the four-chamber view and outflow tracts in 80% of a series of 12,793 patients and make an effective diagnosis of cardiac abnormality in 55% of affected cases [75]. Since these early reports, many groups have focused attention of the efficacy of formal fetal echocardiography before 18 weeks' gestation.

i. Screening Performance in Low Risk or Unselected Groups

We have identified 28 studies that report the screening performance of a first-trimester anomaly scan for detection of major cardiac abnormalities in an unselected population (Table **3**). These include a contribution of a total of 171,540 pregnancies with total of 486 infants affected by major cardiac defect; giving a prevalence of 2.8/1,000 livebirths. 164 (34%) of these cardiac defects were detected in the first trimester [76 - 103]. Twenty-two studies were done prospectively, six were retrospective and there was one prospective randomised controlled trial. Three studies exclusively involved transvaginal assessment whilst the remainder used a transabdominal approach which was supplemented by a transvaginal scan if transabdominal views were inadequate. The prevalence of the cardiac defects varied from 0.5-6.1/1,000 livebirths, suggesting that there was incomplete outcome ascertainment in some studies and inclusion of minor cardiac defects in other studies. There was a wide range of variation in first-trimester detection of cardiac abnormality.

Studies that exclusively used a transvaginal approach reported detection rates of 4-33%, contrary to early reports of better visualisation of fetal anatomy using this methodology [76, 78, 82]. Whilst the transvaginal probe has the advantage of being a higher-frequency - giving better resolution, there is the disadvantage of limited ability to manipulate the probe to develop planes for visualisation. Complete visualisation of heart structures and correct interpretation of anatomy is the prerequisite for the potentially detectable cardiac anomaly. D'Ottavio *et al*. who completed a prospective study of 4,050 patients, demonstrated that the lower rate of visualisation of cardiac anatomy was related to both the operator's experience and technical difficulties with respect to restriction of the imaging plane [76]. The authors concluded that further operator training and an increase in available examination time would increase the detection rate. Studies by other groups had similar conclusions [78, 82].

Table 3. Twenty-eight first trimester screening studies reporting the diagnosis of major congenital heart disease (CHD) in low risk or unselected populations.

Author	N	Design	Population	Scan route	Gestation weeks	Cases and prevalence of CHD	Early detection of CHD
D Ottavia*et al.* 1998 [76]	4,050	prospective	unselected	TV	14	9 (2.2/1,000)	3 (33%)
Hafner *et al.* 1999 [77]	4,233	prospective	unselected	TA	11-13	14 (4.6/1,000)	1 (7%)
Rustico *et al.* 2000 [78]	4,785	prospective	unselected	TV	13-15	41 (0.8/1,000)	4 (10%)
Mavrides *et al.* 2001 [79]	7,339	prospective	unselected	TA	11-14	26 (3.5/1,000)	4 (23%)
Michailidis *et al.* 2001 [80]	6,650	prospective	unselected	TA/TV	11-14	8 (1.2/1,000)	1 (13%)
Carvalho *et al.* 2002 [81]	2,853	prospective	unselected	TA/TV	11-14	16 (5.6/1,000)	9 (56%)
Taipale *et al.* 2004 [82]	4,073	prospective	unselected	TV	13-14	25 (6.1/1,000)	1 (4%)
Chen *et al.* 2004 [83]	1,599	prospective	unselected	TA/TV	11-14	3 (1.9/1,000)	0
Becker *et al.* 2006 [84]	3,008	prospective	unselected	TA/TV	11-13	11 (3.6/1,000)	6 (55%)
Westin *et al.* 2006 [85]	18,148	RCT	unselected	TA	12-14	61 (3.3/1,000)	7 (11%)
McAuliffe *et al.* 2005 [86]	300	prospective	unselected	TA/TV	11-14	1 (3.3/1,000)	0
Souka *et al.* 2006 [87]	1,148	prospective	unselected	TA/TV	11-14	4 (3.5/1,000)	3 (75%)
Cedergren *et al.* 2006 [88]	2,708	prospective	unselected	TA/TV	11-14	9 (3.3/1,000)	0
Dane *et al.* 2007 [89]	1,274	prospective	unselected	TA/TV	11-14	4 (3.1/1,000)	1 (25%)
Lombardi *et al.* 2007 [90]	606	prospective	unselected	TA	11-14	1 (1.7/1,000)	1 (100%)

(Table 3) cont.....

Author	N	Design	Population	Scan route	Gestation weeks	Cases and prevalence of CHD	Early detection of CHD
Oztekin *et al.* 2009 [91]	1,085	prospective	unselected	TA/TV	11-14	3 (2.7/1,000)	0
Ebrashy *et al.* 2010 [92]	2,876	prospective	unselected	TA/TV	13-14	4(1.4/1,000)	1 (25%)
Abu - Rustum *et al.* 2010 [93]	1,370	retrospective	unselected	TA/TV	11-14	8 (5.8/1,000)	6 (75%)
Hartge *et al.* 2011 [94]	3,166	retrospective	unselected	TA/TV	11-14	22 (6.9/1,000)	15 (68%)
Volpe *et al.* 2011 [95]	4,435	prospective	unselected	TA/TV	11-14	12 (2.7/1,000)	4 (33%)
Jakobson *et al.* 2011 [96]	9,324	retrospective	unselected	TA/TV	11-14	12(1.3/1,000)	3 (25%)
Vavilala *et al.* 2011 [97]	7,916	prospective	unselected	TA/TV	11-14	4 (0.5/1,000)	0
Syngelaki *et al.* 2011 [98]	44,859	retrospective	unselected	TA	11-14	85 (1.9/1,000)	28 (33%)
Eleftheriades *et al.* 2012 [99]	3,759	prospective	unselected	TA/TV	11-14	14 (3.7/1,000)	5 (36%)
Grande *et al.* 201 [100]	13,723	retrospective	unselected	TA/TV	11-14	44 (3.2/1,000)	25 (57%)
Becker *et al.* 2012 [101]	6,879	prospective	unselected	TA/TV	11-14	15 (2.2/1,000)	7 (47%)
Pilas *et al.* 2012 [102]	3,902	retrospective	unselected	TA/TV	11-14	11(2.8/1,000)	2 (18%)
Iliescu *et al.* 2013 [103]	5,472	prospective	unselected	TA/TV	12-14	30 (5.4/1,000)	27 (90%)
Total	**171,540**					**486 (2.8/1,000)**	**164 (34%)**

TA: transabdominal; TV: transvaginal; RCT: randomized controlled trial.

There was a significant association between the sensitivity of screening and the level of detail included in the anatomical protocol described by the authors. The studies achieving high detection rates included both the four-chamber view and examination of great arteries in their protocol. Iliescu *et al.* reported using an extended protocol where the four-chamber view and outflow tracts were examined using 2D grey scale, colour and pulse wave Doppler imaging [103]. This prospective study of 5,472 unselected pregnancies reported a detection rate of nearly 90%. Colour Doppler appears to be of particular importance in first trimester assessment as a 2D grey scale sweep provides a less detailed picture of heart structure and function. It is also worth noting that 35 minutes was allocated to each assessment and, in cases of nonvisualisation of targeted organs, the patient was re-examined after a short break or the examination was rescheduled in the next few days. The examinations were also performed by operators who had five years' experience in anomaly screening and echocardiography.

Some of the other studies that achieved a high detection rate offered detailed early fetal echocardiography to a subgroup of women defined as being high-risk based on increased nuchal translucency; highlighting the potential importance of markers for population assessment.

ii. Diagnostic Performance in High-risk Groups

Thirteen studies have reported the detection rate of cardiac abnormalities in high-risk fetuses in the first trimester (Table **4**) [104 - 116]. These patients were referred due to fetal or maternal factors defining them as being at high-risk of having a cardiac abnormality. Detailed fetal echocardiography was performed by experienced subspecialists and sonographers. These authors reported a total of 2,431 pregnancies with a prevalence of major cardiac abnormalities approaching 10%. Nearly 83% of the anomalies were detected in the first trimester. The majority of these fetuses also had chromosomal aberrations leading to early termination of pregnancy and there is minimal validation of the sonographic findings.

Table 4. Series reporting first trimester detection cardiac abnormalities in pregnancies recognised to be at high-risk.

Author	Study type	Cases scanned (n)	GA (weeks)	Scan route	Affected cases (n)	Early diagnosis
Gembruch *et al.* 1993 [104]	Prospective	114	11-14	TV	13	12 (92%)
Carvalho *et al.* 1998 [105]	Prospective	15	12-14	TA	4	1 (25%)
Zosmer *et al.* 1999 [106]	Prospective	323	13-17	TA/TV	27	24 (88%)
Simpson *et al.* 2000 [107]	Retrospective	229	12-15	TA	13	11 (84%)
Gabriel *et al.* 2002 [108]	Prospective	330	12-17	TA/TV	48	38 (79%)
Haak *et al.* 2003 [109]	Prospective	45	11-14	TV	10	10 (100%)

(Table 4) cont.....

Author	Study type	Cases scanned (n)	GA (weeks)	Scan route	Affected cases (n)	Early diagnosis
Lopes *et al.* 2003 [110]	Prospective	275	11-14	TV	37	33 (89%)
McAuliffe *et al.* 2005 [111]	Retrospective and prospective	160	11-16	TA/TV	20	14 (70%)
Galindo *et al.* 2005 [112]	Prospective	138	12-14	TA/TV	18	17 (94%)
Weiner *et al.* 2008 [113]	Prospective	200	12 -13	TA/TV	19	13 (68%)
Belloti *et al.* 2010 [114]	Prospective	121	12-14	TA	23	20 (87%)
Mirza *et al.* 2012 [115]	Retrospective	81	12-16	TA/TV	6	4 (66%)
Mogra *et al.* 2015 [116]	Retrospective	400	13-16	TA/TV	15	14 (93%)
Total		2,431			253 (10%)	211 (83%)

GA: gestational age; TA: transabdominal; TV: transvaginal;

Gembruch *et al.* described a transvaginal approach in a mixed risk population of 114 patients including 13 cardiac malformations which were later confirmed at autopsy using stereo-microscopic examination [104]. Cardiac anatomy (four-chamber view and great arteries) was visualised in all cases at 13-14 weeks' gestation. In three cases, the diagnosis was precisely the same; in eight cases, additional cardiovascular malformations were seen on autopsy. In one case, a complex cardiac abnormality was missed until later in pregnancy, and in two other cases, the presence of visceral situs and dextrocardia was overlooked. The authors concluded that whilst transvaginal scanning provides good resolution, there are some limitations in achieving all imaging planes and spatial orientation was more difficult; they therefore felt there should also be a transabdominal scan in every case. Haak *et al.* examined 45 high risk cases using transvaginal ultrasound and cardiac anatomy was successfully visualised in 95% of cases [109]. All 10 cardiac defects were identified with no major discrepancies at postmortem.

The lowest detection rate from a formal first trimester echo was reported by Carvalho *et al.* in 1998; the authors identified 1 in 4 (25%) cardiac anomalies in small series of 15 first trimester scans [105]. This was one of the first series reporting transabdominal assessment and the resolution of machines was more limited at this time. The three cardiac abnormalities that were missed were ventricular septal defects - which are frequently missed at later gestations. Lopes *et al.* also described a transabdominal series completing a very detailed assessment protocol using 2D-grey scale, colour Doppler imaging and pulse wave interrogation of the aortic and pulmonary valves [110]. There was no time limit set for the examination and examinations were rescheduled until all anatomy was evaluated. 33/37 (89%) cardiac defects were diagnosed. Three of the four missed diagnoses involved isolated ventricular septal defects - reinforcing the difficulty in making this diagnosis at early gestations.

Recently Zidere *et al.* reported findings in a comprehensive series of 1200 patients who had both a first and a second trimester echo [117]. They described high sensitivity (85%) and specificity (95%) for the diagnosis of cardiac defects at 12 weeks. There was discordance in the first and second trimester findings in 29 (2.4%) cases; including 14 cases where a minor finding was missed at 12 weeks' (*e.g.* an ARSA, a ventricular septal defect or a persistent left superior vena cava). In the remaining 15 cases (1% of the total population) more significant diagnoses were missed including two cases of tetralogy of Fallot, two cases of atrioventricular septal defect and a case of Ebstein's anomaly with pulmonary atresia. These authors also noted that minor functional anomalies (seen in 50 cases - with features such as tricuspid regurgitation) frequently resolved between the first and second trimester scans. There were also three false positive diagnoses - two cases of AVSD and one case of coarctation of the aorta that were either found to be inappropriately categorised or found to be normal at the second scan. Interestingly, AVSDs are harder to diagnose at 12 weeks as the offset in the crux is typically less apparent at this stage. It is also important to note that as some pathologies are progressive (for example hypoplastic left heart) the findings at 12 weeks' may be different to those used to identify the lesion at a later gestation.

Rasiah *et al.* presented a meta-analysis that included an assessment of the efficacy of transabdominal and transvaginal approaches and found a significant higher sensitivity using transabdominal ultrasound (96% *vs.* 62%) [118]. As transabdominal imaging has continued to improve through the development of high frequency transducers with amplified spatial and axial resolution, it has become possible to obtain all standardized sections for a detailed cardiac examination in the first trimester. Lombardi and Ebrashy have pioneered the use of high frequency linear transducers for first trimester fetal echocardiography demonstrating high resolution to a depth of at least 8cm from the maternal abdominal wall [119, 120]. The linear transducer also enables high spatial resolution with colour Doppler allowing clear demonstration of forward flow through both ventricles, exclusion of large ventricular septal defects and assessment of the outflow tracts. The convex probe most commonly used in obstetric ultrasound has been designed for second-trimester imaging because it provides a large field of view and deep penetration to allow visualization of fetal organs many of which are often >8 cm away from the transducer. However, the consequence of the divergent ultrasound beams produced by the convex probe is a decrease in image line density and therefore lower resolution in both B-mode and colour flow imaging with increasing depth.

THE OPTIMAL GESTATIONAL AGE FOR EARLY FETAL ECHO

A complete evaluation of heart for detection of CHD includes an examination of situs, the four-chamber view, outflow tracts and pulmonary and systemic venous circulations. By 10 completed weeks of gestation the fetal heart has reached its complete anatomic form. With the introduction of high-frequency transvaginal probes in the early 1990s, many research groups looked at the feasibility of visualising cardiac structures at an early gestation. Allan *et al.* compared the results of transvaginal ultrasound at 5-12 weeks' with anatomic structures of the micro-dissected heart. They found that at nine weeks' gestation the fetal heart is centrally placed in the chest and by ten weeks the heart position changes to the left-sided orientation as seen in later pregnancy [119]. At 11 weeks' gestation, the four-chamber view and outflow tract are identifiable. Mean heart diameter increased linearly with gestational age and ranged from approximately 2 mm at seven weeks' to 7 mm at 13 weeks' gestation. Gestational age plays a determinant role in the early heart scan. Dolkart *et al.* also examined the feasibility of early fetal echocardiography [120]. They examined 52 patients transvaginally between 10 and 15 weeks' gestation and concluded that the four-chamber view and aorta (long axis) could be visualised in 100% and 40% of cases respectively by 13 weeks' gestation. This study of normal cardiac anatomy suggested that there may be significant potential for the diagnosis of many fetal cardiac anomalies during the late first and early second trimesters of pregnancy.

Achrion *et al.* evaluated the feasibility of early echocardiography in 660 patients considered to be at low risk for CHD and were successful in obtaining the four-chamber view in 100% of cases and outflow tracts in 98% of cases at 13-15 week gestation using a high frequency (6.5-7.5 MHz) transvaginal probe [121]. Much of this success appears to be operator dependent as other experienced fetal cardiologists reported much lower success rates in establishing a four-chamber (70%) and outflow tract (43%) views before 14 weeks' gestation [122]. This may, in part, reflect the fact that cardiologists are less used to manipulating a transvaginal probe to obtain the required planes and views. Gembruch *et al.*, using a combined transabdominal and transvaginal technique and reported that adequate views of the four-chamber view and outflow tracts were always obtainable from 13 weeks' onwards [123]. This contrasted with Rustico *et al.* who demonstrated only 48% visualisation rate of full cardiac anatomy in the unselected population and emphasized that the operator's experience is important [78].

Few studies have looked at transabdominal route for visualisation of cardiac anatomy. Huggon *et al*. demonstrated that full cardiac anatomy was visualised in 90% of cases with crown-rump length (CRL) >60mm. Technical failure was attributed to maternal obesity, persistently unfavourable fetal position or a retroverted uterus [124]. Similarly, Simpson *et al*. were able to visualise cardiac anatomy in >98% of referred cases transabdominally after 13 weeks' gestation [107]. The cases with incomplete visualisation were rescheduled for a repeat examination. This highlighted the difference between the referred and unselected population as every attempt is made to complete the anatomy in the referred group. Aortic, ductal arches and systemic and pulmonary veins were particularly difficult to visualise at an early gestation. Smrcek *et al*. suggested a high success rate for visualisation of these structures can be obtained by using colour and power Doppler [125]. McAulife *et al*. in a study of 160 high-risk patient at 11-16 weeks demonstrated that the pulmonary veins were visualised in only 16% of cases and the aortic and ductal arches in 45% of cases using colour Doppler [111].

With the improvement in technology modern ultrasound machines are offering greater image resolution with better grey scale definition. Therefore, by utilizing harmonic imaging and power Doppler facility the cardiac anatomy can be better visualised by the transabdominal route. Most recent studies have used mainly transabdominal route and have supplemented transvaginal route for the difficult fetal position or maternal factors such as obesity.

It seems clear that to maximize the visualisation of cardiac anatomy the best gestational age for an early cardiac assessment is 13-14 weeks (Table **5**). Evaluation of cardiac anatomy should include assessment of situs, four-chamber view, both great arteries, and pulmonary and systemic venous circulation by using both 2D and colour Doppler technology and utilising both transabdominal and transvaginal route.

A SIMPLIFIED PROTOCOL FOR EARLY FETAL ECHO AND DETECTION RATE

The fetal echocardiography at early gestation is challenging and requires a specialised skill. A couple of studies have looked at if detection of a cardiac abnormality can be improved by using a simplified protocol in the low-risk population. Wiecheic *et al*. analysed the diagnostic performance of the combined four chambers, three vessel and tracheal view in colour mapping at the time of NT scan for the detection of cardiac abnormality in the unselected population [126]. The simplified protocol included visualisation of the fetal chest with the fetal spine in a 6 or 12 o'clock position and with an insonation angle of 45 degrees to the interventricular septum allowing a smooth transition between the four-chamber, three vessel and three vessel tracheal views. Colour flow was used for the shortest time possible. This approach gave a sensitivity of 85% and specificity of 100% for the diagnosis of CHD at the time of the first-trimester scan [126]. The technique was simple and easy to reproduce. The technique allowed identification of most cases with a univentricular heart, AVSD, coarctation of the aorta, pulmonary stenosis, pulmonary atresia, and conotruncal defects.

Table 5. Proportion of scans (four chamber view and outflow tracts) successfully completed by gestational age.

Author	Scan Route	11-11^{+6} (%)	12-12^{+6} (%)	13-13^{+6} (%)
Dolkart *et al.* 1991 [120]	TV	20	40	46
Johnson *et al.* 1992 [122]	TV	0	59	62
Gembruch *et al.* 1993 [104]	TV	67	80	100
Achrion *et al.* 1994 [121]	TV			95
Gembruch *et al.* 2000 [123]	TV	75	93	100
Haak *et al.* 2002 [109]	TV	75	89	98
Huggon *et al.* 2002 [124]	TA			84
Carvalho *et al.* 1998 [105]	TA			73
Simpson *et al.* 2005 [107]	TA			98
McAuliffe *et al.* 2005 [111]	TV/TA			95

TA: transabdominal; TV: transvaginal.

Quarello *et al.* reported a short study of demonstrating the feasibility of simplified fetal echocardiography in a low-risk population [127]. This basic heart assessment used cross-sections of the four-chamber view and the three vessel tracheal view, using colour or directional power Doppler. The studies were completed at the time of the first-trimester nuchal translucency scan without modifying the allocated time for the scan. Sixty observers participated in the study and performed a total of 597 examinations. Most of the examinations were done by the transabdominal route. The four-chamber view was obtained in 94% of cases and the three vessel tracheal view in 87% of cases.

De Robertis *et al.* also evaluated the feasibility of using the three vessel tracheal view at the time of the first trimester NT scan, reporting a prospective study including 5,343 fetuses. Sonographers were instructed to take images/clips of abdominal situs, the four-chamber view and the three vessel tracheal view in 2D and colour Doppler [128]. The three vessel tracheal view was demonstrated in 94% of cases. Suspicion of a cardiac abnormality included detection of abnormal vessel number, abnormal vessel size or abnormal spatial relationship. An abnormal three vessel tracheal view was suspected in 22 cases and was confirmed in 21 of these. The detection rate of cardiac abnormality using the complete protocol was 75.8%. This simple method allows the identification of a 'high-risk' group which can then be targeted through specialist echocardiography for further clarification of the cardiac defect.

THE LEARNING CURVE

Performing extended echocardiography at the time of the first trimester scan is based on sonographer's skill, knowledge and understanding of cardiac defects. It is difficult to establish how many ultrasound scans are necessary to obtain the expertise. Tegnander *et al.* demonstrated, in a second trimester screening study, that sonographers with previous experience of more than 2000 scans had a detection rate of 54% as compare to 32% detection for operators performing less than 2000 cardiac examinations [129].

Abu Rustum *et al.* prospectively examined the learning curve of early fetal echo in the first trimester [130]. All examinations were done transabdominally by a sonologist who already had performed more than 1,500 first trimester scans and had a thorough knowledge of second trimester fetal echocardiography. The learning curve was evaluated in progressing from obtaining a four-chamber view to extended views including the outflow tracts, ductal and aortic arches and the vena cavae. The mean time allocated for the fetal echo was 9 minutes. A complete examination was possible in 94% of cases after the operator had completed 50 examinations.

The baseline level of a sonographer's experience also affects the learning curve. Nemescu *et al.* reported the learning curve for early fetal echo for sonographers at the beginning of their training [131]. Sonographers were asked to take a colour sweep of the heart including the four-chamber view and the outflow tracts. The cine loop facility was then used to check anatomical views. Mean examination time was only 2.7 min, but a sonographer at the beginning of their training needed to complete at least 180 examinations before they could successfully examine the heart in 80% of cases. After 500 cases the heart could be successfully examined in nearly 100% of cases. Significant factors that increased the probability of a successful examination were the length of the examination and the experience of the sonographer. Gestation (CRL), maternal body mass index (BMI) and restrictive fetal position did not affect the adequacy of the examination.

WHAT CONSTITUTES AN EARLY FETAL ECHO

The approach to scanning the fetal heart in early pregnancy is the same as that used in the second trimester. Operators performing early fetal echo should intend to obtain all standard views recommended for a standard (20 week) fetal echo using sequential segmental analysis in both 2D and colour Doppler [132, 133].

Operators should optimize the image by appropriate adjustment of technical settings, such as image magnification, signal gain, acoustic focus, frequency selection and harmonic imaging. Images should be magnified until the heart fills at least a third/half of the display screen. System settings should highlight a high frame rate, with increased contrast and high resolution. Low persistence, a single acoustic focal zone and a relatively narrow image field should also be used. A narrow field of view has the additional benefit of improving the frame rate, which is essential for obtaining high resolution fetal heart images in the first trimester. If a cine-loop storage feature is available, this is very useful as it allows the operator to retrospectively evaluate anomalous cases later.

The transverse plane is used for the assessment of abdominal situs, the four-chamber view, three vessel and three vessel tracheal views (Fig. **6**). The sagittal plane can be utilized to assess the aortic and ductal arches, and superior and inferior vena cava. Colour and pulsed-Doppler assessments should be made of ventricular inflows, outflow tracts, aortic and ductal arches, systemic and pulmonary veins.

From an anatomical perspective, the fetal heart essentially looks the same in the first trimester as it does at the time of the 18-23 week fetal morphology scan. At the start of the examination, abdominal situs should be assessed. The four-chamber view of the heart then becomes easily visible by moving the transducer cranially from the axial abdominal view. A normal heart occupies approximately one third of the thorax and the cardiac axis lies at 45 degrees to the left of the midline. Two thirds of the heart are in the left hemithorax. The descending aorta is located anterior and to the left of the spine behind the left atrium. The two atria and ventricles are roughly equal in size. The moderator band is within the right ventricle. Even minimal ventricular disproportion is indicative of pathology such as coarctation of aorta. The two atrioventricular valves are equally opened and differentially inserted; offset of the AV valve can be very subtle before 12 weeks' gestation. Blood flow across both the valves should be evaluated by colour Doppler imaging to ensure that both ventricles fill equally in diastole without regurgitation. At least two pulmonary veins can be seen entering in to the left atrium- this can be the most challenging part of the early fetal echo but can be clearly visualised from 13 weeks' onwards.

From the four-chamber view, the transducer is moved upward and towards the right shoulder of the fetus to obtain the left ventricular outflow tract and the aorta (branching at a wide angle far from the semilunar valve). The semilunar valve should open freely and completely disappear during systole. Septo-aortic continuity should also be assessed in this view. Blood flow across the aortic valve should be laminar with no evidence of turbulence or regurgitation.

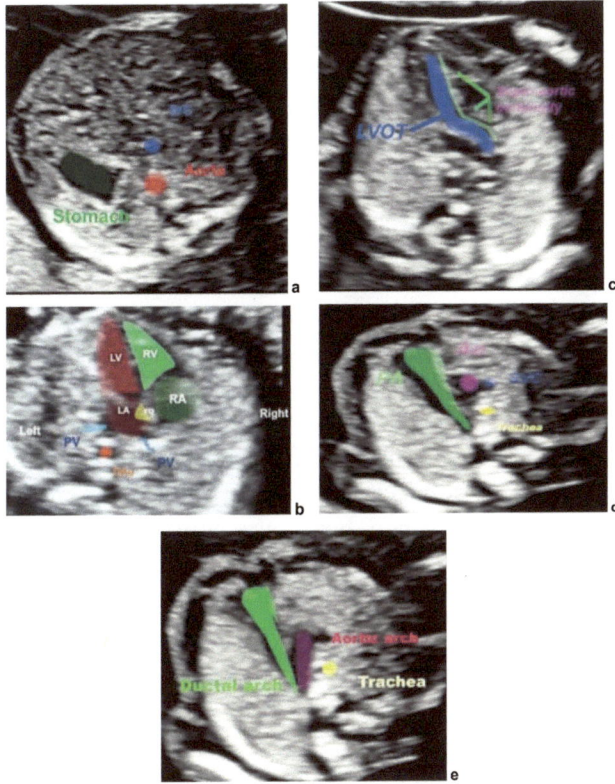

Fig. (6). (**a**) Abdominal situs; (**b**) 4 chamber view {(Left atrium (LA), Left ventricle (LV), Right ventricle (RV), Right atrium (RA), FO (Foramen ovale), PV (Pulmonary vein), Dao (Descending aorta)}; (**c**) LVOT (Left ventricle outflow tract) view; (**d**) 3 Vessel view {(Aorta (Ao), Pulmonary artery (PA), Superior vena cava (SVC); (**e**) 3 Vessel tracheal view.

Further upward movement of the probe reveals the three vessel and three vessel tracheal view. An oblique section of the pulmonary trunk and cross section of the aorta and superior vena cava are seen. The three vessels are arranged in a straight line from left/anterior to right/posterior with decreasing order of size. The pulmonary artery is largest in size followed by the ascending aorta and superior vena cava (SVC). A slight upward movement shows the three vessel tracheal view where both the aortic and ductal arches can be seen to form a "V" shape confluence at the descending aorta. Colour Doppler shows blood flow in the same direction in both arches. If only one great artery can be identified or if there is a size discrepancy or abnormal flow on colour or pulse Doppler, this strongly suggest the possibility of a cardiac defect. Some examples of common cardiac abnormalities that can be detected in the first trimester are shown.

CONCLUSION

A variety of extracardiac tools as well as direct cardiac assessment can be used to screen low risk populations for cardiac abnormalities. Combinations of screening tools will likely identify the majority of major cardiac defects but further prospective studies are needed to demonstrate precise efficacy. A complete fetal echo is more difficult to perform, requires technical skill and is most readily completed beyond 13 weeks' gestation. The optimal time for a transabdominal study appears to be 13-15 weeks' gestation. A completed study does, however, appear to have high sensitivity, specificity and negative predictive value for structural cardiac defects. The early diagnosis of a cardiac defect allows further investigation to determine association with chromosomal abnormality and, if necessary, safer access to termination of pregnancy. In circumstances where anomalies are isolated and parents chose to continue, early identification of an anomaly allows parents to gain as much information as possible during the course of pregnancy. As cardiac anomalies evolve through pregnancy, any suspected structural defect should be reassessed during the course of the pregnancy.

CONSENT FOR PUBLICATION

Not applicable.

CONFLICT OF INTEREST

The authors confirm that the contents of this chapter have no conflict of interest.

ACKNOWLEDGEMENTS

Declare none.

REFERENCES

[1] van der Linde D, Konings EE, Slager MA, *et al.* Birth prevalence of congenital heart disease worldwide: a systematic review and meta-analysis. J Am Coll Cardiol 2011; 58(21): 2241-7.
      [http://dx.doi.org/10.1016/j.jacc.2011.08.025] [PMID: 22078432]

[2] Bernier PL, Stefanescu A, Samoukovic G, Tchervenkov CI. The challenge of congenital heart disease worldwide: epidemiologic and demographic facts. Semin Thorac Cardiovasc Surg Pediatr Card Surg Annu 2010; 13(1): 26-34.
      [http://dx.doi.org/10.1053/j.pcsu.2010.02.005] [PMID: 20307858]

[3] Jorgensen M, McPherson E, Zaleski C, Shivaram P, Cold C. Stillbirth: the heart of the matter. Am J Med Genet A 2014; 164A(3): 691-9.
      [http://dx.doi.org/10.1002/ajmg.a.36366] [PMID: 24459042]

[4] Marelli AJ, Ionescu-Ittu R, Mackie AS, Guo L, Dendukuri N, Kaouache M. Lifetime prevalence of

congenital heart disease in the general population from 2000 to 2010. Circulation 2014; 130(9): 749-56.
[http://dx.doi.org/10.1161/CIRCULATIONAHA.113.008396] [PMID: 24944314]

[5]   Gilboa SM, Salemi JL, Nembhard WN, Fixler DE, Correa A. Mortality resulting from congenital heart disease among children and adults in the United States, 1999 to 2006. Circulation 2010; 122(22): 2254-63.
[http://dx.doi.org/10.1161/CIRCULATIONAHA.110.947002] [PMID: 21098447]

[6]   Mahle WT, Clancy RR, McGaurn SP, Goin JE, Clark BJ. Impact of prenatal diagnosis on survival and early neurologic morbidity in neonates with the hypoplastic left heart syndrome. Pediatrics 2001; 107(6): 1277-82.
[http://dx.doi.org/10.1542/peds.107.6.1277] [PMID: 11389243]

[7]   Verheijen PM, Lisowski LA, Stoutenbeek P, *et al.* Prenatal diagnosis of congenital heart disease affects preoperative acidosis in the newborn patient. J Thorac Cardiovasc Surg 2001; 121(4): 798-803.
[http://dx.doi.org/10.1067/mtc.2001.112825] [PMID: 11279423]

[8]   Bonnet D, Coltri A, Butera G, *et al.* Detection of transposition of the great arteries in fetuses reduces neonatal morbidity and mortality. Circulation 1999; 99(7): 916-8.
[http://dx.doi.org/10.1161/01.CIR.99.7.916] [PMID: 10027815]

[9]   Viñals F, Tapia J, Giuliano A. Prenatal detection of ductal-dependent congenital heart disease: how can things be made easier? Ultrasound Obstet Gynecol 2002; 19(3): 246-9.
[http://dx.doi.org/10.1046/j.1469-0705.2002.00651.x] [PMID: 11896944]

[10]   Tuuli MG, Dicke JM, Stamilio DM, *et al.* Prevalence and likelihood ratios for aneuploidy in fetuses diagnosed prenatally with isolated congenital cardiac defects. Am J Obstet Gynecol 2009; 201(4): 390.e1-5.
[http://dx.doi.org/10.1016/j.ajog.2009.06.035] [PMID: 19716116]

[11]   Hartman RJ, Rasmussen SA, Botto LD, *et al.* The contribution of chromosomal abnormalities to congenital heart defects: a population-based study. Pediatr Cardiol 2011; 32(8): 1147-57.
[http://dx.doi.org/10.1007/s00246-011-0034-5] [PMID: 21728077]

[12]   Pollex RL, Hegele RA. Copy number variation in the human genome and its implications for cardiovascular disease. Circulation 2007; 115(24): 3130-8.
[http://dx.doi.org/10.1161/CIRCULATIONAHA.106.677591] [PMID: 17576883]

[13]   Thienpont B, Mertens L, de Ravel T, *et al.* Submicroscopic chromosomal imbalances detected by array-CGH are a frequent cause of congenital heart defects in selected patients. Eur Heart J 2007; 28(22): 2778-84.
[http://dx.doi.org/10.1093/eurheartj/ehl560] [PMID: 17384091]

[14]   Jansen FA, Blumenfeld YJ, Fisher A, *et al.* Array comparative genomic hybridization and fetal congenital heart defects: a systematic review and meta-analysis. Ultrasound Obstet Gynecol 2015; 45(1): 27-35.
[http://dx.doi.org/10.1002/uog.14695] [PMID: 25319878]

[15]   Dugoff L, Mennuti MT, McDonald-McGinn DM. The benefits and limitations of cell-free DNA screening for 22q11.2 deletion syndrome. Prenat Diagn 2017; 37(1): 53-60.
[http://dx.doi.org/10.1002/pd.4864] [PMID: 27329064]

[16]   Myers A, Bernstein JA, Brennan ML, *et al.* Perinatal features of the RASopathies: Noonan syndrome, cardiofaciocutaneous syndrome and Costello syndrome. Am J Med Genet A 2014; 164A(11): 2814-21.
[http://dx.doi.org/10.1002/ajmg.a.36737] [PMID: 25250515]

[17]   Gaudineau A, Doray B, Schaefer E, *et al.* Postnatal phenotype according to prenatal ultrasound features of Noonan syndrome: a retrospective study of 28 cases. Prenat Diagn 2013; 33(3): 238-41.
[http://dx.doi.org/10.1002/pd.4051] [PMID: 23345196]

[18]   Azamian M, Lalani SR. Cytogenomic aberrations in congenital cardiovascular malformations. Mol

Syndromol 2016; 7(2): 51-61.
[http://dx.doi.org/10.1159/000445788] [PMID: 27385961]

[19] Pavlicek J, Gruszka T, Polanska S, *et al.* Parents' request for termination of pregnancy due to a congenital heart defect of the fetus in a country with liberal interruption laws. J Matern Fetal Neonatal Med 2019; 1-9. Epub ahead of print
[http://dx.doi.org/10.1080/14767058.2018.1564029] [PMID: 30646776]

[20] Maxwell S, Bower C, O'Leary P. Impact of prenatal screening and diagnostic testing on trends in Down syndrome births and terminations in Western Australia 1980 to 2013. Prenat Diagn 2015; 35(13): 1324-30.
[http://dx.doi.org/10.1002/pd.4698] [PMID: 26411476]

[21] Kornman LH, Wortelboer MJ, Beekhuis JR, Morssink LP, Mantingh A. Women's opinions and the implications of first- *versus* second-trimester screening for fetal Down's syndrome. Prenat Diagn 1997; 17(11): 1011-8.
[http://dx.doi.org/10.1002/(SICI)1097-0223(199711)17:11<1011::AID-PD193>3.0.CO;2-1] [PMID: 9399348]

[22] Daugirdaitė V, van den Akker O, Purewal S. Posttraumatic stress and posttraumatic stress disorder after termination of pregnancy and reproductive loss: a systematic review. J Pregnancy 2015; 2015646345
[http://dx.doi.org/10.1155/2015/646345] [PMID: 25734016]

[23] Davies V, Gledhill J, McFadyen A, Whitlow B, Economides D. Psychological outcome in women undergoing termination of pregnancy for ultrasound-detected fetal anomaly in the first and second trimesters: a pilot study. Ultrasound Obstet Gynecol 2005; 25(4): 389-92.
[http://dx.doi.org/10.1002/uog.1854] [PMID: 15791695]

[24] Germanakis I, Sifakis S. The impact of fetal echocardiography on the prevalence of liveborn congenital heart disease. Pediatr Cardiol 2006; 27(4): 465-72.
[http://dx.doi.org/10.1007/s00246-006-1291-6] [PMID: 16830077]

[25] Allan L. Fetal cardiac scanning today. Prenat Diagn 2010; 30(7): 639-43.
[http://dx.doi.org/10.1002/pd.2540] [PMID: 20572107]

[26] Cardiac screening examination of the fetus: guidelines for performing the 'basic' and 'extended basic' cardiac scan. Ultrasound Obstet Gynecol 2006; 27(1): 107-13.
[PMID: 16374757]

[27] https://assets.publishing.service.gov.uk/government/uploads/system/uploads/attachment_data/file/7497 42/NHS_fetal_anomaly_screening_programme_handbook_FINAL1.2_18.10.18.pdf

[28] Wright D, Kagan KO, Molina FS, Gazzoni A, Nicolaides KH. A mixture model of nuchal translucency thickness in screening for chromosomal defects. Ultrasound Obstet Gynecol 2008; 31(4): 376-83.
[http://dx.doi.org/10.1002/uog.5299] [PMID: 18383462]

[29] Spencer K. Aneuploidy screening in the first trimester. Am J Med Genet C Semin Med Genet 2007; 145C(1): 18-32.
[http://dx.doi.org/10.1002/ajmg.c.30119] [PMID: 17290444]

[30] Snijders RJM, Thom EA, Zachary JM, *et al.* First-trimester trisomy screening: nuchal translucency measurement training and quality assurance to correct and unify technique. Ultrasound Obstet Gynecol 2002; 19(4): 353-9.
[http://dx.doi.org/10.1046/j.1469-0705.2002.00637.x] [PMID: 11952964]

[31] Small M, Copel JA, Copel JA. Indications for fetal echocardiography. Pediatr Cardiol 2004; 25(3): 210-22.
[http://dx.doi.org/10.1007/s00246-003-0587-z] [PMID: 15360114]

[32] Friedberg MK, Silverman NH. Changing indications for fetal echocardiography in a University Center population. Prenat Diagn 2004; 24(10): 781-6.

[http://dx.doi.org/10.1002/pd.981] [PMID: 15503290]

[33]   Simpson LL. Indications for fetal echocardiography from a tertiary-care obstetric sonography practice. J Clin Ultrasound 2004; 32(3): 123-8.
[http://dx.doi.org/10.1002/jcu.20007] [PMID: 14994252]

[34]   Sharony R, Fejgin MD, Biron-Shental T, Hershko-Klement A, Amiel A, Levi A. Who should be offered fetal echocardiography? One center's experience with 3965 cases. Isr Med Assoc J 2009; 11(9): 542-5.
[PMID: 19960848]

[35]   Hyett J, Perdu M, Sharland G, Snijders R, Nicolaides KH. Using fetal nuchal translucency to screen for major congenital cardiac defects at 10-14 weeks of gestation: population based cohort study. BMJ 1999; 318(7176): 81-5.
[http://dx.doi.org/10.1136/bmj.318.7176.81] [PMID: 9880278]

[36]   Mavrides E, Cobian-Sanchez F, Tekay A, *et al.* Limitations of using first-trimester nuchal translucency measurement in routine screening for major congenital heart defects. Ultrasound Obstet Gynecol 2001; 17(2): 106-10.
[http://dx.doi.org/10.1046/j.1469-0705.2001.00342.x] [PMID: 11251916]

[37]   Michailidis GD, Economides DL. Nuchal translucency measurement and pregnancy outcome in karyotypically normal fetuses. Ultrasound Obstet Gynecol 2001; 17(2): 102-5.
[http://dx.doi.org/10.1046/j.1469-0705.2001.00341.x] [PMID: 11251915]

[38]   Hafner E, Schuller T, Metzenbauer M, Schuchter K, Philipp K. Increased nuchal translucency and congenital heart defects in a low-risk population. Prenat Diagn 2003; 23(12): 985-9.
[http://dx.doi.org/10.1002/pd.721] [PMID: 14663835]

[39]   Bahado-Singh RO, Wapner R, Thom E, *et al.* Elevated first-trimester nuchal translucency increases the risk of congenital heart defects. Am J Obstet Gynecol 2005; 192(5): 1357-61.
[http://dx.doi.org/10.1016/j.ajog.2004.12.086] [PMID: 15902108]

[40]   Bruns RF, Moron AF, Murta CG, Gonçalves LF, Zamith MM. The role of nuchal translucency in the screening for congenital heart defects. Arq Bras Cardiol 2006; 87(3): 307-14.
[PMID: 17057931]

[41]   Westin M, Saltvedt S, Bergman G, Almström H, Grunewald C, Valentin L. Is measurement of nuchal translucency thickness a useful screening tool for heart defects? A study of 16,383 fetuses. Ultrasound Obstet Gynecol 2006; 27(6): 632-9.
[http://dx.doi.org/10.1002/uog.2792] [PMID: 16715530]

[42]   Müller MA, Clur SA, Timmerman E, Bilardo CM. Nuchal translucency measurement and congenital heart defects: modest association in low-risk pregnancies. Prenat Diagn 2007; 27(2): 164-9.
[http://dx.doi.org/10.1002/pd.1643] [PMID: 17238215]

[43]   Chelemen T, Syngelaki A, Maiz N, Allan L, Nicolaides KH. Contribution of ductus venosus Doppler in first-trimester screening for major cardiac defects. Fetal Diagn Ther 2011; 29(2): 127-34.
[http://dx.doi.org/10.1159/000322138] [PMID: 21160164]

[44]   Matias A, Huggon I, Areias JC, Montenegro N, Nicolaides KH. Cardiac defects in chromosomally normal fetuses with abnormal ductus venosus blood flow at 10-14 weeks. Ultrasound Obstet Gynecol 1999; 14(5): 307-10.
[http://dx.doi.org/10.1046/j.1469-0705.1999.14050307.x] [PMID: 10623988]

[45]   Bilardo CM, Müller MA, Zikulnig L, Schipper M, Hecher K. Ductus venosus studies in fetuses at high risk for chromosomal or heart abnormalities: relationship with nuchal translucency measurement and fetal outcome. Ultrasound Obstet Gynecol 2001; 17(4): 288-94.
[http://dx.doi.org/10.1046/j.1469-0705.2001.00387.x] [PMID: 11339183]

[46]   Murta CG, Moron AF, Avila MA, Weiner CP. Application of ductus venosus Doppler velocimetry for the detection of fetal aneuploidy in the first trimester of pregnancy. Fetal Diagn Ther 2002; 17(5):

308-14.
[http://dx.doi.org/10.1159/000063185] [PMID: 12169818]

[47] Zoppi MA, Putzolu M, Ibba RM, Floris M, Monni G. First-trimester ductus venosus velocimetry in relation to nuchal translucency thickness and fetal karyotype. Fetal Diagn Ther 2002; 17(1): 52-7.
[http://dx.doi.org/10.1159/000048007] [PMID: 11803218]

[48] Favre R, Cherif Y, Kohler M, *et al.* The role of fetal nuchal translucency and ductus venosus Doppler at 11-14 weeks of gestation in the detection of major congenital heart defects. Ultrasound Obstet Gynecol 2003; 21(3): 239-43.
[http://dx.doi.org/10.1002/uog.51] [PMID: 12666217]

[49] Haak MC, Twisk JW, Bartelings MM, Gittenberger-de Groot AC, van Vugt JM. Ductus venosus flow velocities in relation to the cardiac defects in first-trimester fetuses with enlarged nuchal translucency. Am J Obstet Gynecol 2003; 188(3): 727-33.
[http://dx.doi.org/10.1067/mob.2003.157] [PMID: 12634648]

[50] Toyama JM, Brizot ML, Liao AW, *et al.* Ductus venosus blood flow assessment at 11 to 14 weeks of gestation and fetal outcome. Ultrasound Obstet Gynecol 2004; 23(4): 341-5.
[http://dx.doi.org/10.1002/uog.1025] [PMID: 15065182]

[51] Maiz N, Plasencia W, Dagklis T, Faros E, Nicolaides K. Ductus venosus Doppler in fetuses with cardiac defects and increased nuchal translucency thickness. Ultrasound Obstet Gynecol 2008; 31(3): 256-60.
[http://dx.doi.org/10.1002/uog.5262] [PMID: 18307193]

[52] Timmerman E, Clur SA, Pajkrt E, Bilardo CM. First-trimester measurement of the ductus venosus pulsatility index and the prediction of congenital heart defects. Ultrasound Obstet Gynecol 2010; 36(6): 668-75.
[http://dx.doi.org/10.1002/uog.7742] [PMID: 20617506]

[53] Martínez JM, Comas M, Borrell A, *et al.* Abnormal first-trimester ductus venosus blood flow: a marker of cardiac defects in fetuses with normal karyotype and nuchal translucency. Ultrasound Obstet Gynecol 2010; 35(3): 267-72.
[http://dx.doi.org/10.1002/uog.7544] [PMID: 20052662]

[54] Borrell A, Grande M, Bennasar M, *et al.* First-trimester detection of major cardiac defects with the use of ductus venosus blood flow. Ultrasound Obstet Gynecol 2013; 42(1): 51-7.
[http://dx.doi.org/10.1002/uog.12349] [PMID: 23152003]

[55] Edwards JE. Malformations of the aortic arch system manifested as vascular rings. Lab Invest 1953; 2(1): 56-75.
[PMID: 13036024]

[56] Weinberg P. Aortic arch anomalies.Moss and Adams heart disease in infants, children, and adolescents including the fetus and young adult. Baltimore, MD: Williams & Wilkins 1998; pp. 810-37.

[57] Goldstein WB. Aberrant right subclavian artery in Mongolism. Am J Roentgenol Radium Ther Nucl Med 1965; 95: 131-4.
[http://dx.doi.org/10.2214/ajr.95.1.131] [PMID: 14344351]

[58] Chaoui R, Thiel G, Heling KS. Prevalence of an aberrant right subclavian artery (ARSA) in normal fetuses: a new soft marker for trisomy 21 risk assessment. Ultrasound Obstet Gynecol 2005; 26: 356.
[http://dx.doi.org/10.1002/uog.2167]

[59] Willruth AM, Dwinger N, Ritgen J, *et al.* Fetal aberrant right subclavian artery (ARSA) - a potential new soft marker in the genetic scan? Ultraschall Med 2012; 33(7): E114-8.
[http://dx.doi.org/10.1055/s-0029-1245935] [PMID: 21614745]

[60] Fehmi Yazıcıoğlu H, Sevket O, Akın H, Aygün M, Özyurt ON, Karahasanoğlu A. Aberrant right subclavian artery in Down syndrome fetuses. Prenat Diagn 2013; 33(3): 209-13.
[http://dx.doi.org/10.1002/pd.4042] [PMID: 23319208]

[61]   Zalel Y, Achiron R, Yagel S, Kivilevitch Z. Fetal aberrant right subclavian artery in normal and Down syndrome fetuses. Ultrasound Obstet Gynecol 2008; 31(1): 25-9.
[http://dx.doi.org/10.1002/uog.5230] [PMID: 18098348]

[62]   Borenstein M, Minekawa R, Zidere V, Nicolaides KH, Allan LD. Aberrant right subclavian artery at 16 to 23 + 6 weeks of gestation: a marker for chromosomal abnormality. Ultrasound Obstet Gynecol 2010; 36(5): 548-52.
[http://dx.doi.org/10.1002/uog.7683] [PMID: 20503237]

[63]   Gul A, Corbacioglu A, Bakirci IT, Ceylan Y. Associated anomalies and outcome of fetal aberrant right subclavian artery. Arch Gynecol Obstet 2012; 285(1): 27-30.
[http://dx.doi.org/10.1007/s00404-011-1907-9] [PMID: 21487731]

[64]   Rembouskos G, Passamonti U, De Robertis V, et al. Aberrant right subclavian artery (ARSA) in unselected population at first and second trimester ultrasonography. Prenat Diagn 2012; 32(10): 968-75.
[http://dx.doi.org/10.1002/pd.3942] [PMID: 22847746]

[65]   Sinkovskaya E, Horton S, Berkley EM, Cooper JK, Indika S, Abuhamad A. Defining the fetal cardiac axis between 11 + 0 and 14 + 6 weeks of gestation: experience with 100 consecutive pregnancies. Ultrasound Obstet Gynecol 2010; 36(6): 676-81.
[http://dx.doi.org/10.1002/uog.8814] [PMID: 20814876]

[66]   Bennasar M, Martínez JM, Gómez O, et al. Intra- and interobserver repeatability of fetal cardiac examination using four-dimensional spatiotemporal image correlation in each trimester of pregnancy. Ultrasound Obstet Gynecol 2010; 35(3): 318-23.
[http://dx.doi.org/10.1002/uog.7570] [PMID: 20127758]

[67]   McBrien A, Howley L, Yamamoto Y, et al. Changes in fetal cardiac axis between 8 and 15 weeks' gestation. Ultrasound Obstet Gynecol 2013; 42(6): 653-8.
[http://dx.doi.org/10.1002/uog.12478] [PMID: 24273201]

[68]   Wolter A, Kawecki A, Stressig R, et al. Fetal cardiac axis in fetuses with conotruncal anomalies. Ultraschall Med 2017; 38(2): 198-205.
[PMID: 26425859]

[69]   Zheng MM, Tang HR, Zhang Y, et al. Contribution of the Fetal Cardiac Axis and V-Sign Angle in First-Trimester Screening for Major Cardiac Defects. J Ultrasound Med 2019; 38(5): 1179-87.
[http://dx.doi.org/10.1002/jum.14796] [PMID: 30208223]

[70]   Falcon O, Faiola S, Huggon I, Allan L, Nicolaides KH. Fetal tricuspid regurgitation at the 11 + 0 to 13 + 6-week scan: association with chromosomal defects and reproducibility of the method. Ultrasound Obstet Gynecol 2006; 27(6): 609-12.
[http://dx.doi.org/10.1002/uog.2736] [PMID: 16526003]

[71]   Huggon IC, DeFigueiredo DB, Allan LD. Tricuspid regurgitation in the diagnosis of chromosomal anomalies in the fetus at 11-14 weeks of gestation. Heart 2003; 89(9): 1071-3.
[http://dx.doi.org/10.1136/heart.89.9.1071] [PMID: 12923032]

[72]   Faiola S, Tsoi E, Huggon IC, Allan LD, Nicolaides KH. Likelihood ratio for trisomy 21 in fetuses with tricuspid regurgitation at the 11 to 13 + 6-week scan. Ultrasound Obstet Gynecol 2005; 26(1): 22-7.
[http://dx.doi.org/10.1002/uog.1922] [PMID: 15937972]

[73]   Pereira S, Ganapathy R, Syngelaki A, Maiz N, Nicolaides KH. Contribution of fetal tricuspid regurgitation in first-trimester screening for major cardiac defects. Obstet Gynecol 2011; 117(6): 1384-91.
[http://dx.doi.org/10.1097/AOG.0b013e31821aa720] [PMID: 21606749]

[74]   Gembruch U, Knöpfle G, Chatterjee M, Bald R, Hansmann M. First-trimester diagnosis of fetal congenital heart disease by transvaginal two-dimensional and Doppler echocardiography. Obstet Gynecol 1990; 75(3 Pt 2): 496-8.

[PMID: 2304721]

[75]   Bronshtein M, Siegler E, Yoffe N, Zimmer EZ. Prenatal diagnosis of ventricular septal defect and overriding aorta at 14 weeks' gestation, using transvaginal sonography. Prenat Diagn 1990; 10(11): 697-702.
[http://dx.doi.org/10.1002/pd.1970101103] [PMID: 2284272]

[76]   Bronshtein M, Zimmer EZ, Gerlis LM, Lorber A, Drugan A. Early ultrasound diagnosis of fetal congenital heart defects in high-risk and low-risk pregnancies. Obstet Gynecol 1993; 82(2): 225-9.
[PMID: 8336869]

[77]   D'Ottavio G, Mandruzzato G, Meir YJ, *et al.* Comparisons of first and second trimester screening for fetal anomalies. Ann N Y Acad Sci 1998; 847: 200-9.
[http://dx.doi.org/10.1111/j.1749-6632.1998.tb08941.x] [PMID: 9668713]

[78]   Hafner E, Scholler J, Schuchter K, Sterniste W, Philipp K. Detection of fetal congenital heart disease in a low-risk population. Prenat Diagn 1998; 18(8): 808-15.
[http://dx.doi.org/10.1002/(SICI)1097-0223(199808)18:8<808::AID-PD359>3.0.CO;2-K]   [PMID: 9742568]

[79]   Rustico MA, Benettoni A, D'Ottavio G, *et al.* Early screening for fetal cardiac anomalies by transvaginal echocardiography in an unselected population: the role of operator experience. Ultrasound Obstet Gynecol 2000; 16(7): 614-9.
[http://dx.doi.org/10.1046/j.1469-0705.2000.00291.x] [PMID: 11169366]

[80]   Mavrides E, Cobian-Sanchez F, Tekay A, *et al.* Limitations of using first-trimester nuchal translucency measurement in routine screening for major congenital heart defects. Ultrasound Obstet Gynecol 2001; 17(2): 106-10.
[http://dx.doi.org/10.1046/j.1469-0705.2001.00342.x] [PMID: 11251916]

[81]   Michailidis GD, Economides DL. Nuchal translucency measurement and pregnancy outcome in karyotypically normal fetuses. Ultrasound Obstet Gynecol 2001; 17(2): 102-5.
[http://dx.doi.org/10.1046/j.1469-0705.2001.00341.x] [PMID: 11251915]

[82]   Carvalho MH, Brizot ML, Lopes LM, Chiba CH, Miyadahira S, Zugaib M. Detection of fetal structural abnormalities at the 11-14 week ultrasound scan. Prenat Diagn 2002; 22(1): 1-4.
[http://dx.doi.org/10.1002/pd.200] [PMID: 11810640]

[83]   Taipale P, Ammälä M, Salonen R, Hiilesmaa V. Two-stage ultrasonography in screening for fetal anomalies at 13-14 and 18-22 weeks of gestation. Acta Obstet Gynecol Scand 2004; 83(12): 1141-6.
[http://dx.doi.org/10.1111/j.0001-6349.2004.00453.x] [PMID: 15548146]

[84]   Chen M, Lam YH, Lee CP, Tang MH. Ultrasound screening of fetal structural abnormalities at 12 to 14 weeks in Hong Kong. Prenat Diagn 2004; 24(2): 92-7.
[http://dx.doi.org/10.1002/pd.798] [PMID: 14974113]

[85]   Becker R, Wegner RD. Detailed screening for fetal anomalies and cardiac defects at the 11-13-week scan. Ultrasound Obstet Gynecol 2006; 27(6): 613-8.
[http://dx.doi.org/10.1002/uog.2709] [PMID: 16570262]

[86]   Westin M, Saltvedt S, Bergman G, *et al.* Routine ultrasound examination at 12 or 18 gestational weeks for prenatal detection of major congenital heart malformations? A randomised controlled trial comprising 36,299 fetuses. BJOG 2006; 113(6): 675-82.
[http://dx.doi.org/10.1111/j.1471-0528.2006.00951.x] [PMID: 16709210]

[87]   McAuliffe FM, Fong KW, Toi A, Chitayat D, Keating S, Johnson JA. Ultrasound detection of fetal anomalies in conjunction with first-trimester nuchal translucency screening: a feasibility study. Am J Obstet Gynecol 2005; 193(3 Pt 2): 1260-5.
[http://dx.doi.org/10.1016/j.ajog.2005.06.075] [PMID: 16157148]

[88]   Souka AP, Pilalis A, Kavalakis I, *et al.* Screening for major structural abnormalities at the 11- to 14-week ultrasound scan. Am J Obstet Gynecol 2006; 194(2): 393-6.

[http://dx.doi.org/10.1016/j.ajog.2005.08.032] [PMID: 16458635]

[89]   Cedergren M, Selbing A. Detection of fetal structural abnormalities by an 11-14-week ultrasound dating scan in an unselected Swedish population. Acta Obstet Gynecol Scand 2006; 85(8): 912-5.
[http://dx.doi.org/10.1080/00016340500448438] [PMID: 16862467]

[90]   Dane B, Dane C, Sivri D, Kiray M, Cetin A, Yayla M. Ultrasound screening for fetal major abnormalities at 11-14 weeks. Acta Obstet Gynecol Scand 2007; 86(6): 666-70.
[http://dx.doi.org/10.1080/00016340701253405] [PMID: 17520396]

[91]   Lombardi CM, Bellotti M, Fesslova V, Cappellini A. Fetal echocardiography at the time of the nuchal translucency scan. Ultrasound Obstet Gynecol 2007; 29(3): 249-57.
[http://dx.doi.org/10.1002/uog.3948] [PMID: 17318942]

[92]   Oztekin O, Oztekin D, Tinar S, Adibelli Z. Ultrasonographic diagnosis of fetal structural abnormalities in prenatal screening at 11-14 weeks. Diagn Interv Radiol 2009; 15(3): 221-5.
[PMID: 19728272]

[93]   Ebrashy A, El Kateb A, Momtaz M, et al. 13-14-week fetal anatomy scan: a 5-year prospective study. Ultrasound Obstet Gynecol 2010; 35(3): 292-6.
[http://dx.doi.org/10.1002/uog.7444] [PMID: 20205205]

[94]   Abu-Rustum RS, Daou L, Abu-Rustum SE. Role of ultrasonography in early gestation in the diagnosis of congenital heart defects. J Ultrasound Med 2010; 29(5): 817-21.
[http://dx.doi.org/10.7863/jum.2010.29.5.817] [PMID: 20427794]

[95]   Hartge DR, Weichert J, Krapp M, Germer U, Gembruch U, Axt-Fliedner R. Results of early foetal echocardiography and cumulative detection rate of congenital heart disease. Cardiol Young 2011; 21(5): 505-17.
[http://dx.doi.org/10.1017/S1047951111000345] [PMID: 21733344]

[96]   Volpe P, Ubaldo P, Volpe N, et al. Fetal cardiac evaluation at 11-14 weeks by experienced obstetricians in a low-risk population. Prenat Diagn 2011; 31(11): 1054-61.
[http://dx.doi.org/10.1002/pd.2831] [PMID: 21800333]

[97]   Jakobsen TR, Søgaard K, Tabor A. Implications of a first trimester Down syndrome screening program on timing of malformation detection. Acta Obstet Gynecol Scand 2011; 90(7): 728-36.
[http://dx.doi.org/10.1111/j.1600-0412.2011.01156.x] [PMID: 21504413]

[98]   Syngelaki A, Chelemen T, Dagklis T, Allan L, Nicolaides KH. Challenges in the diagnosis of fetal non-chromosomal abnormalities at 11-13 weeks. Prenat Diagn 2011; 31(1): 90-102.
[http://dx.doi.org/10.1002/pd.2642] [PMID: 21210483]

[99]   Eleftheriades M, Tsapakis E, Sotiriadis A, Manolakos E, Hassiakos D, Botsis D. Detection of congenital heart defects throughout pregnancy; impact of first trimester ultrasound screening for cardiac abnormalities. J Matern Fetal Neonatal Med 2012; 25(12): 2546-50.
[http://dx.doi.org/10.3109/14767058.2012.703716] [PMID: 22712625]

[100]   Grande M, Arigita M, Borobio V, Jimenez JM, Fernandez S, Borrell A. First-trimester detection of structural abnormalities and the role of aneuploidy markers. Ultrasound Obstet Gynecol 2012; 39(2): 157-63.
[http://dx.doi.org/10.1002/uog.10070] [PMID: 21845742]

[101]   Becker R, Schmitz L, Kilavuz S, Stumm M, Wegner RD, Bittner U. 'Normal' nuchal translucency: a justification to refrain from detailed scan? Analysis of 6858 cases with special reference to ethical aspects. Prenat Diagn 2012; 32(6): 550-6.
[http://dx.doi.org/10.1002/pd.3854] [PMID: 22517407]

[102]   Pilalis A, Basagiannis C, Eleftheriades M, et al. Evaluation of a two-step ultrasound examination protocol for the detection of major fetal structural defects. J Matern Fetal Neonatal Med 2012; 25(9): 1814-7.
[http://dx.doi.org/10.3109/14767058.2012.664199] [PMID: 22348739]

[103] Iliescu D, Tudorache S, Comanescu A, *et al.* Improved detection rate of structural abnormalities in the first trimester using an extended examination protocol. Ultrasound Obstet Gynecol 2013; 42(3): 300-9.
[http://dx.doi.org/10.1002/uog.12489] [PMID: 23595897]

[104] Gembruch U, Knöpfle G, Bald R, Hansmann M. Early diagnosis of fetal congenital heart disease by transvaginal echocardiography. Ultrasound Obstet Gynecol 1993; 3(5): 310-7.
[http://dx.doi.org/10.1046/j.1469-0705.1993.03050310.x] [PMID: 12797253]

[105] Carvalho JS, Moscoso G, Ville Y. First-trimester transabdominal fetal echocardiography. Lancet 1998; 351(9108): 1023-7.
[http://dx.doi.org/10.1016/S0140-6736(97)08406-7] [PMID: 9546509]

[106] Zosmer N, Souter VL, Chan CS, Huggon IC, Nicolaides KH. Early diagnosis of major cardiac defects in chromosomally normal fetuses with increased nuchal translucency. Br J Obstet Gynaecol 1999; 106(8): 829-33.
[http://dx.doi.org/10.1111/j.1471-0528.1999.tb08405.x] [PMID: 10453834]

[107] Simpsom JM, Jones A, Callaghan N, Sharland GK. Accuracy and limitations of transabdominal fetal echocardiography at 12-15 weeks of gestation in a population at high risk for congenital heart disease. BJOG 2000; 107(12): 1492-7.
[http://dx.doi.org/10.1111/j.1471-0528.2000.tb11673.x] [PMID: 11192105]

[108] Comas Gabriel C, Galindo A, Martínez JM, *et al.* Early prenatal diagnosis of major cardiac anomalies in a high-risk population. Prenat Diagn 2002; 22(7): 586-93.
[http://dx.doi.org/10.1002/pd.372] [PMID: 12124694]

[109] Haak MC, Bartelings MM, Gittenberger-De Groot AC, Van Vugt JM. Cardiac malformations in first-trimester fetuses with increased nuchal translucency: ultrasound diagnosis and postmortem morphology. Ultrasound Obstet Gynecol 2002; 20(1): 14-21.
[http://dx.doi.org/10.1046/j.1469-0705.2002.00739.x] [PMID: 12100412]

[110] Lopes LM, Brizot ML, Lopes MA, Ayello VD, Schultz R, Zugaib M. Structural and functional cardiac abnormalities identified prior to 16 weeks' gestation in fetuses with increased nuchal translucency. Ultrasound Obstet Gynecol 2003; 22(5): 470-8.
[http://dx.doi.org/10.1002/uog.905] [PMID: 14618659]

[111] McAuliffe FM, Trines J, Nield LE, Chitayat D, Jaeggi E, Hornberger LK. Early fetal echocardiography--a reliable prenatal diagnosis tool. Am J Obstet Gynecol 2005; 193(3 Pt 2): 1253-9.
[http://dx.doi.org/10.1016/j.ajog.2005.05.086] [PMID: 16157147]

[112] Galindo A, Comas C, Martínez JM, *et al.* Cardiac defects in chromosomally normal fetuses with increased nuchal translucency at 10-14 weeks of gestation. J Matern Fetal Neonatal Med 2003; 13(3): 163-70.
[PMID: 12820838]

[113] Weiner Z, Weizman B, Beloosesky R, Goldstein I, Bombard A. Fetal cardiac scanning performed immediately following an abnormal nuchal translucency examination. Prenat Diagn 2008; 28(10): 934-8.
[http://dx.doi.org/10.1002/pd.2071] [PMID: 18702103]

[114] Bellotti M, Fesslova V, De Gasperi C, *et al.* Reliability of the first-trimester cardiac scan by ultrasound-trained obstetricians with high-frequency transabdominal probes in fetuses with increased nuchal translucency. Ultrasound Obstet Gynecol 2010; 36(3): 272-8.
[http://dx.doi.org/10.1002/uog.7685] [PMID: 20499407]

[115] Mirza FG, Bauer ST, Williams IA, Simpson LL. Early fetal echocardiography: ready for prime time? Am J Perinatol 2012; 29(4): 313-8.
[http://dx.doi.org/10.1055/s-0031-1295640] [PMID: 22143968]

[116] Mogra R, Saaid R, Kesby G, Hayward J, Malkoun J, Hyett J. Early fetal echocardiography: Experience of a tertiary diagnostic service. Aust N Z J Obstet Gynaecol 2015; 55(6): 552-8.

[http://dx.doi.org/10.1111/ajo.12379] [PMID: 26223960]

[117] Zidere V, Bellsham-Revell H, Persico N, Allan LD. Comparison of echocardiographic findings in fetuses at less than 15 weeks' gestation with later cardiac evaluation. Ultrasound Obstet Gynecol 2013; 42(6): 679-86.
[http://dx.doi.org/10.1002/uog.12517] [PMID: 23703918]

[118] Rasiah SV, Publicover M, Ewer AK, Khan KS, Kilby MD, Zamora J. A systematic review of the accuracy of first-trimester ultrasound examination for detecting major congenital heart disease. Ultrasound Obstet Gynecol 2006; 28(1): 110-6.
[http://dx.doi.org/10.1002/uog.2803] [PMID: 16795132]

[119] Allan LD, Santos R, Pexieder T. Anatomical and echocardiographic correlates of normal cardiac morphology in the late first trimester fetus. Heart 1997; 77(1): 68-72.
[http://dx.doi.org/10.1136/hrt.77.1.68] [PMID: 9038698]

[120] Dolkart LA, Reimers FT. Transvaginal fetal echocardiography in early pregnancy: normative data. Am J Obstet Gynecol 1991; 165(3): 688-91.
[http://dx.doi.org/10.1016/0002-9378(91)90310-N] [PMID: 1892198]

[121] Achiron R, Weissman A, Rotstein Z, Lipitz S, Mashiach S, Hegesh J. Transvaginal echocardiographic examination of the fetal heart between 13 and 15 weeks' gestation in a low-risk population. J Ultrasound Med 1994; 13(10): 783-9.
[http://dx.doi.org/10.7863/jum.1994.13.10.783] [PMID: 7823340]

[122] Johnson P, Sharland G, Maxwell D, Allan L. The role of transvaginal sonography in the early detection of congenital heart disease. Ultrasound Obstet Gynecol 1992; 2(4): 248-51.
[http://dx.doi.org/10.1046/j.1469-0705.1992.02040248.x] [PMID: 12796949]

[123] Gembruch U, Shi C, Smrcek JM. Biometry of the fetal heart between 10 and 17 weeks of gestation. Fetal Diagn Ther 2000; 15(1): 20-31.
[http://dx.doi.org/10.1159/000020970] [PMID: 10705210]

[124] Huggon IC, Ghi T, Cook AC, Zosmer N, Allan LD, Nicolaides KH. Fetal cardiac abnormalities identified prior to 14 weeks' gestation. Ultrasound Obstet Gynecol 2002; 20(1): 22-9.
[http://dx.doi.org/10.1046/j.1469-0705.2002.00733.x] [PMID: 12100413]

[125] Smrcek JM, Gembruch U, Krokowski M, *et al.* The evaluation of cardiac biometry in major cardiac defects detected in early pregnancy. Arch Gynecol Obstet 2003; 268(2): 94-101.
[http://dx.doi.org/10.1007/s00404-002-0358-8] [PMID: 12768297]

[126] Wiechec M, Knafel A, Nocun A. Prenatal detection of congenital heart defects at the 11- to 13-week scan using a simple color Doppler protocol including the 4-chamber and 3-vessel and trachea views. J Ultrasound Med 2015; 34(4): 585-94.
[http://dx.doi.org/10.7863/ultra.34.4.585] [PMID: 25792573]

[127] Quarello E, Lafouge A, Fries N, Salomon LJ. Basic heart examination: feasibility study of first-trimester systematic simplified fetal echocardiography. Ultrasound Obstet Gynecol 2017; 49(2): 224-30.
[http://dx.doi.org/10.1002/uog.15866] [PMID: 26799640]

[128] De Robertis V, Rembouskos G, Fanelli T, Volpe G, Muto B, Volpe P. The three-vessel and trachea view (3VTV) in the first trimester of pregnancy: an additional tool in screening for congenital heart defects (CHD) in an unselected population. Prenat Diagn 2017; 37(7): 693-8.
[http://dx.doi.org/10.1002/pd.5067] [PMID: 28505706]

[129] Tegnander E, Eik-Nes SH. The examiner's ultrasound experience has a significant impact on the detection rate of congenital heart defects at the second-trimester fetal examination. Ultrasound Obstet Gynecol 2006; 28(1): 8-14.
[http://dx.doi.org/10.1002/uog.2804] [PMID: 16736449]

[130] Abu-Rustum RS, Ziade MF, Abu-Rustum SE. Learning curve and factors influencing the feasibility of

performing fetal echocardiography at the time of the first-trimester scan. J Ultrasound Med 2011; 30(5): 695-700.
[http://dx.doi.org/10.7863/jum.2011.30.5.695] [PMID: 21527618]

[131] Nemescu D, Onofriescu M. Factors affecting the feasibility of routine first-trimester fetal echocardiography. J Ultrasound Med 2015; 34(1): 161-6.
[http://dx.doi.org/10.7863/ultra.34.1.161] [PMID: 25542952]

[132] Allan L. Technique of fetal echocardiography. Pediatr Cardiol 2004; 25(3): 223-33.
[http://dx.doi.org/10.1007/s00246-003-0588-y] [PMID: 15360115]

[133] Yoo SJ, Lee YH, Cho KS, Kim DY. Sequential segmental approach to fetal congenital heart disease. Cardiol Young 1999; 9(4): 430-44.
[http://dx.doi.org/10.1017/S1047951100005266] [PMID: 10476836]

CHAPTER 7

Normal Fetal Cardiac Rhythm and Arrhythmias

Ganesh Acharya[1,2,3,*] and **Agata Wloch**[4]

[1] *Division of Obstetrics and Gynecology, Department of Clinical Science, Intervention and Technology, Karolinska Institutet, Stockholm, Sweden*

[2] *Center for Fetal Medicine, Karolinska University Hospital, Stockholm, Sweden*

[3] *Women's Health and Perinatology Research Group, Department of Clinical Medicine, UiT-The Artic University of Norway, Tromsø, Norway*

[4] *Department of Obstetrics and Gynecology, Woman's Health Chair, Medical University of Silesia, Katowice, Poland*

Abstract: Fetal arrhythmias are rare but they are an important avoidable cause of perinatal mortality. Timely diagnosis is therefore crucial, as treatment can be life saving. Careful evaluation of cardiac structure and function using different echocardiographic modalities can exclude structural cardiac anomalies as well as provide accurate information about the atrial and ventricular contraction rates, their relationship, conduction pattern and hemodynamic consequences of arrhythmia. Although observation and reassurance will suffice in a substantial proportion of pregnancies complicated by fetal arrhythmia, some will require intrauterine therapy or early delivery followed by postnatal treatment to prevent heart failure and fetal/neonatal demise. Fortunately, most common fetal arrhythmias are few of those conditions that can be managed successfully *in utero* with good results. In this chapter, we describe the normal and abnormal fetal cardiac rhythms, their diagnosis and prenatal management.

Keywords: Arrhythmia, Bradycardia, Fetal cardiology, Fetal cardiac rhythm, Fetal echocardiography, Fetal heart, Tachycardia.

INTRODUCTION

There are substantial differences between the adult and fetal heart both with regard to its structure and function [1]. Fetal cardiovascular system undergoes continuous changes throughout the gestation as it matures. Being aware of these physiological changes is important to be able to diagnose and manage disturbances in fetal heart rate and rhythm *in utero*.

* **Corresponding author Ganesh Acharya:** Department of Clinical Science, Intervention and Technology, Division of Obstetrics and Gynecology, Karolinska Institutet, Stockholm, Sweden; E-mail: ganesh.acharya@ki.se

Edward Araujo Júnior, Nathalie Jeanne M. Bravo-Valenzuela and Alberto Borges Peixoto (Eds.)

NORMAL FETAL CARDIAC RHYTHM AND HEART RATE

After 5 weeks of gestation (postmenstrual age), the heart rhythm is generally regular and the ventricular contraction is normally preceded by an atrial contraction. The basal fetal heart rate (FHR) varies with gestation. The normal embryonic heart rate ranges between 110-180 beats per minute (bpm) with a mean of approximately 115 bpm at 6 weeks and 170 bpm at 10 weeks of gestation [2 - 7]. In the fetal period, the heart rate decreases with advancing gestation. Between 11^{+0}-13^{+6} weeks, the FHR decreases significantly with increasing crown-rump length (CRL) and ranges between 144 and 176 bpm [8].

In the second and third trimester, when the conduction system is relatively mature, the normal range for FHR is considered to be 110 to 160 bpm. Von Steinburg *et al.* [9] analysed baseline FHR from 78 852 carditocographic (CTG) recordings obtained between 24 and 42 weeks of gestation confirming the normal range to be between 120 to 160 bpm with a decreasing trend as gestation advances.

FHR is relatively easy to measure using a variety of techniques. In clinical practice, auscultation using a stethoscope, and handheld continuous-wave (CW) Doppler device or CTG recording are most commonly used. External electrocardiogram (ECG) recording has been shown to be feasible in the third trimester of pregnancy to evaluate fetal cardiac time intervals [10 - 13]. External ECG has also been occasionally used for home fetal monitoring and internal ECG electrode attached to the fetal scalp is frequently used for intrapartum FHR monitoring. Different components of fetal cardiac cycle can be identified, and their sequence and duration can be measured using some of these modalities that allow delineating electrical (ECG), mechanical (M-mode echocardiography and tissue Doppler) or hemodynamic (spectral pulsed-wave Doppler) events within the cardiac cycle. This allows confirmation of normal fetal cardiac rhythm and rate as well as screening and diagnosis of arrhythmias antenatally.

METHODS OF DETECTING FETAL ARRHYTHMIAS

Fetal arrhythmias are generally detected by the midwives and obstetricians when they listen to the fetal heart sounds during the routine antenatal care, or by ultrasonographers during prenatal ultrasound scanning. An abnormal fetal heart rate or irregular rhythm usually leads to referral to a fetal medicine specialist or a perinatal cardiologist for fetal echocardiography. However, an initial ultrasound evaluation should be able to differentiate the benign rhythm disturbances from sustained significant arrhythmias that requires accurate diagnosis and expert management.

CTG is a widely used method for FHR monitoring both antenatally and during labor. However, it does not allow accurate diagnosis of arrhythmias. CTG monitoring functions poorly with FHR >200 bpm and <60 bpm and in cases with irregular fetal heart rhythm. Incorrect interpretation of CTG in fetuses with arrhythmias can lead to unnecessary cesarean section and premature delivery.

The postnatal diagnosis of cardiac rhythm disturbances is based on a 12-lead ECG. Noninvasive fetal ECG obtained through maternal abdomen allows evaluation of P-waves and QRS complexes during stable cardiac rhythm [14]. However, it but does not have the same diagnostic capacity as the conventional neonatal ECG as it is based on signal averaging and does not allow analysis of each cardiac cycle separately. Fetal magnetocardiography (fMCG) is another noninvasive technique that has been shown to be useful in the assessment of fetal cardiac electrophysiology allowing the analysis of the P-wave, QRS complex, T-wave and measurement of the QT-interval. fMCG is especially useful for elucidating the mechanisms of tachyarrhythmias and identifying long-QT syndrome [15 - 17], but it is expensive, cumbersome, and has limited availability. Therefore, fetal echocardiography continues to be the main diagnostic tool for assessing cardiac arrhythmias prenatally, and the diagnostic basis is visualization of the mechanical or hemodyamic events as the surrogates of electrical activity.

The standard assessment of the fetus with arrhythmia in a referral center includes:

a. A detailed fetal ultrasonography to assess fetal size/growth (biometry), placental location and structure, amniotic fluid volume and fetal anatomy.
b. Doppler ultrasonography to access blood flow in the umbilical artery (UA), middle cerebral artery (MCA), umbilical vein (UV), and ductus venosus (DV).
c. Echocardiography to evaluate fetal cardiac rate, rhythm, structure and function.

Fetal arrhythmias can be associated with structural cardiac defects, and evaluation of fetal visceral situs and cardiac structure is important to exclude major abnormalities such as, left or right atrial isomerism, congenitally corrected transposition of great arteries, atrioventricular septal defect *etc.* Additionally, it is important to evaluate fetal cardiac function looking for signs of heart failure. Most importantly, evaluation should include whether the cardiac rhythm is regular or irregular, followed by separate measurements of atrial and ventricular rates, assessment of atrioventricular sequence and timing of atrial and ventricular contractions and measurement of atrioventricular (AV) and ventriculo-atrial (VA) time intervals.

Although a majority of fetal arrhythmias are benign, they can lead to fetal cardiac dysfunction, heart failure, hydrops and fetal demise. Their accurate timely diagnosis followed by appropriate management can be life saving.

Motion Mode (M-mode) Echocardiography

M-mode has excellent temporal resolution and this technique allows visualization of the timing of motion of various parts of the fetal myocardium. By placing the M-mode sampling line across the atrial and ventricular walls, atrial and ventricular contractions can be recorded simultaneously and the sequence of contractions and their relationship to each other can be assessed [18, 19] (Fig. **1**). It is possible to measure the atrial and ventricular rates, AV and VA intervals, and AV conduction using M-mode [20, 21] (Fig. **2**).

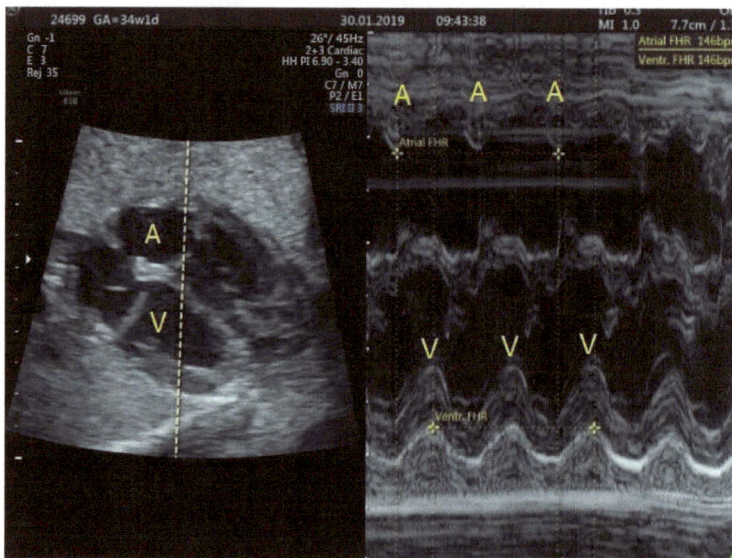

Fig. (1). M-mode ultrasound technique in which the beam is directed through the right atrium (**A**) and left ventricle (**V**) showing the 1:1 mechanical atrial and ventricular relationship (**A**) atrial wall movement (= atrial contraction); (**V**) ventricular wall movement (=ventricular contraction).

Use of color M-mode can further enhance the ability to identify direction of cardiac wall motion and anatomical M-mode can help more accurate placement of the M-mode cursor [22]. However, M-mode assessment may be difficult in some occasions, such as cursor placement may be difficult during the first trimester due to poor resolution of the two-dimensional images of cardiac chambers, or when visualization is poor due to unfavorable fetal position. It may be difficult to record and identify myocardial contractions in hydropic fetuses with cardiac contractile dysfunction.

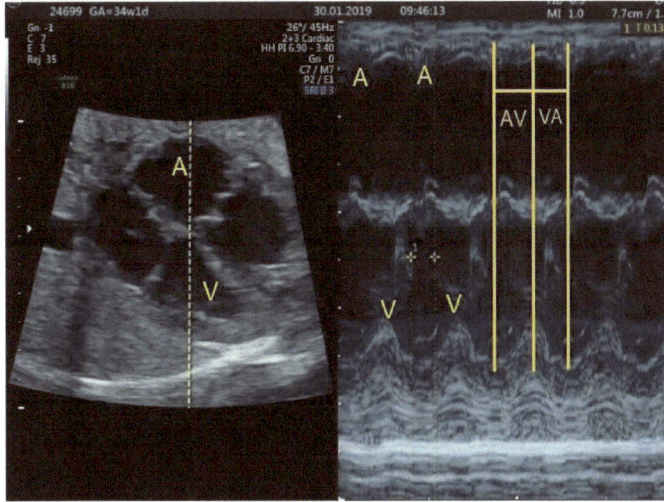

Fig. (2). M-mode ultrasound recording showing how to measure the AV and VA time intervals using atrial and ventricular wall motions. (**A**) atrial wall movement (=atrial contraction); (**V**) ventricular wall movement (=ventricular contraction); AV: atrioventricular time interval; VA: ventriculoatrial time interval.

Pulsed-wave (PW) Doppler

This technique allows simultaneous recording of blood flow during atrial and ventricular contractions from a variety of sites. Conventionally, a relatively large Doppler gate (sample volume) is placed in the ventricular inflow and outflow tracts to record the blood flow velocity waveforms simultaneously (Fig. **3**). PW-Doppler interrogation of the left ventricular inflow (mitral valve) and aortic outflow (MV-Ao Doppler), with evaluation of the relationship between the A-wave of the mitral valve inflow during atrial contraction and the aortic outflow waveform occurring during the ventricular contraction can provide essential information required to evaluate AV conduction and chronology [23]. The AV interval, which is the time between atrial and ventricular contractions, can be measured from the onset of the A-wave to the onset of the outflow ventricular wave (V-wave). The VA interval is the time from the onset of the V-wave to the onset of the A wave. The AV and VA intervals represent hemodynamic surrogates of the electrical PR and RP intervals of the ECG, respectively. These intervals are particularly important for analyzing AV conduction when assessing fetal cardiac rhythm.

However, the information is limited when atrial contraction occurs against a closed AV valve such as may occur in AV block [24]. Fouron *et al.* [25] have described the use of superior vena cava and ascending aorta (SVC-Ao) Doppler blood flow velocity waveforms obtained simultaneously to assess AV conduction (Fig. **4**). Similarly, blood flow velocity waveforms recorded simultaneously from the pulmonary artery and pulmonary vein (Fig. **5**) has also been shown to be useful for this purpose [26, 27]. With these techniques, which demonstrate the relationship between atrial contraction (A-wave of the central venous waveform characterized by very low velocity or reversal of blood flow) and ventricular contraction (characterized by forward flow in the arterial waveform), AV and VA time intervals can be defined [28]. Measurement of the time interval between atrial and ventricular systoles permits indirect assessment of cardiac AV conduction.

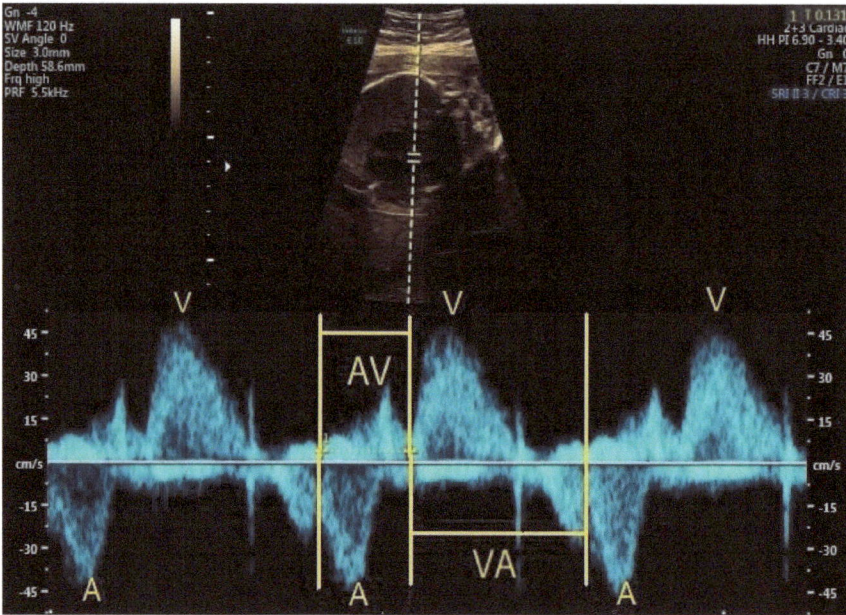

Fig. (3). Doppler assessment of fetal heart rhythm with simultaneous sampling of the left ventricular inflow (**A**: flow during atrial systole) and outflow (**V**: ventricular outflow). Doppler recording of mitral and aortic flow demonstrating how to measure the AV and VA intervals. AV: atrioventricular time interval; VA: ventriculoatrial time interval.

Tissue Doppler Imaging

Both color tissue Doppler imaging (TDI) (Fig. **6**) and spectral PW TDI (Fig. **7**) can be used to assess the cardiac wall motion with the waveforms representing mechanical events during the whole cardiac cycle [29].

TDI-derived AV interval measured as the time interval from atrial contraction (A′-wave) to isovolumic contraction velocity (ICV) rather than to the beginning myocardial systolic (S′-velocity) has been shown to track ECG derived PR interval more closely compared to PW Doppler derived AV intervals that include isovolumic contraction time (ICT) in the measurement of AV interval [10].

However, it may not always be easy to identify isovolumic contraction velocity (especially when using color TDI).

TDI is a reliable diagnostic tool for accurate diagnosis of the arrhythmias [30]. AV conduction time as well as other cardiac cycle time intervals can be measured using TDI techniques [10, 29, 30].

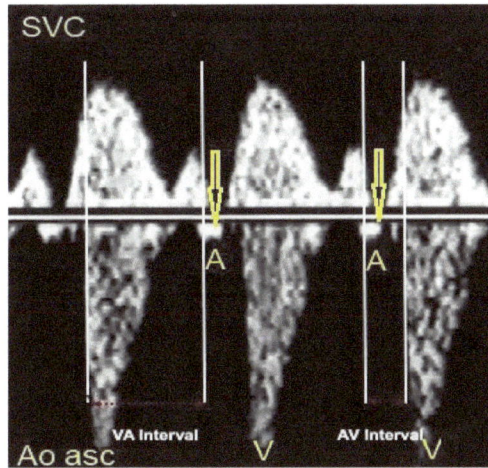

Fig. (4). Simultaneous Doppler recording of SVC (superior vena cava) and aortic (Ao asc - ascending aorta) flow demonstrating how to measure the AV and VA intervals (analogous to the electrical PR and RP intervals, respectively recorded by an ECG). AV: atrioventricular time interval; VA: ventriculoatrial time interval. A: reversed A-wave in SCV waveform during atrial contraction (arrows). V: forward flow in the ascending aorta during ventricular contraction. Note: Doppler waveforms are inverted.

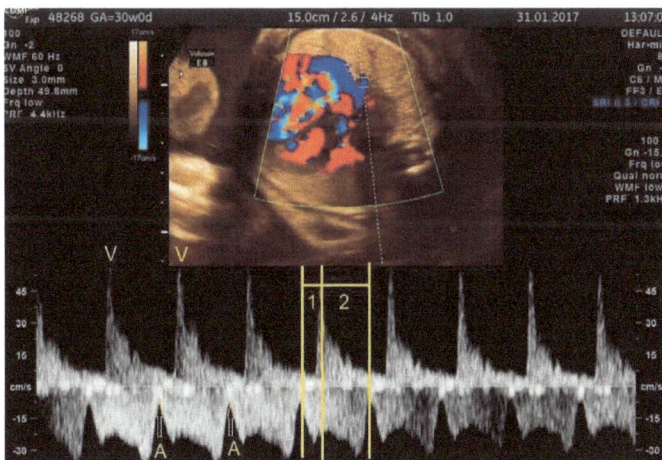

Fig. (5). Simultaneous Doppler recording of pulmonary artery and pulmonary vein flow showing how to measure the AV and VA intervals. A: atrial contraction; V: ventricular contraction; AV: atrioventricular time interval; VA: ventriculoatrial time interval.

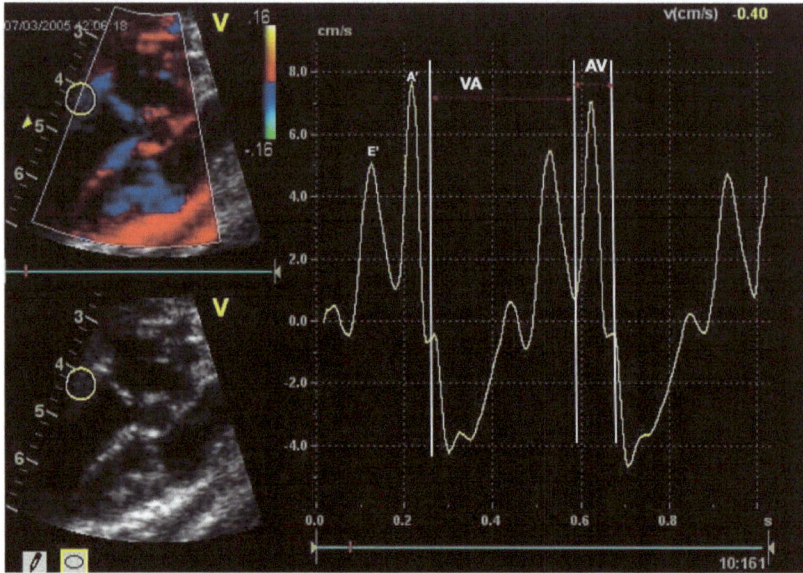

Fig. (6). Measurement of AV and VA time intervals using color tissue Doppler imaging. AV: atrioventricular time interval; VA: ventriculoatrial time interval; E′: myocardial velocity during early filling of ventricle; A: myocardial velocity during atrial contraction phase of ventricular filling.

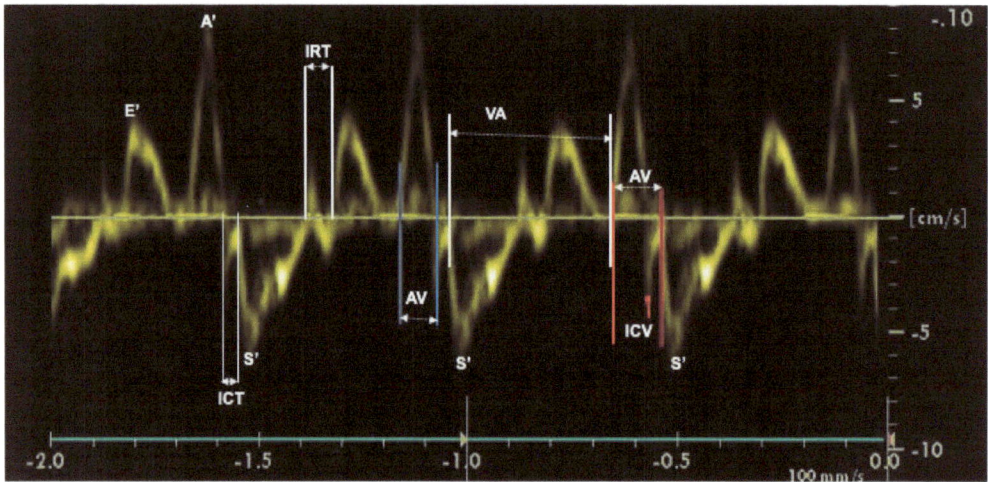

Fig. (7). Measurement of AV and VA time intervals using spectral Pulses-wave (PW) tissue Doppler imaging. AV: atrioventricular time interval ; VA: ventriculoatrial time interval; E′: myocardial velocity during early filling of ventricle; A′: myocardial velocity during atrial contraction phase of ventricular filling. ICT: isovolumic contraction time; ICV: isovolumic contraction velocity; S′: systolic myocardial velocity. Note: AV interval measured as the time between the start of A′ velocity waveform to the beginning of ICV (between two blue lines) is shorter than AV interval measured as the time between the start of A′ velocity to the beginning of S′ velocity (between two red lines). This methodological difference is important to consider when making a diagnosis and appropriate references should be used.

NORMAL REFERENCE RANGES FOR CARDIAC TIME INTERVALS

Reference ranges for fetal cardiac cycle time intervals are available based on ECG [31] and magnetocardiography [32]. Normograms for AV interval based on simultaneous interrogation of a variety of arterial and central venous blood flow waveforms using PW Doppler also have been established and their positive association with gestational age has been confirmed [28, 33 - 35].

TDI derived reference values for cardiac time intervals are available and shown to reflect ECG derived time intervals [10]. However, there is a scarcity of reference ranges based on adequate sample size and longitudinal observations. Furthermore, the focus of most studies have been AV (PR) interval rather than VA (RP) interval. Mossiman *et al.* reported the median [IQR] AV time of 122 [112-130], VA time of 298 [283-317] and AV:VA ratio of 0.40 [0.37-0.44] by MV-Ao Doppler technique, and 129 [118-140], 293 [277-311], 0.44 [0.38-0.49], respectively by TDI technique [35].

A recently published systematic review showed that noninvasive fetal ECG derived average PR interval varies between 93 and 135 ms [36]. The PR interval measured by ECG appears to be the shortest followed by that measured by SVC-Ao Doppler, MV-Ao Doppler, pulmonary artery-vein Doppler and TDI, respectively.

Cut-off value for diagnosing abnormal AV conduction in the fetuses remains controversial. However, Doppler derived fetal PR interval (AV interval) is generally below 145 ms (95th percentile), and AV intervals >150 ms measured are considered prolonged, consistent with first-degree AV block [37]. Doppler derived AV interval is significantly influenced by gestational age (GA) and FHR. The AV interval increases with advancing gestational age, but decreases with increasing FHR [28].

FETAL ARRHYTHMIAS

The real incidence of fetal arrhythmia is unknown, but it is generally accepted that 1%-3% of pregnancies develop cardiac rhythm disturbances. Fortunately, the vast majority of arrhythmias are transient and benign with no major hemodynamic consequences. These are mostly atrial ectopic beats and transient fetal sinus bradycardia observed between 16-24 weeks of pregnancy. However, in approximately 10% of pregnancies complicated by fetal rhythm disturbances, the arrhythmia may be potentially life threatening [15, 38, 39]. Recently, the problem of "hidden" or "silent" arrhythmias has been highlighted and it has been suggested to be responsible for up to 10% of unexplained fetal demise [40]. This is usually due to cardiac channelopathies that are very difficult to diagnose *in utero*.

Common Types of Fetal Arrhythmias, their Diagnosis and Management

Irregular Fetal Cardiac Rhythm

The most common forms of irregular rhythm are premature atrial contractions (PACs, atrial ectopy) and premature ventricular contractions (PVCs, ventricular ectopy). They are reported to occur in up to 3% of all pregnancies [41].

PACs usually are detected in the late second trimester or the third trimester of pregnancy. PACs are much more common than PVCs [39] with atrial ectopic beats occurring in up to 90% cases. PACs originate from the atria and influence the sinus node. Therefore, there is a pause in atrial activity after the premature ectopic beat and atrial rate is irregular. PACs may be conducted to the ventricle or blocked. Blocked atrial extrasystoles cause incomplete compensatory pause in ventricular contraction. In general, PACs are benign and isolated, although a small proportion (approximately 2%) of fetuses with atrial ectopic beats may have prolongation of PR interval which can be associated with QT syndrome, fetal/neonatal tachycardia and second degree AV block [42]. PACs may also occasionally occur in fetuses with cardiac tumors, such as rhabdomyoma [43], congenital heart defects and aneurysmal and redundant of atrial septum. The risk of fetal tachycardia with PACs is about 0.5% to 1%, the risk increases to 10% when they occur in couplets such as bigeminy or trigeminy. Blocked atrial bigeminy causes fetal bradycardia with a regular ventricular rhythm and FHR of approximately 70-90 bpm [44, 45].

PVCs originate from the ventricle, they are not conducted to the atria, and don't influence the sinus node. Therefore, a pause in atrial activity doesn't occur and the atrial contractions are regular. However, the ventricular contractions are irregular and there is a complete compensatory pause after a PVC in contrast to an incomplete compensatory pause in case of a conducted atrial PAC. No association between PVCs and SVT has been found.

Diagnosis

Fetal echocardiography using PW Doppler and M-mode technique is the best tool for diagnosing PAC and PVC. PACs can be demonstrated as irregular atrial contractions with premature atrial beats conducted or blocked with subsequently occuring compensatory pause in the ventricular activity leading to slower ventricular rate (Figs. **8** and **9**). With PVCs, the atrial contractions are regular with irregular ventricular rate due to premature ventricular contractions (Fig. **10**).

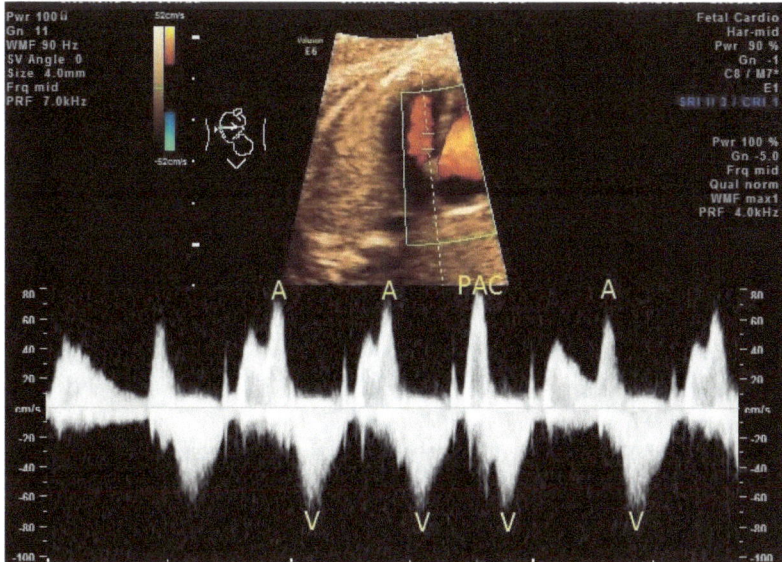

Fig. (8). Conducted premature atrial contraction (PAC). Irregular atrial rhythm (**A**) and irregular ventricular rhythm (**V**).

Management

In general, isolated PACs or PVCs have a benign course, good outcome and do not require any antiarrhythmic therapy. In the majority of cases, these arrhythmias resolve spontaneously before birth. Detailed fetal echocardiography is recommended if the irregular beats are more frequent than 1 in 5-10, persist longer than 1-2 weeks, or if the fetus develops tachy- or bradycardia. CTG monitoring is not recommended. PAC may result in small ventricular stroke volume that may not be recorded as a heartbeat by the CTG. This may lead to misinterpretation and erroneous diagnosis. In a small minority of cases with multiple extrasystoles (couplets), the risk for a sustained SVT is high. In these cases, weekly FHR auscultation by a midwife or obstetrician is recommended until arrhythmia resolves [39, 41].

Fetal Bradyarrhythmias

Brief episodes of fetal bradycardia (transient fetal decelerations) that resolve within minutes, are frequent in the second trimester, and are generally benign and have no clinical significance. Fetal sinus bradycardia is defined as a sustained FHR <110 bpm over at least a 10 min period. However, consideration should be given to the facts that FHR is gestational age-dependent and long duration of bradycardia can have adverse effect on fetal wellbeing.

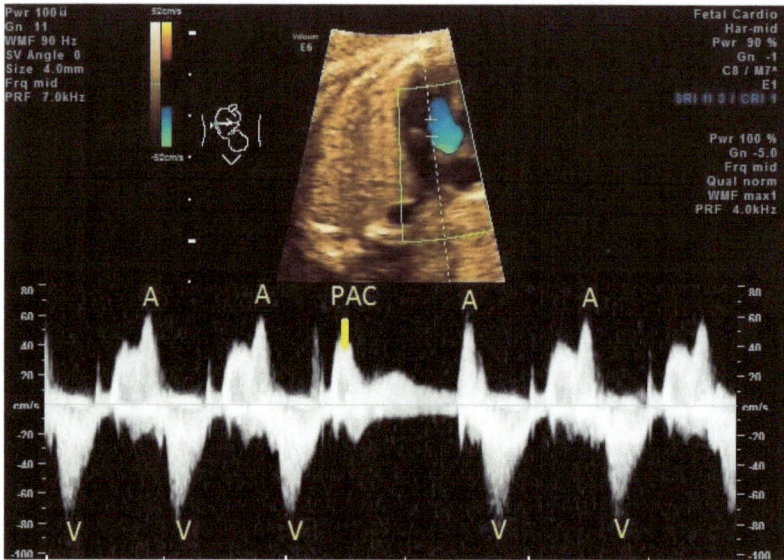

Fig. (9). Blocked premature atrial contraction (PAC) with a compensatory pause in ventricular activity (V). A: atrial contractions.

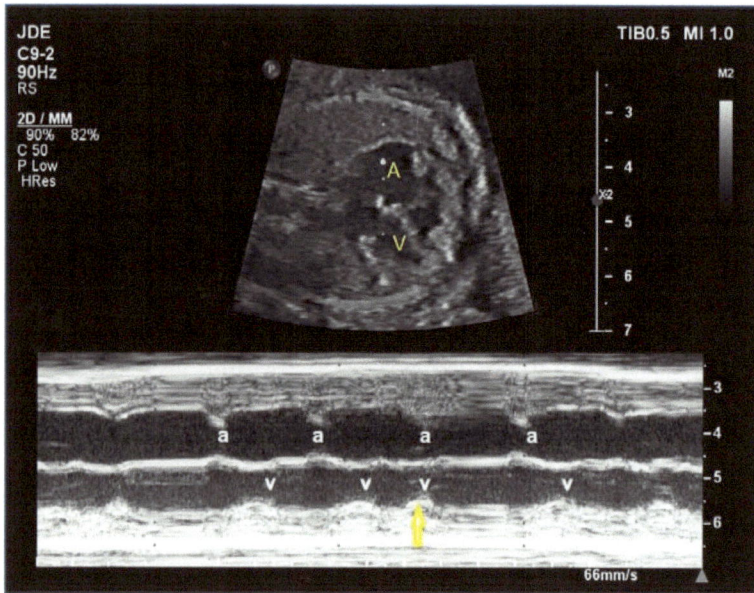

Fig. (10). Premature ventricular contraction (PVC - arrow). Regular atrial rhythm, irregular ventricular rhythm (courtesy of J. Szymkiewicz-Dangel, MD).

Persistent FHR below the third percentile can be normal, but can also be a sign of conduction disease [13]. Mitchel *et al.* analyzed the reason for referral of fetuses diagnosed as long QT group and 40% of them presented with sinus bradycardia [46 - 49]. Serra *et al.* analyzed the electronic CTG records from 4412 healthy singleton fetuses, and obtained percentiles for FHR from 25 weeks' gestation onward. On average, ventricular rates were below the fifth percentile if they were <130 bpm at 25 weeks of gestation, <120 bpm at 30 weeks gestation, or <110 bpm at term [21].

Fetal Sinus and Low-atrial Bradycardias

Persistent fetal bradycardia occurs rarely. The basic mechanisms include congenital displacement of atrial activation, acquired damage of the sinoatrial node (SA), ion channel dysfunction, and secondary suppression of the sinus node rate.

Both left and right atrial isomerism can result in bradycardia as a result of low atrial rhythm or dual sinoatrial nodes. FHR ranges between 90 and 130 bpm in these conditions. Fetal sinus node can be suppressed due to inflammation and fibrosis due to viral myocarditis, in pregnant women with anti-Ro/SSA or anti-La/SSB antibodies, in pregnancies treated with beta-blockers, sedatives or other drugs, in rare metabolic disorders (*e.g.* Pompes disease), and autonomic disorders.

Diagnosis

In fetal sinus bradycardia, echocardiography demonstrates that the atrial and ventricular contractions are equally slow and occur with a normal 1:1 AV conduction and AA intervals are constant (Fig. **11**). In low-atrial bradycardia, the PR (AV) interval is shorter (Fig. **12**).

Management

No intrauterine fetal therapy is recommended. However, neonatal ECG is recommended due to high risk of associated long-QT syndrome [11, 49], especially in cases with persistent bradycardia <110 bpm.

Fetal sinus and low-atrial bradycardias usually demonstrate FHR reactivity even in the presence of serious underlying conditions; however, this reactivity may be blunted due to a reduction in the autonomic influences [50]. Intermittent CTG monitoring can be reassuring and useful in this pathology.

Long QT Syndrome and Other Ion Channelopathies

Long QT syndrome is the most lethal cardiac rhythm disturbance occuring with normal heart rate. It can be suspected when the FHR persists at lower limits of normal rate (below third percentile) for the given gestational age. A family history of unexplained fetal/neonatal demise or sudden death in young age may provide a clue to such channelopathies.

Diagnosis

Measurement of the QTc by fetal magnetocardiography or fetal ECG is possible when the index of suspicion is high and these diagnostic modalities and expertise to interpret the findings are available. Otherwise, close observation and postnatal evaluation are recommended. When fetal sinus bradycardia was a reason for referral to a tertiary center, subsequent evaluation of heart rhythm using fetal magnetocardiography revealed long QT syndrome in 40% of cases [49].

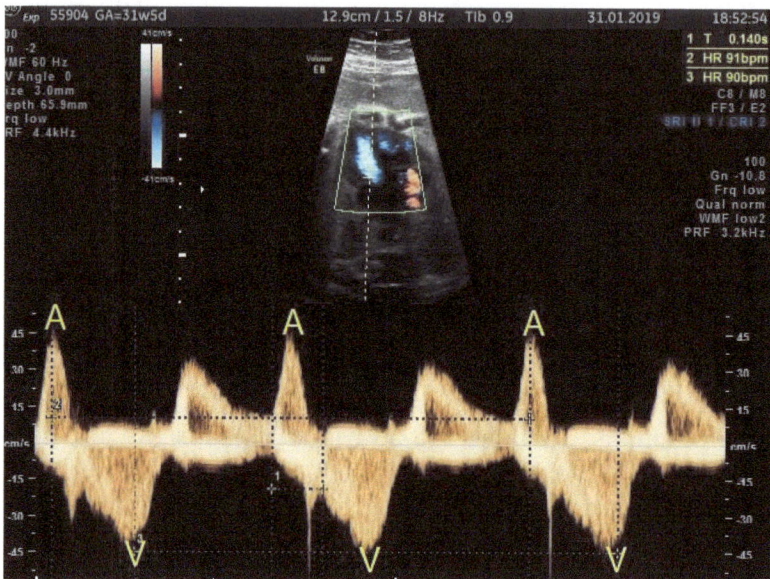

Fig. (11). Sinus bradycardia with slow regular atrial and slow regular ventricular rate. A:V conduction is 1:1. AV (mechanical PR) interval is in normal range.

Management

Prenatal treatment is not recommended for bradycardia at lower limits of normal FHR. Hypomagnesemia and hypocalcemia should be avoided, as well as the drugs that lengthen the QT interval [46].

Blocked Atrial Bigeminy

Blocked atrial bigeminy when AV conduction is 2:1, produces bradycardia in the range of 70-90 bpm.

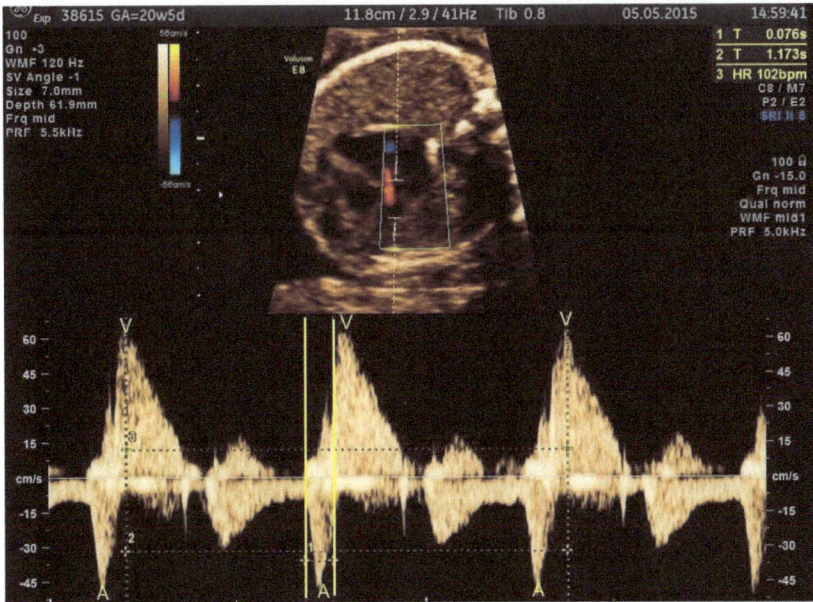

Fig. (12). Low atrial bradycardia with short AV interval (AV interval is 76 milliseconds). Slow atrial and ventricular rhythm with 1:1 AV conduction (AV: atrioventricular).

Diagnosis

Fetal echocardiography will demonstrate that every second atrial contraction is premature and is not conducted to the ventricle. There is irregular atrial rhythm in the normal range and slow regular ventricular rhythm (Fig. **13**).

Management

Weekly auscultation of FHR is recommended due to associated higher risk of SVT. CTG monitoring can also be useful as it allows longer periods of continuous FHR recording. No intrauterine treatment is needed if FHR is stable and sustained SVT does not develop.

Fetal Congenital Atrioventricular Block

The incidence of congenital atrioventricular block (AVB) is between 1 in 15,000 and 1 in 20,000 births [50]. Three types of congenital heart block (CHB) have been described based on their etiology. CHB due to congenitally malformed conduction system with complex structural cardiac defects, occurs in about 50-55% of all CHB detected in fetal life. Immune-mediated CHB associated with maternal Sjogren anti-Ro/SSA and anti-La/SSB antibodies occurs in 40% and rest of the CHB are of undetermined origin and unclear etiology.

Clinically, there are three grades of CHB: First degree (prolonged AV conduction time), second degree (incomplete AVB), and third degree (complete AVB) [22].

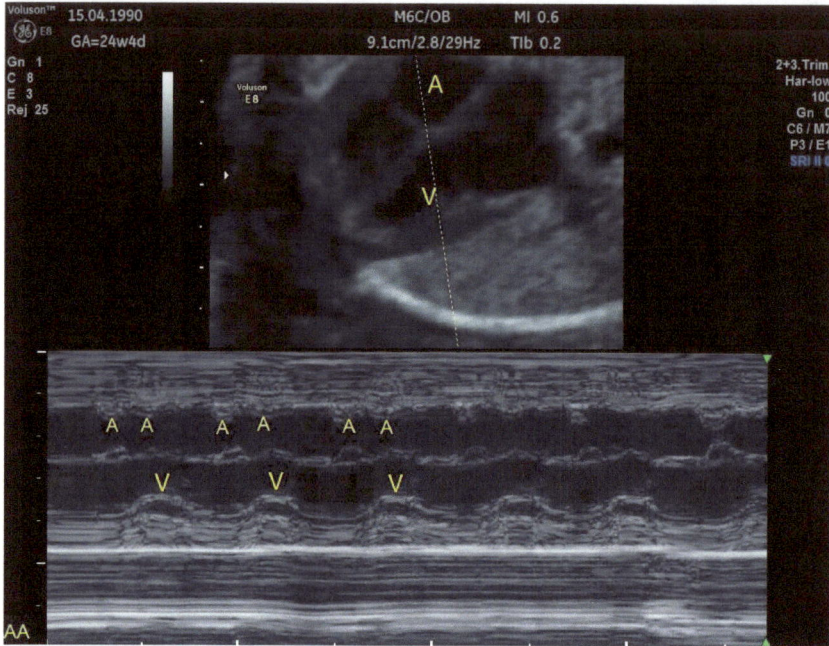

Fig. (13). Blocked atrial bigeminy, every second premature atrial beat is blocked and not conducted to ventricle. Atrial rhythm (A) is irregular and faster (140 bpm) than regular slower (70 bpm) ventricular rhythm (V). There is a ventricular bradycardia.

First-degree Atrioventricular Block

In first-degree AVB, all atrial contractions are conducted from the atria to the ventricles, but AV conduction time is prolonged beyond the upper limit of normal.

Diagnosis

MV-Ao or SVC-Ao Doppler are the most widely used modalities for detecting prolonged AV conduction. Increased FHR >160 bpm or prolonged AV time interval in first degree AV block leading to fusion of mitral early filing (E) wave and atrial contraction (A) wave can cause difficulties in correctly identifying the starting point of the AV interval measurement using MV-Ao Doppler, making the SVC-Ao Doppler a superior technique in these fetuses [37].

Second-degree Atrioventricular Block

Second-degree AVB is rare in fetal life. It is caused by failure to conduct some atrial impulses (contractions) to the ventricles. Second-degree AVB, is typically associated with structural heart disease or maternal anti-Ro/SSA and anti-La/SSB autoantibodies [51] and does not usually resolve spontaneously.

Diagnosis

The atrial rhythm is regular with constant AA intervals, and atrial rate is faster than the ventricular rate [23, 51]. Second degree AVB should be distinguished from blocked atrial premature beats, which are characterized by short and long (not constant) AA intervals.

hird-degree Atrioventricular Block

Third-degree AVB or complete heart block is a condition where there is no AV conduction and the atria and ventricle contract with their own rates (complete AV dissociation).

Diagnosis

In third-degree AV block, fetal echocardiology shows that the atria and ventricles beat independently of each other. The atrial rhythm is regular, AA intervals are constant and in normal range. The ventricular rhythm is regular and slow. CTG is not useful as a diagnostic or monitoring tool as it does not usually record the ventricular rates below 60 bpm. Noninvasive fetal ECG and magnetocardiography can also be helpful in making accurate diagnosis.

Atrioventricular Block Associated with Congenital Cardiac Defects

Congenital cardiac defects associated with AVB mainly include heterotaxy syndromes, discordant AV connection and atrioventricular septal defect. These cardiac defects are usually complex. In left atrial isomerism, the absence of a sino-arterial node can lead to low-atrial bradycardia. The right and left chambers are misaligned with the inflow and outflow portions of the heart, resulting in a discontinuity between the AV node and the conduction system. The prognosis for fetal AVB associated with congenital heart defects remains extremely poor, with a combined fetal and neonatal mortality >80% [38]. When hydrops is present lethality is almost 100%. When the CHB is diagnosed in the first trimester, it is a marker of complex congenital heart defect [52].

Immune-mediated Atrioventricular Block

When the fetal heart is structurally normal, AVB is mainly secondary to immune-mediated inflammation and fibrosis of the fetal conduction system. Most commonly it is caused by maternal anti-Ro/SSA and/or anti-La/SSB antibodies that can cross the placenta [47, 51]. These antibodies enter the fetal circulation in mid-gestation and may cause a progressive destruction of the fetal AV node, myocardial inflammation, and endocardial fibroelastosis in the fetus [51]. Other manifestations of immune-mediated cardiac disease include sinus node dysfunction, bundle branch block, and late-onset rupture of the AV valve chordae [53].

The incidence of congenital heart block in patients with anti-Ro/SSA and antiLa/SSB antibodies is approximately 2%-5% but up to one-third of fetuses of pregnant women who are positive for anti-Ro/SSA 52 kD antibodies may show signs of first degree CHB [54]. Approximately 50% of these women are asymptomatic concerning their rheumatologic disorder and may be unaware that they carry the antibodies. AVB is generally not seen before 18 weeks gestation, and rarely occurs after 28 weeks gestation [47]. The risk of recurrence for CHB when a fetus in a previous pregnancy has been affected is 12-25% [55].

Nonisoimmune Atrioventricular Block

Isolated AVB without positive anti-Ro/SSA or anti-La/SSB antibodies or structural cardiac malformations is rare [50]. The long-term prognosis seems to be better in isolated AVB than in other types of CHB [45, 50, 56]. Lopes *et al.* [56] reported that spontaneous regression of AVB *in utero* is possible in fetuses whose mothers remained seronegative for antinuclear antibodies throughout pregnancy (Fig. **14**).

Management of AV Block

Anti-Ro/SSA antibody positive pregnant women should be recommended to have weekly echocardiograms to measure AV interval serially and see if CHB develops during 16-18 to 26-28 weeks of gestation. However, some fetuses with normal AV intervals can develop complete CHB within days with no preceding first-degree AVB [57]. On the other hand, when first-degree AVB is detected, it rarely progresses to CHB [54, 56 - 58]. Prolongation of the AV interval does not always precede more advanced congenital AVB and it cannot be considered as a definitive predictor of early signs of immune CHB. Nevertheless, moderate-to-severe tricuspid regurgitation and increased endocardial echodensity are signs of cardiac injury associated with development of advanced AVB [57]. Thus, these findings especially in conjunction with prolongation of AV interval may indicate a need for closer surveillance and/or treatment. The etiology of CHB, ventricular rate, gestational age at diagnosis and the presence of heart failure or hydrops should be taken into account when deciding the management.

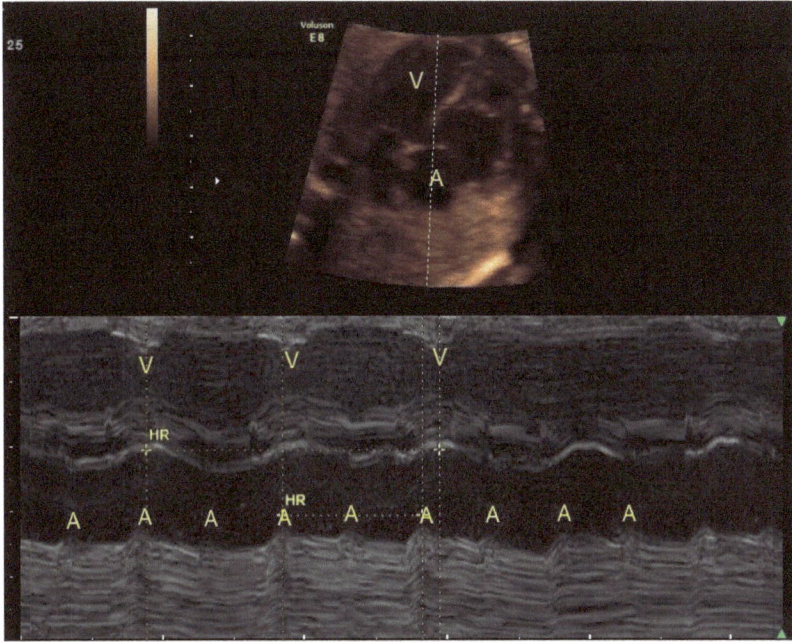

Fig. (14). Complete atrioventricular (AV) block with normal heart anatomy. Atrial rhythm is in normal range. There is an ectopic slow ventricular rhythm. There is lack of AV synchrony with an atrial rate of 122 bpm and ventricular rate of 58 bpm. A: atrial systole; V: ventricular systole.

AVB related to maternal anti-Ro/SSA antibodies has substantial, perinatal mortality of around 15%. Outcome is worse in cases diagnosed in early gestation, with hydrops, and low heart rate. Presence of dilated cardiomyopathy or endocardial fibroelastosis further increase the risk. Maternal treatment with fluorinated steroids may inhibit the progression, or even reverse incomplete AVB, especially when it is immune mediated [59, 60]. Although there is limited evidence [61] and continuing debate regarding effectiveness and safety of fluorinated steroids, Dexamethsone 4-8 mg daily has been used in many centres to treat recent onset first or second degree AVB. It is important to monitor fetal growth and amniotic fluid volume when Dexamethasone is used for a longer time. The dose can be reduced to 2 mg daily after 30-32 weeks of gestation if the amniotic fluid volume and/or fetal growth is reduced. Intravenous immunoglobulin G (IVIG) in combination with or without steroid therapy has been used to treat fetuses with complete heart block with signs of cardiac dysfunction, endocardial fibroelastosis or fetal hydrops with the hope of preventing cardiomyopathy and fetal death. Many centers offer transplacental steroid treatment in third degree AV Block when there are risk factors for an adverse outcome (*i.e.* very low heart rate, presence of dilated cardiomyopathy, endocardial fibroelastosis or hydrops). A retrospective multicenter study [62] has demonstrated survival benefit when IVIG was used with dexamethasone to treat complete CHB associated with signs of endocardial fibroelastosis or systolic dysfunction.

Beta-adrenergic drugs, *e.g.* salbutamol, terbutaline, isoprenaline, administered to mother have been shown to effectively increase the fetal ventricular rate by approximately 10%-20% and reverse hydrops in some fetuses with AVB [58]. These drugs are frequently used in clinical practice when the fetal ventricular rate is <55 bpm. Salbutamol and terbutaline are normally well tolerated *in utero*, but do cause maternal tachycardia (around 100-120 bpm) and benign ectopic beats. Unfortunately, no studies have demonstrated a survival benefit.

Fetal Tachycardia

Fetal tachycardia is diagnosed when the FHR (ventricular rate) exceeds 180 bpm. Tachyarrhythmias can occur at any gestational age and they may be intermittent or incessant. When tachycardia is present more than 50% of the observed evaluation time (during echocardiographic examination, CTG monitoring or intermittent auscultation) it is considered to be incessant. Sustained fetal tachyarrhythmias occur rarely, but are an important cause of fetal heart failure, hydrops, intrauterine death, perinatal morbidity and mortality. Most of the intermittent tachyarrhythmias remain intermittent and fetuses do not lead to fetal congestive heart failure. However, occasionally intermittent tachycardia become sustained. Therefore, close observation and follow-up is recommended although treatment may not be required. The management of incessant fetal tachyarrhythmia depends on gestational age, severity of hemodynamic changes leading to cardiac failure, maternal condition and potential maternal and fetal of risk from fetal therapy vs. early delivery. Tachyarrhythmias can originate at different levels of the heart's pacemaker and conduction pathway and can be associated with a variety of electrophysiological mechanisms. However, for clinical purpose they can be divided into: sinus tachycardia (ST), supraventricular tachycardia (SVT) and ventricular tachycardia (VT).

Sinus Tachycardia (ST)

ST is characterized by FHR between 180 - 200 bpm and mostly, with normal AV conduction (1:1). It can be related to several causes, such as maternal-fetal infection, rheumatic disease, thyrotoxicosis, drugs (*e.g.* beta-sympathomimetics), fetal hypoxemia, anemia *etc.*

Diagnosis

Atrial and ventricular rates are similar with normal 1:1 AV conduction

Management

Anti-arrhythmic therapy is not indicated. The underlying cause of ST should be identified and treated. Pregnant women should be advised to avoid stimulants such as caffeine, nicotine and drugs that may increase the heart rate.

Sustained Supraventricular Tachycardia (SVT)

SVT is the most common form of fetal tachycardia that accounts for 70%-75% of all tachyarrhythmias [63]. Sustained SVT includes atrioventricular re-entrant tachycardia (AVRT), atrial flutter (AF) and other rare tachyarrhythmias, such as junctional ectopic tachycardia (JET), permanent junctional reciprocating tachycardia and atrial ectopic tachycardia including chaotic multifocal tachycardia [64].

Atrioventricular Re-entrant Tachycardia (AVRT)

AVRT is the most common SVT type. It is associated with a fast conducting accessory pathway and, in general, is initiated by an ectopic cardiac beat. Conduction of the electrical pulse by the accessory pathway controls the cardiac rhythm with a fast heart rate. In AVRT, the electrical circuit uses retrograde accessory ventriculoatrial (VA) conduction pathway, whereas the normal electrical conduction uses the antegrade AV node conduction pathway. Due to the immaturity of the fetal myocardium, accessory pathways occur more frequently *in utero* and may occur in different locations [39]. In AV nodal re-entry tachycardia, the circuit forms within or immediately adjacent to the AV node [39].

Diagnosis

The rhythm is regular and FHR usually ranges between 220 and 300 bpm, with a 1:1 AV relationship (atrial rate equals to ventricular rate) (Fig. **15**). As the retrograde accessory pathway conduction is faster than the normal AV conduction pathway, the atrium is excited shortly after the ventricle, and AVRT is characterized by a short VA interval (VA < AV). Signs of fetal congestive heart failure and hydrops may be present.

Management

The prenatal management of fetal tachycardias remains controversial and varies from centre to centre [65]. The recent statements from the American Heart Association acknowledged the lack of consensus on the most effective and best tolerated first-line agent for fetal SVT or AF [64]. In many centers, the drug of first choice used to treat fetal AVRT (short VA SVT) is transplacental Digoxin [41, 64]. Digoxin can be administred intravenously, intramuscularly or orally. Usually an oral loading dose of 1.5 mg (0.5 mg thrice a day) in the first 24 hours followed by a maintenance dose of 0.5 mg per day (0.25 mg twice a day) can be given to keep maternal serum Digoxin levels in the range of 1.5-2 ng/ml. Flecainide or Sotalol are added after 3-5 days, if the heart rate remains high despite therapeutic Digoxin levels.

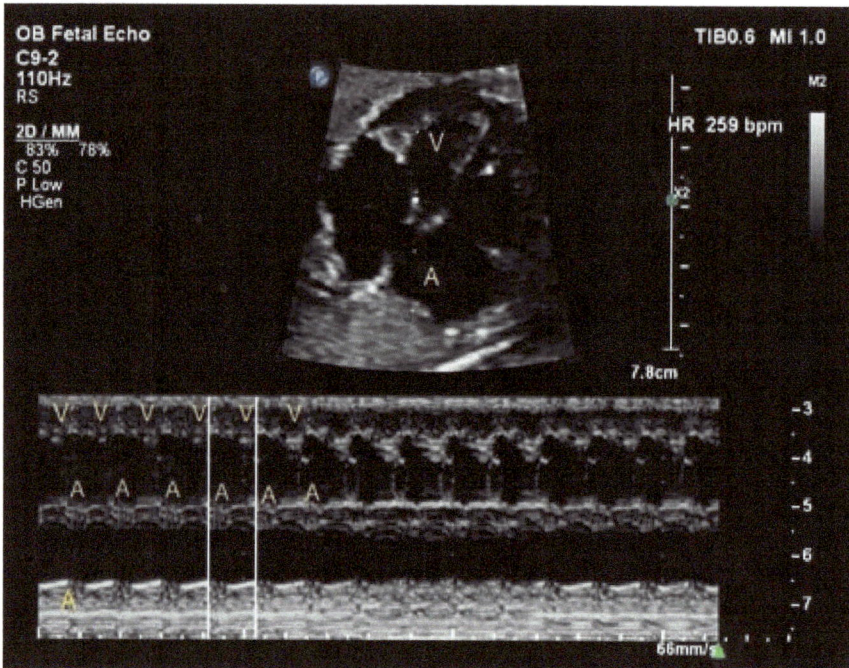

Fig. (15). M-mode tracing obtained in a 32 week fetus with supraventricular tachycardia (SVT) with an atrial (A) rate of 259 bpm and a ventricular (V) rate of 259 bpm. There was AV conduction 1:1.

Some centers prefer Flecainide or Sotalol as the first-line therapy [66, 67]. Flecainide is given orally in a dose of 100 mg 2-3 times daily (maximum dose 400 mg per day). Sotalol is started at an oral dose of 80 mg twice daily and increased to 160 mg twice daily within 3 days (maximum dose 160 mg 3 times a day). Sotalol or Flecainide are preferred over Digoxin as single agent therapy in cases with hydrops as transplacental transfer of Digoxin is less efficient in hydropic fetuses. Sotalol or Flecainide can also be given in combination with Digoxin as the first line treatment.

For refractory tachycardia Amiodarone has been used alone or in combination with Digoxin as a second or third line drug [64, 68]. However, one serious effect of its long-term use is fetal and neonatal hypothyroidism. As Digoxin, Flecainide, Sotalol, and Amiodarone are associated with maternal proarrhythmic risk, maternal ECG should be monitored during the treatment.

Fetal hydrops reduces the transplacental transfer of drugs, therefore in hydropic fetuses direct fetal treatment concomitantly with transplacental therapy has been used to restore sinus rhythm faster [64, 69, 70]. Direct treatment can be intramuscular to the fetal buttock or thigh or to fetal umbilical vein. Adenosine has not been effective in maintaining sinus rhythm in fetuses with SVT, therefore it is not recommended [64].

Recently published two systematic reviews on treatment of fetal tachyarrhythmias were concordant in their conclusion that Flecainide is more effective as a first-line treatment for fetal SVT compared to Digoxin and the maternal side effects and the rate of fetal demise were not increased in the Flecainide group. Therefore, Digoxin should not be first-line therapy for fetal tachycardia, particularly in the presence of hydrops fetalis [71, 72].

Vaginal delivery with continuous FHR monitoring is not contraindicated after conversion to normal sinus rhythm has occurred spontaneously or following transplacental therapy. All newborns treated with antiarrhythmic therapy *in utero* should be evaluated at birth with a 12-lead ECG and need to continue medical treatment must be reassessed relative to antiarrhythmic drugs used *in utero* and mechanism of tachycardia. Postnatal recurrence of SVT is observed in approximately 50% of AVRT [73].

Atrial Flutter

Atrial Flutter (AF) occurs at a frequency of 25%-30% among all types of tachyarrhythmia [45, 63, 67]. AF is caused by an intra-atrial re-entry circuit. AF can be associated with myocarditis, anti-Ro/SSA or anti-La/SSB antibodies, and congenital heart diseases, such as Ebstein's anomaly. AF is observed only in the third trimester, which is probably related to the large atrial size at 27-30 weeks of gestation, with high vulnerability to atrial extrasystoles [50, 66].

Diagnosis

In AF, the atrial rate is usually >350 bpm (350 - 480 bpm). The AF always results in functional AV block and ventricular rate is slower and half or one-third of the atrial rate depending on whether the AV conduction is 2:1 or 3:1 (Fig. **16**).

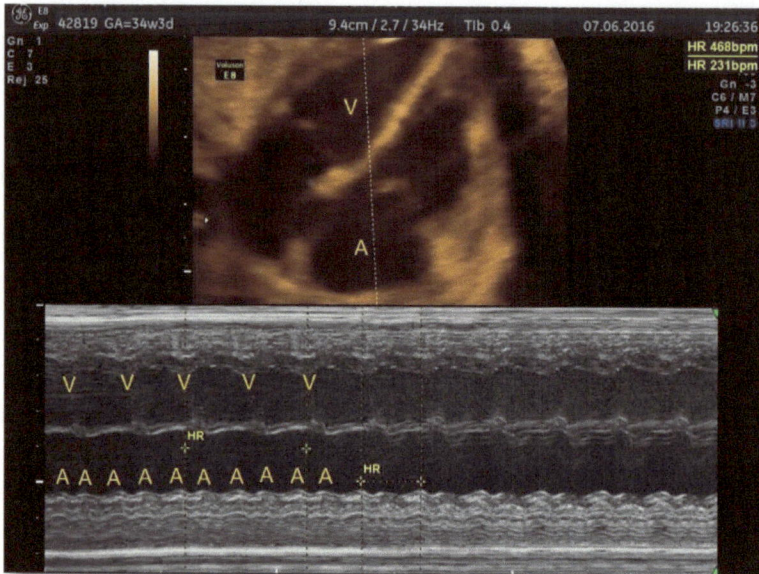

Fig. (16). M mode tracing obtained in a 34^{+3} week fetus with incessant atrial flutter and normal heart anatomy. The atrial (**A**) rate is 468 bpm and the ventricular (**V**) rate is 231 bpm. There is 2:1 AV block and the ventricular rate is approximately half of the atrial rate.

Management

Sotalol is recommended as the first line treatment in AF especially in cases with hydrops [45, 64]. Digoxin can be used in combination with Sotolol, and Amiodarone may be considered [64, 68]. Flecainide should be avoided as a single agent therapy in AF as it does not block the AV node like Digoxin or Sotalol. Therefore, a reduction of atrial rate <300 bpm may lead to conduction of all atrial contractions to ventricle resulting in sustained SVT. Procainamide is contraindicated in AF.

A meta-analysis of the two studies compared the efficacy of different medications used for AF showed no significant difference between Digoxin and Sotalol in the conversion to sinus rhythm [72].

Other Fetal Tachyarrhythmias

Atrial Ectopic Tachycardia and Chaotic Multifocal Atrial Tachycardia

In this type of SVT one or more atrial ectopic foci exist. The FHR (ventricular rate) ranges between 160 and 250 bpm and VA interval is longer than AV interval [40]. When atrial ectopic tachycardia occurs in a multifocal form it creates chaotic ventricular rhythm, frequently with brief periods of AF, and it is referred to as chaotic multifocal atrial tachycardia. It is a rare tachycardia that is usually seen late in the second or third trimester of pregnancy and can be associated with Costello syndrome. Increased nuchal thickness, polyhydramnios, short femurs and humeri, and myocardial hypertrophy associated with atrial tachycardia should raise suspicion of Costello syndrome [74, 75].

Diagnosis

Detailed fetal scanning may show abnormal fetal anatomy. Echocardiographic evaluation demonstrates long VA tachycardia with an atrial rate of about 180-220 bpm and 1:1 AV conduction. Long VA tachycardia with chaotic ventricular rhythm and brief periods of AF is characteristic to multifocal atrial ectopic tachycardia.

Management

Atrial ectopic tachycardias are difficult to treat. Digoxin is generally used as the first-line therapy in fetuses without hydrops or ventricular dysfunction. Sotalol or Fecainide may be considered if fetal hydrops is present.

Junctional Ectopic Tachycardia (JET)

JET is a very rare type of fetal SVT characterized by retrograde VA conduction. It is generally caused by an automatic ectopic focus in the AV junction. Fetal JET has been associated with anti-Ro/SSA antibodies isoimmunization [57, 64, 66]. Fetal hydrops is quite common with JET despite moderate tachycardia. In JET, atrial contractions arise from AV node rather than from accessory pathway.

Diagnosis

FHR ranges typically from 160 to 210 bpm. There is AV dissociation with a ventricular rate exceeding that in the atria. JET is characterized by simultaneous onset of atrial and ventricular contractions which can be recorded using SVC-Ao or MV-Ao Doppler. Diagnosis can be confirmed by fMCG.

Management

The *in utero* treatment of JET is similar to most of other SVT, but it can be quite refractory to therapy. Transplacental therapy with Digoxin, Sotalol, Flecainide or Amiodarone have been used to treat JET. Dexamethasone may be considered if anti-SSA/SSB antibodies are present.

Permanent Junctional Reciprocating Tachycardia (PJRT) or Coumel Tachycardia

PJRT is another rare form of incessant SVT. It is caused by an AV re-entry using the AV node as the antegrade limb and a slowly conducting accessory pathway as the retrograde limb. The usual location of the accessory pathway is right posteroseptal.

Diagnosis

In PJRT, FHR is in the range of 160 and 240 bpm, with 1:1 AV relationship. PJRT is characterized by a long VA interval. A slow conducting re-entry pathway back to the atrium explains the long VA interval. Signs of congestive heart failure and cardiomyopathy are frequently observed.

Management

Commonly used drugs for *in utero* transplacental treatment are Flecainide, Sotalol and Digoxin. PJRT can be refractory to transplacental therapy. Postnatally radiofrequency ablation can be performed if pharmacological therapy fails to restore normal rhythm.

Ventricular Tachycardia

Ventricular tachycardia (VT) is extremely rare during fetal life. VT has been observed in underlying cardiac diseases such as cardiac tumors, myocarditis, ventricular aneurysm, long QT syndrome, unstable AV block, myocardial hypertrophy due to AV valve stenosis. The electrophysiological mechanism of VT is an ectopic ventricular focus due to inflammation (cardiomyopathy) or abnormalities of the myocardial oxygen supply.

Diagnosis

Ventricular rates range from 180 to 300 bpm, with AV dissociation. Atrial rate is usually lower than the ventricular rate, however if there is a retrograde 1:1 VA conduction, the ventricular and atrial rates can be similar (1:1), making it almost impossible to differentiate these types of VT from SVT by fetal echocardiography. VA interval is shorter than AV interval (VA < AV). VT is associated with long-QT syndrome, and it should be strongly suspected when the tachycardia occurs in combination with periods of bradycardia and AV block. However, the prenatal measurement of QT interval is only possible by fMCG.

Management

In sustained VT, maternal intravenous magnesium sulfate therapy for less than 48 hours duration is recommended as the first-line treatment if FHR is >200 bpm. In addition to short-term magnesium, treatment for VT may include intravenous Lidocaine (especially when hydrops occurs) or oral Propranolol or Mexiletine [57, 64, 76, 77]. Dexamethasone and IVIG are recommended if there is evidence of myocarditis or isoimmunization [50, 74]. Sotalol, Amiodarone and Flecainide can be used if the long QT syndrome is excluded [57, 76].

FIRST TRIMESTER FETAL ARRHYTHMIAS

First trimester fetal arrhythmias are not studied well. They occur much more rarely than later in pregnancy. Some of them have never been described in the literature. However, the reference ranges for FHR during 6-14 weeks are established [5, 6, 8]. It is known, that bradycardia <80-90 bpm in 6-8 weeks of gestation is associated with a higher rate of adverse pregnancy outcome by the end of the first trimester as well as increased risk of fetal abnormalities [78 - 80]. However, reference ranges for AV and VA time intervals in the first trimester are lacking. Many reports are available on FHR as a first trimester marker of chromosomal abnormalities while none has focused on the arrhythmias as an issue [81, 82].

The most common arrythmia in the 2nd and 3rd trimester is the irregular rhythm caused by PACs. However, in the first trimester, PAC is an extremely rare rhythm disturbance. To our knowledge, only one case of PAC with the fetal bradycardia in the first trimester has been published so far [83]. We have observed a similar case at 12+6 weeks of gestation. No cases of PVC in the first trimester have been reported yet.

The SVT is also extremely rare in the first trimester; only several cases of fetal tachycardia >200 bpm have been reported [84]. We have observed a rare case with a FHR of 292 bpm at 13 weeks of gestation which resolved spontaneously within 24 hours and the fetus showed no pathology on further follow up.

No cases of AF, VT, or JET have been reported in the first trimester. Persistent fetal bradycardia in the first trimester is usually associated with complete AV block and heart defects (atrial isomerism, L-TGA) and is associated with adverse outcome. In left atrial isomerism, the absence of a sinus node can lead to low-atrial bradycardia that is possible to diagnose in the first trimester. When the CHB is diagnosed in the first trimester it is generally a marker of complex congenital heart defect [51, 85]. Immune-mediated atrioventricular blocks are not observed in the first trimester since the maternal antibodies do not cross the placenta until 16 weeks of gestation.

CONCLUSION

When an abnormality in fetal cardiac rhythm is detected, the primary goal should be to identify its cause if possible, establish its mechanism and hemodynamic consequences that have an effect on fetal wellbeing. This helps to determine whether arrhythmia should be treated *in utero* or expectant management will suffice. Delivery and postnatal management is an option close to term.

CONSENT FOR PUBLICATION

Not applicable.

CONFLICT OF INTEREST

The authors confirm that the contents of this chapter have no conflict of interest.

ACKNOWLEDGEMENTS

Declared none.

REFERENCES

[1]   Acharya G, Rasanen J, Kiserud T, Huhta JC. The fetal cardiac function. Curr Cardiol Rev 2006; 2: 41-53.
        [http://dx.doi.org/10.2174/157340306775515362]

[2]   Włoch A, Rozmus-Warcholinska W, Czuba B, *et al.* Doppler study of the embryonic heart in normal pregnant women. J Matern Fetal Neonatal Med 2007; 20(7): 533-9.
        [http://dx.doi.org/10.1080/14767050701434747] [PMID: 17674267]

[3]   Doubilet PM, Benson CB. Embryonic heart rate in the early first trimester: what rate is normal? J Ultrasound Med 1995; 14(6): 431-4.
        [http://dx.doi.org/10.7863/jum.1995.14.6.431] [PMID: 7658510]

[4]   Stefos TI, Lolis DE, Sotiriadis AJ, Ziakas GV. Embryonic heart rate in early pregnancy. J Clin Ultrasound 1998; 26(1): 33-6.
        [http://dx.doi.org/10.1002/(SICI)1097-0096(199801)26:1<33::AID-JCU7>3.0.CO;2-K]   [PMID: 9475206]

[5]   Levi CS, Lyons EA, Zheng XH, Lindsay DJ, Holt SC. Endovaginal US: demonstration of cardiac activity in embryos of less than 5.0 mm in crown-rump length. Radiology 1990; 176(1): 71-4.

[http://dx.doi.org/10.1148/radiology.176.1.2191372] [PMID: 2191372]

[6]   Tezuka N, Sato S, Kanasugi H, Hiroi M. Embryonic heart rates: development in early first trimester and clinical evaluation. Gynecol Obstet Invest 1991; 32(4): 210-2.
        [http://dx.doi.org/10.1159/000293033] [PMID: 1778511]

[7]   Acharya G, Gui Y, Cnota W, Huhta J, Wloch A. Human embryonic cardiovascular function. Acta Obstet Gynecol Scand 2016; 95(6): 621-8.
        [http://dx.doi.org/10.1111/aogs.12860] [PMID: 26830850]

[8]   Rozmus-Warcholinska W, Wloch A, Acharya G, *et al.* Reference values for variables of fetal cardiocirculatory dynamics at 11-14 weeks of gestation. Ultrasound Obstet Gynecol 2010; 35(5): 540-7.
        [http://dx.doi.org/10.1002/uog.7595] [PMID: 20178107]

[9]   Pildner von Steinburg S, Boulesteix AL, Lederer C, *et al.* What is the "normal" fetal heart rate? PeerJ 2013; 1: e82.
        [http://dx.doi.org/10.7717/peerj.82] [PMID: 23761161]

[10]   Nii M, Hamilton RM, Fenwick L, Kingdom JC, Roman KS, Jaeggi ET. Assessment of fetal atrioventricular time intervals by tissue Doppler and pulse Doppler echocardiography: normal values and correlation with fetal electrocardiography. Heart 2006; 92(12): 1831-7.
        [http://dx.doi.org/10.1136/hrt.2006.093070] [PMID: 16775085]

[11]   Pasquini L, Seale AN, Belmar C, *et al.* PR interval: a comparison of electrical and mechanical methods in the fetus. Early Hum Dev 2007; 83(4): 231-7.
        [http://dx.doi.org/10.1016/j.earlhumdev.2006.05.020] [PMID: 16828991]

[12]   Arya B, Govindan R, Krishnan A, Duplessis A, Donofrio MT. Feasibility of noninvasive fetal electrocardiographic monitoring in a clinical setting. Pediatr Cardiol 2015; 36(5): 1042-9.
        [http://dx.doi.org/10.1007/s00246-015-1118-4] [PMID: 25608698]

[13]   Wacker-Gussmann A, Plankl C, Sewald M, Schneider KM, Oberhoffer R, Lobmaier SM. Fetal cardiac time intervals in healthy pregnancies - an observational study by fetal ECG (Monica Healthcare System). J Perinat Med 2018; 46(6): 587-92.
        [http://dx.doi.org/10.1515/jpm-2017-0003] [PMID: 28453441]

[14]   Taylor MJ, Smith MJ, Thomas M, *et al.* Non-invasive fetal electrocardiography in singleton and multiple pregnancies. BJOG 2003; 110(7): 668-78.
        [http://dx.doi.org/10.1046/j.1471-0528.2003.02005.x] [PMID: 12842058]

[15]   Zhao H, Strasburger JF, Cuneo BF, Wakai RT. Fetal cardiac repolarization abnormalities. Am J Cardiol 2006; 98(4): 491-6.
        [http://dx.doi.org/10.1016/j.amjcard.2006.03.026] [PMID: 16893703]

[16]   Parilla B, Strasburger J. Fetal Arrhythmias. Glob. Libr. Women's Med. (ISSN: 1756-2228) 2008.
        [http://dx.doi.org/10.3843/GLOWM.10200]

[17]   Strand SA, Strasburger JF, Wakai RT. Fetal magnetocardiogram waveform characteristics. Physiol Meas 2019; 40(3): 035002.
        [http://dx.doi.org/10.1088/1361-6579/ab0a2c] [PMID: 30802886]

[18]   Allan LD, Anderson RH, Sullivan ID, Campbell S, Holt DW, Tynan M. Evaluation of fetal arrhythmias by echocardiography. Br Heart J 1983; 50(3): 240-5.
        [http://dx.doi.org/10.1136/hrt.50.3.240] [PMID: 6193800]

[19]   DeVore GR, Siassi B, Platt LD. Fetal echocardiography. III. The diagnosis of cardiac arrhythmias using real-time-directed M-mode ultrasound. Am J Obstet Gynecol 1983; 146(7): 792-9.
        [http://dx.doi.org/10.1016/0002-9378(83)91080-3] [PMID: 6869451]

[20]   Fouron JC, Proulx F, Miró J, Gosselin J. Doppler and M-mode ultrasonography to time fetal atrial and ventricular contractions. Obstet Gynecol 2000; 96(5 Pt 1): 732-6.
        [PMID: 11042309]

[21]   Jaeggi E, Fouron JC, Fournier A, van Doesburg N, Drblik SP, Proulx F. Ventriculo-atrial time interval measured on M mode echocardiography: a determining element in diagnosis, treatment, and prognosis of fetal supraventricular tachycardia. Heart 1998; 79(6): 582-7.
[http://dx.doi.org/10.1136/hrt.79.6.582] [PMID: 10078085]

[22]   Jaeggi ET, Nii M. Fetal brady- and tachyarrhythmias: new and accepted diagnostic and treatment methods. Semin Fetal Neonatal Med 2005; 10(6): 504-14.
[http://dx.doi.org/10.1016/j.siny.2005.08.003] [PMID: 16213203]

[23]   Glickstein JS, Buyon J, Friedman D. Pulsed Doppler echocardiographic assessment of the fetal PR interval. Am J Cardiol 2000; 86(2): 236-9.
[http://dx.doi.org/10.1016/S0002-9149(00)00867-5] [PMID: 10913494]

[24]   Sonesson SE, Acharya G. Hemodynamics in fetal arrhythmia. Acta Obstet Gynecol Scand 2016; 95(6): 697-709.
[http://dx.doi.org/10.1111/aogs.12837] [PMID: 26660845]

[25]   Fouron JC, Fournier A, Proulx F, et al. Management of fetal tachyarrhythmia based on superior vena cava/aorta Doppler flow recordings. Heart 2003; 89(10): 1211-6.
[http://dx.doi.org/10.1136/heart.89.10.1211] [PMID: 12975422]

[26]   DeVore GR, Horenstein J. Simultaneous Doppler recording of the pulmonary artery and vein: a new technique for the evaluation of a fetal arrhythmia. J Ultrasound Med 1993; 12(11): 669-71.
[http://dx.doi.org/10.7863/jum.1993.12.11.669] [PMID: 8264020]

[27]   Carvalho JS, Prefumo F, Ciardelli V, Sairam S, Bhide A, Shinebourne EA. Evaluation of fetal arrhythmias from simultaneous pulsed wave Doppler in pulmonary artery and vein. Heart 2007; 93(11): 1448-53.
[http://dx.doi.org/10.1136/hrt.2006.101659] [PMID: 17164485]

[28]   Wojakowski A, Izbizky G, Carcano ME, Aiello H, Marantz P, Otaño L. Fetal Doppler mechanical PR interval: correlation with fetal heart rate, gestational age and fetal sex. Ultrasound Obstet Gynecol 2009; 34(5): 538-42.
[http://dx.doi.org/10.1002/uog.7333] [PMID: 19731250]

[29]   Rein AJ, O'Donnell C, Geva T, et al. Use of tissue velocity imaging in the diagnosis of fetal cardiac arrhythmias. Circulation 2002; 106(14): 1827-33.
[http://dx.doi.org/10.1161/01.CIR.0000031571.92807.CC] [PMID: 12356637]

[30]   Herling L, Johnson J, Ferm-Widlund K, et al. Automated analysis of fetal cardiac function using color tissue Doppler imaging in second half of normal pregnancy. Ultrasound Obstet Gynecol 2019; 53(3): 348-57.
[http://dx.doi.org/10.1002/uog.19037] [PMID: 29484743]

[31]   Chia EL, Ho TF, Rauff M, Yip WC. Cardiac time intervals of normal fetuses using noninvasive fetal electrocardiography. Prenat Diagn 2005; 25(7): 546-52.
[http://dx.doi.org/10.1002/pd.1184] [PMID: 16032763]

[32]   Stinstra J, Golbach E, van Leeuwen P, et al. Multicentre study of fetal cardiac time intervals using magnetocardiography. BJOG 2002; 109(11): 1235-43.
[http://dx.doi.org/10.1046/j.1471-0528.2002.01057.x] [PMID: 12452461]

[33]   Andelfinger G, Fouron JC, Sonesson SE, Proulx F. Reference values for time intervals between atrial and ventricular contractions of the fetal heart measured by two Doppler techniques. Am J Cardiol 2001; 88(12): 1433-1436, A8.
[http://dx.doi.org/10.1016/S0002-9149(01)02130-0] [PMID: 11741570]

[34]   Anuwutnavin S, Kolakarnprasert K, Chanprapaph P, Sklansky M, Mongkolchat N. Measurement of fetal atrioventricular time intervals: A comparison of 3 spectral Doppler techniques. Prenat Diagn 2018; 38(6): 459-66.
[http://dx.doi.org/10.1002/pd.5261] [PMID: 29633288]

[35]   Mosimann B, Arampatzis G, Amylidi-Mohr S, *et al.* Reference Ranges for Fetal Atrioventricular and Ventriculoatrial Time Intervals and Their Ratios during Normal Pregnancy. Fetal Diagn Ther 2018; 44(3): 228-35.
[http://dx.doi.org/10.1159/000481349] [PMID: 29045943]

[36]   Smith V, Arunthavanathan S, Nair A, Ansermet D, da Silva Costa F, Wallace EM. A systematic review of cardiac time intervals utilising non-invasive fetal electrocardiogram in normal fetuses. BMC Pregnancy Childbirth 2018; 18(1): 370.
[http://dx.doi.org/10.1186/s12884-018-2006-8] [PMID: 30208861]

[37]   Friedman DM, Kim MY, Copel JA, *et al.* Utility of cardiac monitoring in fetuses at risk for congenital heart block: the PR Interval and Dexamethasone Evaluation (PRIDE) prospective study. Circulation 2008; 117(4): 485-93.
[http://dx.doi.org/10.1161/CIRCULATIONAHA.107.707661] [PMID: 18195175]

[38]   Strasburger JF, Cheulkar B, Wichman HJ. Perinatal arrhythmias: diagnosis and management. Clin Perinatol 2007; 34(4): 627-652, vii-viii.
[http://dx.doi.org/10.1016/j.clp.2007.10.002] [PMID: 18063110]

[39]   Bravo-Valenzuela NJ, Rocha LA, Machado Nardozza LM, Araujo Júnior E. Fetal cardiac arrhythmias: Current evidence. Ann Pediatr Cardiol 2018; 11(2): 148-63.
[http://dx.doi.org/10.4103/apc.APC_134_17] [PMID: 29922012]

[40]   Crotti L, Tester DJ, White WM, *et al.* Long QT syndrome-associated mutations in intrauterine fetal death. JAMA 2013; 309(14): 1473-82.
[http://dx.doi.org/10.1001/jama.2013.3219] [PMID: 23571586]

[41]   Hornberger LK, Sahn DJ. Rhythm abnormalities of the fetus. Heart 2007; 93(10): 1294-300.
[http://dx.doi.org/10.1136/hrt.2005.069369] [PMID: 17890709]

[42]   Cuneo BF, Strasburger JF, Wakai RT, Ovadia M. Conduction system disease in fetuses evaluated for irregular cardiac rhythm. Fetal Diagn Ther 2006; 21(3): 307-13.
[http://dx.doi.org/10.1159/000091362] [PMID: 16601344]

[43]   Atalay S, Aypar E, Uçar T, *et al.* Fetal and neonatal cardiac rhabdomyomas: clinical presentation, outcome and association with tuberous sclerosis complex. Turk J Pediatr 2010; 52(5): 481-7.
[PMID: 21434532]

[44]   Wiggins DL, Strasburger JF, Gotteiner NL, Cuneo B, Wakai RT. Magnetophysiologic and echocardiographic comparison of blocked atrial bigeminy and 2:1 atrioventricular block in the fetus. Heart Rhythm 2013; 10(8): 1192-8.
[http://dx.doi.org/10.1016/j.hrthm.2013.04.020] [PMID: 23619035]

[45]   Bravo-Valenzuela NJ, Lopes LM. Inappropriate Fetal Sinus Tachycardia. Cardiol Young 2010; 20: 71.

[46]   Baruteau AE, Schleich JM. Antenatal presentation of congenital long QT syndrome: A prenatal diagnosis not to be missed. Pediatr Cardiol 2008; 29(6): 1131-2.
[http://dx.doi.org/10.1007/s00246-008-9271-7] [PMID: 18661168]

[47]   Mitchell JL, Cuneo BF, Etheridge SP, Horigome H, Weng HY, Benson DW. Fetal heart rate predictors of long QT syndrome. Circulation 2012; 126(23): 2688-95.
[http://dx.doi.org/10.1161/CIRCULATIONAHA.112.114132] [PMID: 23124029]

[48]   Serra V, Bellver J, Moulden M, Redman CW. Computerized analysis of normal fetal heart rate pattern throughout gestation. Ultrasound Obstet Gynecol 2009; 34(1): 74-9.
[http://dx.doi.org/10.1002/uog.6365] [PMID: 19489020]

[49]   Bordachar P, Zachary W, Ploux S, Labrousse L, Haissaguerre M, Thambo JB. Pathophysiology, clinical course, and management of congenital complete atrioventricular block. Heart Rhythm 2013; 10(5): 760-6.
[http://dx.doi.org/10.1016/j.hrthm.2012.12.030] [PMID: 23276818]

[50] Zhao H, Cuneo BF, Strasburger JF, Huhta JC, Gotteiner NL, Wakai RT. Electrophysiological characteristics of fetal atrioventricular block. J Am Coll Cardiol 2008; 51(1): 77-84.
      [http://dx.doi.org/10.1016/j.jacc.2007.06.060] [PMID: 18174041]

[51] Baschat AA, Gembruch U, Knöpfle G, Hansmann M. First-trimester fetal heart block: a marker for cardiac anomaly. Ultrasound Obstet Gynecol 1999; 14(5): 311-4.
      [http://dx.doi.org/10.1046/j.1469-0705.1999.14050311.x] [PMID: 10623989]

[52] Cuneo BF, Strasburger JF, Yu S, *et al*. In utero diagnosis of long QT syndrome by magnetocardiography. Circulation 2013; 128(20): 2183-91.
      [http://dx.doi.org/10.1161/CIRCULATIONAHA.113.004840] [PMID: 24218437]

[53] Copel JA, Buyon JP, Kleinman CS. Successful *in utero* therapy of fetal heart block. Am J Obstet Gynecol 1995; 173(5): 1384-90.
      [http://dx.doi.org/10.1016/0002-9378(95)90621-5] [PMID: 7503173]

[54] Sonesson SE, Salomonsson S, Jacobsson LA, Bremme K, Wahren-Herlenius M. Signs of first-degree heart block occur in one-third of fetuses of pregnant women with anti-SSA/Ro 52-kd antibodies. Arthritis Rheum 2004; 50(4): 1253-61.
      [http://dx.doi.org/10.1002/art.20126] [PMID: 15077309]

[55] Buyon JP, Hiebert R, Copel J, *et al*. Autoimmune-associated congenital heart block: demographics, mortality, morbidity and recurrence rates obtained from a national neonatal lupus registry. J Am Coll Cardiol 1998; 31(7): 1658-66.
      [http://dx.doi.org/10.1016/S0735-1097(98)00161-2] [PMID: 9626848]

[56] Lopes LM, Tavares GM, Damiano AP, *et al*. Perinatal outcome of fetal atrioventricular block: one-hundred-sixteen cases from a single institution. Circulation 2008; 118(12): 1268-75.
      [http://dx.doi.org/10.1161/CIRCULATIONAHA.107.735118] [PMID: 18765396]

[57] Horigome H, Nagashima M, Sumitomo N, *et al*. Clinical characteristics and genetic background of congenital long-QT syndrome diagnosed in fetal, neonatal, and infantile life: a nationwide questionnaire survey in Japan. Circ Arrhythm Electrophysiol 2010; 3(1): 10-7.
      [http://dx.doi.org/10.1161/CIRCEP.109.882159] [PMID: 19996378]

[58] Maeno Y, Hirose A, Kanbe T, Hori D. Fetal arrhythmia: prenatal diagnosis and perinatal management. J Obstet Gynaecol Res 2009; 35(4): 623-9.
      [http://dx.doi.org/10.1111/j.1447-0756.2009.01080.x] [PMID: 19751319]

[59] Eliasson H, Sonesson SE, Sharland G, *et al*. Isolated atrioventricular block in the fetus: a retrospective, multinational, multicenter study of 175 patients. Circulation 2011; 124(18): 1919-26.
      [http://dx.doi.org/10.1161/CIRCULATIONAHA.111.041970] [PMID: 21986286]

[60] Costedoat-Chalumeau N, Amoura Z, Le Thi Hong D, *et al*. Questions about dexamethasone use for the prevention of anti-SSA related congenital heart block. Ann Rheum Dis 2003; 62(10): 1010-2.
      [http://dx.doi.org/10.1136/ard.62.10.1010] [PMID: 12972484]

[61] Ciardulli A, D'Antonio F, Magro-Malosso ER, *et al*. Maternal steroid therapy for fetuses with second-degree immune-mediated congenital atrioventricular block: a systematic review and meta-analysis. Acta Obstet Gynecol Scand 2018; 97(7): 787-94.
      [http://dx.doi.org/10.1111/aogs.13338] [PMID: 29512819]

[62] Trucco SM, Jaeggi E, Cuneo B, *et al*. Use of intravenous gamma globulin and corticosteroids in the treatment of maternal autoantibody-mediated cardiomyopathy. J Am Coll Cardiol 2011; 57(6): 715-23.
      [http://dx.doi.org/10.1016/j.jacc.2010.09.044] [PMID: 21292131]

[63] Krapp M, Kohl T, Simpson JM, Sharland GK, Katalinic A, Gembruch U. Review of diagnosis, treatment, and outcome of fetal atrial flutter compared with supraventricular tachycardia. Heart 2003; 89(8): 913-7.
      [http://dx.doi.org/10.1136/heart.89.8.913] [PMID: 12860871]

[64] Donofrio MT, Moon-Grady AJ, Hornberger LK, *et al*. Diagnosis and treatment of fetal cardiac

disease: a scientific statement from the American Heart Association. Circulation 2014; 129(21): 2183-242.
[http://dx.doi.org/10.1161/01.cir.0000437597.44550.5d] [PMID: 24763516]

[65]   Skinner JR, Sharland G. Detection and management of life threatening arrhythmias in the perinatal period. Early Hum Dev 2008; 84(3): 161-72.
[http://dx.doi.org/10.1016/j.earlhumdev.2008.01.010] [PMID: 18358642]

[66]   Wacker-Gussmann A, Strasburger JF, Cuneo BF, Wakai RT. Diagnosis and treatment of fetal arrhythmia. Am J Perinatol 2014; 31(7): 617-28.
[http://dx.doi.org/10.1055/s-0034-1372430] [PMID: 24858320]

[67]   Strasburger JF, Wakai RT. Fetal cardiac arrhythmia detection and *in utero* therapy. Nat Rev Cardiol 2010; 7(5): 277-90.
[http://dx.doi.org/10.1038/nrcardio.2010.32] [PMID: 20418904]

[68]   Peyrol M, Lévy S. Clinical presentation of inappropriate sinus tachycardia and differential diagnosis. J Interv Card Electrophysiol 2016; 46(1): 33-41.
[http://dx.doi.org/10.1007/s10840-015-0051-z] [PMID: 26329720]

[69]   Cuneo BF, Strasburger JF. Management strategy for fetal tachycardia. Obstet Gynecol 2000; 96(4): 575-81.
[PMID: 11004362]

[70]   Parilla BV, Strasburger JF, Socol ML. Fetal supraventricular tachycardia complicated by hydrops fetalis: a role for direct fetal intramuscular therapy. Am J Perinatol 1996; 13(8): 483-6.
[http://dx.doi.org/10.1055/s-2007-994432] [PMID: 8989479]

[71]   Hill GD, Kovach JR, Saudek DE, Singh AK, Wehrheim K, Frommelt MA. Transplacental treatment of fetal tachycardia: A systematic review and meta-analysis. Prenat Diagn 2017; 37(11): 1076-83.
[http://dx.doi.org/10.1002/pd.5144] [PMID: 28833310]

[72]   Alsaied T, Baskar S, Fares M, *et al.* First-Line Antiarrhythmic Transplacental Treatment for Fetal Tachyarrhythmia: A Systematic Review and Meta-Analysis. J Am Heart Assoc 2017; 6(12)e007164
[http://dx.doi.org/10.1161/JAHA.117.007164] [PMID: 29246961]

[73]   Naheed ZJ, Strasburger JF, Deal BJ, Benson DW Jr, Gidding SS. Fetal tachycardia: mechanisms and predictors of hydrops fetalis. J Am Coll Cardiol 1996; 27(7): 1736-40.
[http://dx.doi.org/10.1016/0735-1097(96)00054-X] [PMID: 8636562]

[74]   Cuneo BF, Strasburger JF, Niksch A, Ovadia M, Wakai RT. An expanded phenotype of maternal SSA/SSB antibody-associated fetal cardiac disease. J Matern Fetal Neonatal Med 2009; 22(3): 233-8.
[http://dx.doi.org/10.1080/14767050802488220] [PMID: 19330707]

[75]   Lin AE, Alexander ME, Colan SD, *et al.* Clinical, pathological, and molecular analyses of cardiovascular abnormalities in Costello syndrome: a Ras/MAPK pathway syndrome. Am J Med Genet A 2011; 155A(3): 486-507.
[http://dx.doi.org/10.1002/ajmg.a.33857] [PMID: 21344638]

[76]   Cuneo BF, Ovadia M, Strasburger JF, *et al.* Prenatal diagnosis and *in utero* treatment of torsades de pointes associated with congenital long QT syndrome. Am J Cardiol 2003; 91(11): 1395-8.
[http://dx.doi.org/10.1016/S0002-9149(03)00343-6] [PMID: 12767447]

[77]   Simpson JM, Maxwell D, Rosenthal E, Gill H. Fetal ventricular tachycardia secondary to long QT syndrome treated with maternal intravenous magnesium: case report and review of the literature. Ultrasound Obstet Gynecol 2009; 34(4): 475-80.
[http://dx.doi.org/10.1002/uog.6433] [PMID: 19731233]

[78]   Achiron R, Tadmor O, Mashiach S. Heart rate as a predictor of first-trimester spontaneous abortion after ultrasound-proven viability. Obstet Gynecol 1991; 78(3 Pt 1): 330-4.
[PMID: 1876359]

[79]   Merchiers EH, Dhont M, De Sutter PA, Beghin CJ, Vandekerckhove DA. Predictive value of early

embryonic cardiac activity for pregnancy outcome. Am J Obstet Gynecol 1991; 165(1): 11-4.
[http://dx.doi.org/10.1016/0002-9378(91)90214-C] [PMID: 1853885]

[80]   Doubilet PM, Benson CB, Chow JS. Long-term prognosis of pregnancies complicated by slow embryonic heart rates in the early first trimester. J Ultrasound Med 1999; 18(8): 537-41.
[http://dx.doi.org/10.7863/jum.1999.18.8.537] [PMID: 10447078]

[81]   Espinoza AF, Lee W, Belfort MA, Shamshirsaz AA, Mastrobattista J, Espinoza J. Fetal Tachycardia Is an Independent Risk Factor for Chromosomal Anomalies in First-Trimester Genetic Screening. J Ultrasound Med 2019; 38(5): 1327-31.
[http://dx.doi.org/10.1002/jum.14813] [PMID: 30244488]

[82]   Liao AW, Snijders R, Geerts L, Spencer K, Nicolaides KH. Fetal heart rate in chromosomally abnormal fetuses. Ultrasound Obstet Gynecol 2000; 16(7): 610-3.
[http://dx.doi.org/10.1046/j.1469-0705.2000.00292.x] [PMID: 11169365]

[83]   Wong SF, Chau KT, Ho LC. Fetal bradycardia in the first trimester: an unusual presentation of atrial extrasystoles. Prenat Diagn 2002; 22(11): 976-8.
[http://dx.doi.org/10.1002/pd.450] [PMID: 12424759]

[84]   Porat S, Anteby EY, Hamani Y, Yagel S. Fetal supraventricular tachycardia diagnosed and treated at 13 weeks of gestation: a case report. Ultrasound Obstet Gynecol 2003; 21(3): 302-5.
[http://dx.doi.org/10.1002/uog.64] [PMID: 12666229]

[85]   Sciarrone A, Masturzo B, Botta G, Bastonero S, Campogrande M, Viora E. First-trimester fetal heart block and increased nuchal translucency: an indication for early fetal echocardiography. Prenat Diagn 2005; 25(12): 1129-32.
[http://dx.doi.org/10.1002/pd.1286] [PMID: 16231299]

CHAPTER 8

Prenatal Diagnosis of Cardiac Malposition's and *situs* Anomalies

Laudelino M. Lopes[1,2,*], **Michael Tartar**[1], **Sheldon Bailey**[3], **Travis Kowlessar**[4] and **Judy A. Jones**[4]

[1] *London X-Ray Associates, London, Ontario, Canada*

[2] *Department of Obstetrics & Gynaecology, Maternal Fetal Medicine, Schulich School of Medicine & Dentistry - University of Western Ontario, London, Ontario, Canada*

[3] *College of New Caledonia Prince George. Prince George, British Columbia, Canada*

[4] *London Health Sciences Centre, London, Ontario, Canada*

Abstract: Cardiac position refers to the physical location of the heart relative to the thorax irrespective of cardiac axis. Deviation from its normal location can be due to extrinsic factors, embryologic defects, or as a result of structural cardiac abnormalities. In cardiology, *situs* refers to the position, arrangement and orientation of the various organs found in the abdomen (visceral) and thorax (*atrial situs*). In general, more complex congenital heart diseases (CHD) are associated with abnormalities of the *situs* such as *situs ambiguous* (isomerism or 'heterotaxy'). The heterotaxy syndrome has been linked to mutations of different genes and environmental factors (*e.g.* diabetes and retinoic acid exposure *in utero*) during the establishment of left-right asymmetry within earliest embryonic stages. Left atrial isomerism is associated with complete heart block and an increased risk of fetal hydrops, leading to poor *in utero* outcome. Conversely, right isomerism results in poorer postnatal outcomes since anomalous pulmonary venous return and complex cardiac anomalies are common findings in such cases. Prenatal diagnosis of cardiac position and *situs* abnormalities by cardiac ultrasound echocardiography can help guide recommendations concerning *in utero* and postnatal outcome.

Keywords: Abnormal cardiac position, Echocardiography.

ABNORMAL CARDIAC POSITION

Cardiac position refers to the physical location of the heart relative to the thorax irrespective of cardiac axis. Deviation from its normal location can be due to ext-

[*] **Corresponding author Laudelino M. Lopes**: Department of Obstetrics & Gynaecology, Schulich School of Medicine & Dentistry - University of Western Ontario, 104-450 Central Avenue, London, Ontario N6B 2E8, Tel: 519-672-5270; Ext: 7007; Fax: 519-672-2527; E-mail: lopes.laudelino@gmail.com

rinsic factors, embryologic defects, or as a result of structural cardiac abnormalities.

The fetal cardiac position can be assessed most readily in the 4-chamber view. In this view, by tracing sagittal and transverse planes through the center of the thorax, four quadrants can easily be identified. Typically, the majority of the fetal heart (approximately two-thirds) is positioned in the left anterior quadrant of the chest (levoposition) with the axis of its apex approximately 45 degrees to the left. The right ventricle is closest to the left anterior chest wall and the left atrium is closest to the descending aorta and spine. This normal position of the heart is traditionally described as levocardia (Fig. 1).

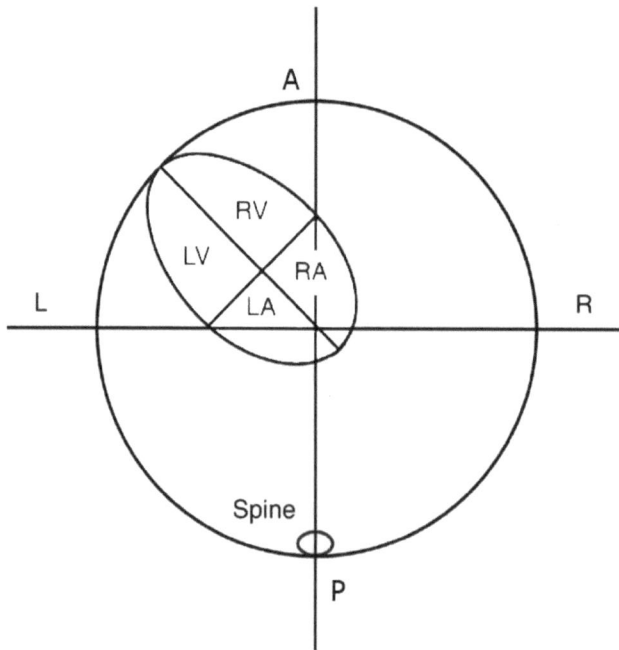

Fig. (1). Diagram depicting the position of the normal fetal heart position from the four-chamber view. A: Anterior; L: Left; LA: left atrium; LV: left ventricle; P: Posterior; R: Right; RA: right atrium; RV: right ventricle.

Whereas an abnormal cardiac axis is frequently associated with a *situs* or an intrinsic cardiac malformation, some abnormal positions of the heart such as dextrocardia are more commonly associated with an extrinsic or extracardiac abnormality such as a space-occupying lesion within the thorax.

Dextrocardia describes a heart located in the right aspect of the thorax while mesocardia refers to a heart positioned within the center thorax. The most extreme abnormal cardiac position is ectopia cordis, which refers to the heart outside of the thorax secondary to a defect during embryologic development.

Descriptive terms such as dextrocardia, dextroposition, or dextroversion are used interchangeably in the literature with no common agreement [1]. In general terms, dextrocardia describes the heart positioned in the right chest regardless of axis. Dextroposition can be thought of as a form of dextrocardia (heart within the right chest) with the heart axis to the left. Another form of dextrocardia is dextroversion where the heart is again located in the right chest, but the heart axis is to the right.

Since there is no definitive consensus regarding this terminology, however, an abnormal heart position should be described separately by its location (*i.e.* within the right chest) and whether the cardiac axis is left, mid, or right. With this terminology in mind, the following are descriptions of abnormal cardiac positions:

Levoposition

As previously mentioned, levocardia indicates the normal position of the heart within the left thorax. Levoposition (or extreme levocardia) signifies that the heart is abnormally shifted to the left usually in the presence of a right-sided space-occupying lesion such as a right lung mass (*e.g.* cystic adenomatoid malformation), a pleural effusion, a right-sided diaphragmatic hernia, or similar extracardiac pathologies (Fig. **2**).

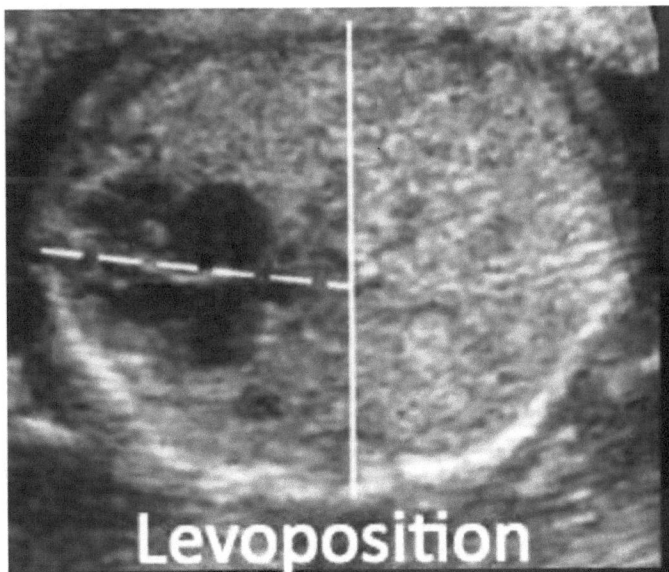

Fig. (2). Levoposition. The heart is abnormally positioned into the left thorax secondary to a cystic adenomatoid malformation.

Dextrocardia with Axis to the Left (Dextroposition)

This describes the heart positioned within the right thorax with a leftward axis and is most commonly due to an extrinsic factor such as a left-sided space-occupying lesion (*e.g.* congenital diaphragmatic hernia, a left lung mass, pleural effusion, bronchopulmonary sequestration, *etc.*) Right lung hypoplasia or agenesis can also produce a shift of the cardiac position to the right.

In most cases the heart is structurally normal and overall this abnormal position may improve in later gestation to the mid or left thorax if the causative lesion regresses (Fig. **3**).

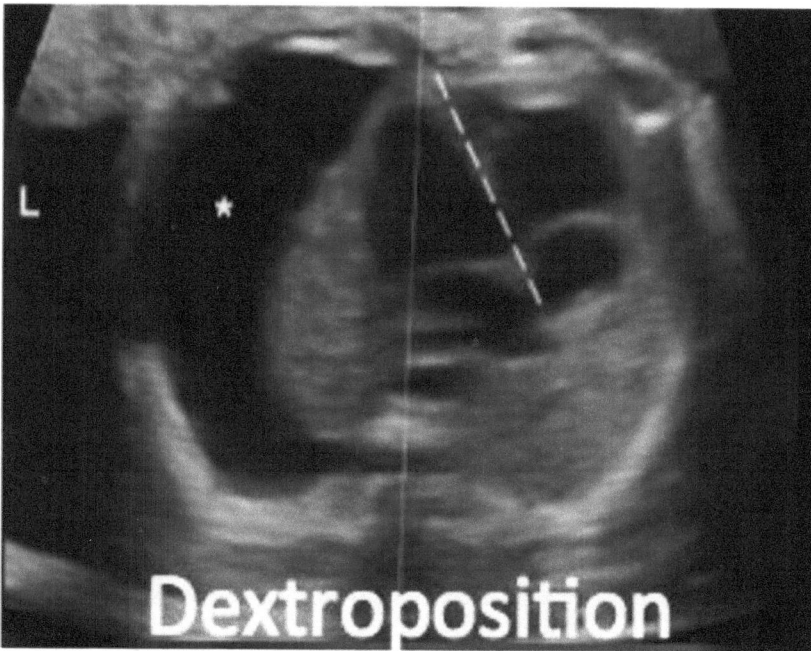

Fig. (3). Dextrocardia with axis to the left. The heart is abnormally positioned into the right thorax due to a left pleural effusion*. L: Left.

Classic Mirror Image Dextrocardia

With this condition the majority of the heart is located within the right chest and the axis of the apex is to the left. Importantly, the chambers are a mirror image of normal. The left atrium and left ventricle are on the patient's right, while the right atrium and right ventricle are on the patient's left. There is also a condition called ventricular inversion where only the ventricles are inverted in position. When abdominal *situs inversus* and mirror image dextrocardia are present together this is known as *situs inversus* totalis. In this condition there are usually no associated structural cardiac abnormalities.

Dextrocardia with Axis to the Right (Dextroversion)

This abnormality describes the heart situated within the right thorax with a rightward axis. It is more commonly associated with intrinsic cardiac anomalies such as atrial or ventricular inversion, congenitally corrected transposition of the great arteries, atrioventricular discordance, and isomerism (most often right-atrial isomerism) (Figs. **4** and **5**).

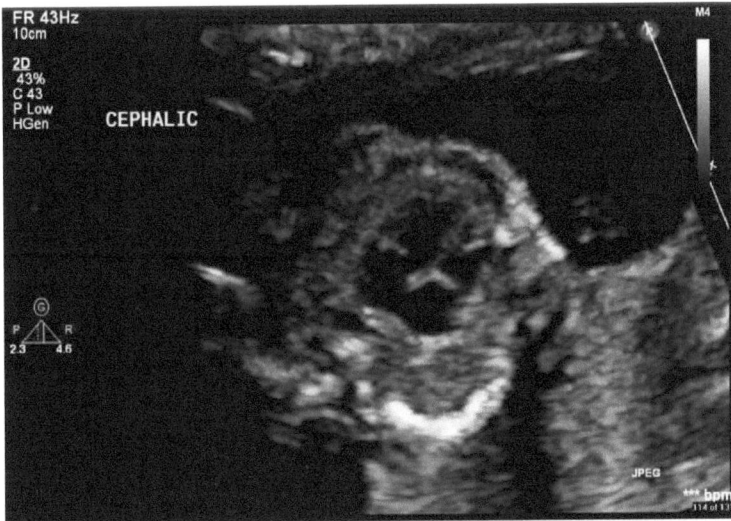

Fig. (4). Dextrocardia with axis to the right. This is a case of *situs inversus* where the heart is abnormally positioned into the right thorax with the axis to the right.

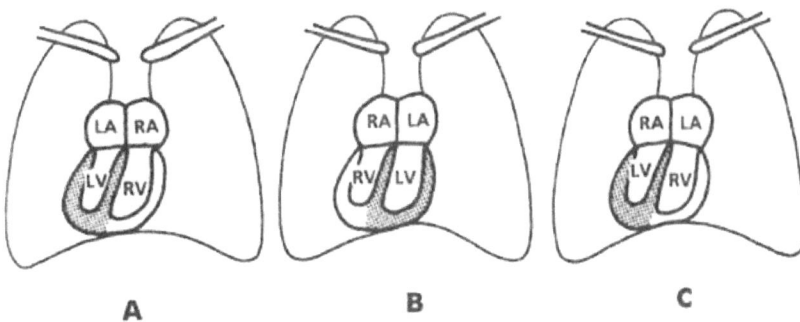

Fig. (5). Common condition in dextrocardia: (**A**) Mirror-image dextrocardia - The RA and RV are leftward and LA and LV are rightward. This can be readily identified with a detailed assessment of the 4-chamber view; (**B**) Dextroversion – The chambers are in the typical positions but with apex to the right; (**C**) Ventricular Inversion- The ventricles are inverted in position. This can also be readily identified with a detailed assessment of the 4-chamber view. RA: right atrium; RV: right ventricle; LA: left atrium; LV: left ventricle.

Mesocardia

Mesocardia describes the heart in the mid thorax with the axis usually directed toward the midline of the chest. It can be associated with heart defects primarily involving the ventriculoarterial connections (*i.e.* transposition of the great arteries and double outlet right ventricle). In addition, single ventricle, common trunk, ventricular septal defect, and pulmonary stenosis have been reported [2]. Enlargement of the lungs, such as the with the condition of laryngeal stenosis or atresia has also been associated with this abnormal cardiac position. Otherwise, the prognosis of mesocardia is generally considered good, but only in its isolated form without chromosomal or associated anomalies (Fig. **6**).

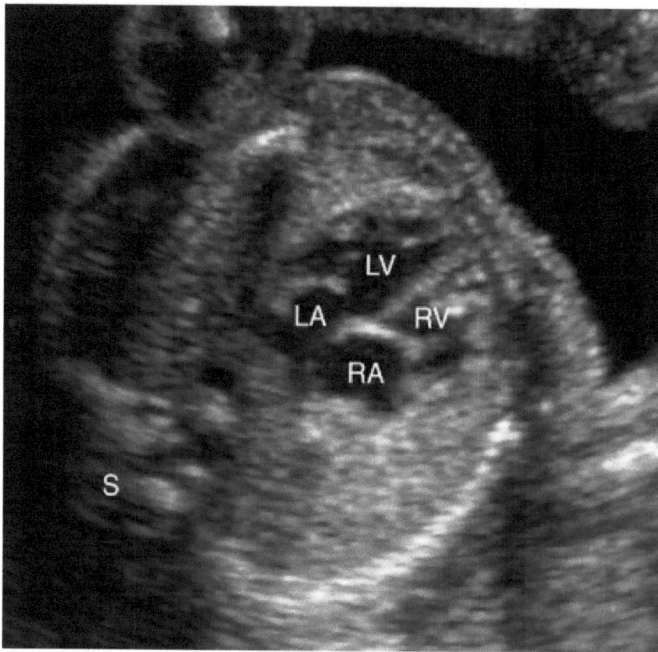

Fig. (6). Mesocardia. The heart is within the central thorax with the apex directed midline. *LA:* left atrium; *LV:* left ventricle; *RA:* right atrium; *RV:* right ventricle; *S:* spine.

Ectopia Cordis

Five types of ectopia cordis are described based on the location of the heart: cervical, thoracocervical, thoracic, thoracoabdominal and abdominal [3]. All classifications of ectopia cordis involve a partial or complete displacement of the heart out of the thoracic cavity [4]. The exact etiology of ectopia cordis is unknown, but it's secondary to defects in the sternum, ventral lower thorax, midepigastrium, diaphragm, or anterior pericardium.

Most incidences of ectopia cordis are isolated, but it can be associated with pentalogy of Cantrell, limb-body wall complex and amniotic band syndrome. Cardiac defects can vary from simple atrial or ventricular septal defects to tetralogy of Fallot or other more complex lesions.

A variety of other cardiac abnormalities can be associated with this condition and although the fetal karyotype is usually normal, trisomy 13 and Turner's syndrome have been described with this condition [5] (Fig. 7).

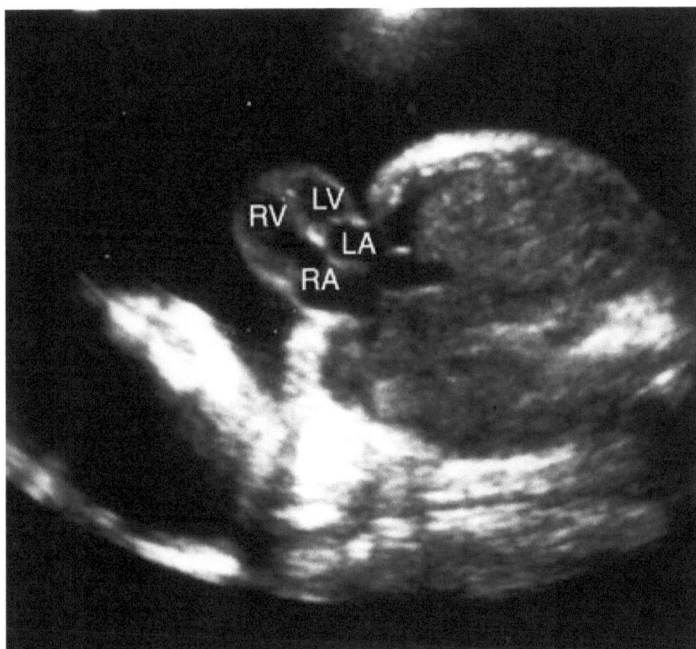

Fig. (7). Thoracoabdominal ectopia cordis in a fetus with pentalogy of Cantrell. The heart lies outside the chest wall in this anomaly due to a sternal defect. *LA:* left atrium; *LV:* left ventricle; *RA:* right atrium; *RV:* right ventricle.

Underscoring the importance of an abnormal cardiac position a retrospective review of 3,556 fetal echocardiograms between 2000 and 2011 revealed an incidence of dextrocardia at 1.1%. Of the 39 fetuses, 22 were primary dextrocardia and 17 were dextroposition. Congenital diaphragmatic hernia was the most common cause of dextroposition with an incidence of 76%. Of the fetuses with dextroposition 35.5% had a cardiac anomaly. The survival rate of dextroposition was only 31.2% and none of the survivors had an associated cardiac anomaly. Primary fetal dextrocardia was most common with *situs solitus* (45.4%), followed by *situs ambiguous* (36.3%) and then *situs inversus* totalis (18.1%). Structural cardiac malformations were found in 100%, 80% and 25% of fetuses with *situs ambiguous*, solitus and inversus, respectively. Of the 17 cases of dextroposition, 47.6% terminated pregnancy, 14.2% resulted in intrauterine death,

9.5% died after birth, and only 28.5% survived [5].

In conclusion, an abnormal cardiac position can be associated with a wide spectrum of complex cardiac malformations potentially signifying a poor prognosis. Whereas an abnormal cardiac axis is associated with a 50% mortality an abnormal cardiac position has an associated 81% mortality [6].

The cardiac position and cardiac axis can be readily identified using the 4-chamber view and is a critically important feature of the fetal heart. When an abnormal cardiac position is identified, a thorough investigation of the cardiac structures as well as any potential underlying, extrinsic anomaly is essential. Proper assessment and classification of the cardiac position with an emphasis on describing the heart's location separately from (and in addition to) its axis are fundamental and vital components of the fetal cardiac evaluation.

CARDIAC MALPOSITIONS AND *SITUS* ANOMALIES

Situs

'*Situs*' is a latin term that refers to the position or place of a particular object. In cardiology, *situs* refers to the position, arrangement and orientation of the various organs found in the abdomen and thorax. This term is further qualified by other latin derivatives to speak to the various visceral arrangements that may be present in the human body. These terms are:

1. *Situs Solitus:* (solitus – normal): the normal and expected arrangement of the thoracic and abdominal organs.
2. *Situs Inversus:* (inversus – inverted): a situation where the positions of the thoracic and abdominal organs are the direct opposite of the normal arrangement – a *mirrored* arrangement.
3. *Situs Ambiguous:* refers to any arrangement of the viscera that does not fit into *situs solitus* or *situs inversus*.

Situs Solitus

When considering *situs* of the fetal thorax and abdomen, it is useful to interrogate each major aspect of the viscera individually. That is, the organs of the abdomen should be examined independent of those in the thorax, and the configuration of the heart separate from both the abdomen and the thorax.

Abdomen

For the purpose of *situs* identification, the fetal abdomen should be examined in the transverse plane. In the normal fetal abdomen, the stomach is to the left of the spine (below the diaphragm) with the liver and gallbladder being predominantly to the right of the spine. The spleen is always adjacent to the greater curvature of the stomach.

Vascular landmarks are also present in the descending aorta (DA) and the inferior vena cava (IVC). The DA should be seen directly in front of the spine in the midline, with the IVC anterior and to the right of the DA (Fig. **8**).

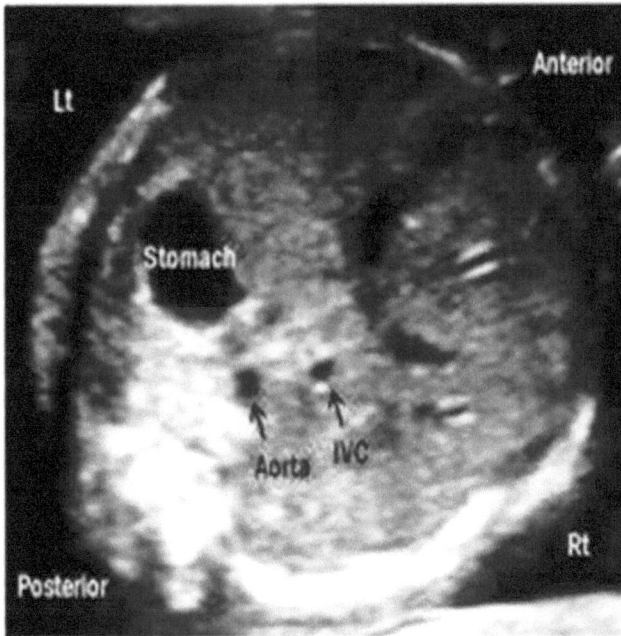

Fig. (8). Transverse view of the fetal abdomen showing the normal location of landmarks. IVC: inferior vena cava.

Thorax

Thoracic *situs* is often difficult to accurately appreciate on a fetal ultrasound but should be considered when doing such an exam. In *situs solitus*, the right lung is tri-lobed, larger and associated with a shorter bronchus than the bilobed left lung. The difference in the size of the lungs is an apparent embryologic facilitation of the size and orientation of the heart [7].

Heart

Fetal cardiac position refers to the position of the heart within the chest and is independent of the fetal cardiac axis [1]. The normal left-sided position of the heart is termed as *levocardia*. *Dextrocardia* describes a heart in the right of the chest and *mesocardia* refers to a heart that is centrally located in the chest. In *ectopia cordis,* the heart is outside of the chest.

It is generally accepted that the most reliable method of determining *situs* of the heart is by the location and correct identification of the atria and their systemic venous connections [8]. In *situs solitus*, the morphologic right atrium is on the same side as the liver, gallbladder and the IVC while the morphologic left atrium, DA, stomach and spleen are ipsilateral.

Situs Inversus

Situs inversus totalis refers to a mirror-image arrangement of the visceral and thoracic structures to that of *situs solitus* [1]. This anomaly may not be diagnosed until late life in some cases and it is associated with primary ciliary dyskinesia and splenic malformations. It may be total or incomplete in 10% of cases. Partial *situs inversus* can either be restricted to to the abdominal organs (*situs inversus* with levocardia) or limited to the chest (dextrocardia) [1].

Situs inversus is rarely symptomatic but may be associated with digestive difficulties [9]. In a fetus with this condition, the arrangement of the abdominal and thoracic organs will be a direct opposite to what is considered normal. That is, the liver, gallbladder, right atrium and IVC will be on the fetal left side, while the stomach, spleen, left atrium and aorta will be on the fetal right side. The apex of the heart commonly points to the right of the thorax, instead of the left (dextrocardia). Additionally, the anatomical right lung will be bilobed while the anatomical left lung will be trilobed.

In general, *situs inversus* is a rare phenomenon, reportedly occuring in 0.00005% of patients [8]. There is concordance between the atrial and visceral *situs* in most of these cases. Occasionally, the apex of the heart will point leftward in *situs inversus*. This is known as levoversion or isolated levocardia – explained in greater detail further on in this chapter. A persistent left superior vena cava can also be present in rare cases [1].

Cardiac anomalies in *situs inversus* are found in 0.3 – 5% of affected patients [1, 8]. Cardiac anomalies associated with *situs inversus* include tetralogy of Fallot, ventricular septal defect and double outlet right ventricle. Complete or corrected transposition of the great arteries have been recorded in *situs inversus*. *Situs inversus* is also commonly associated with Kartagener syndrome, with about 50% of patients with this syndrome having *situs inversus*. However, *situs inversus* frequently remains undetected in life until diagnosed for unrelated reasons, as extracardiac malformations are not typical for this anomaly.

Situs Ambiguous

Any arrangement of the visceral or thoracic organs that do not identify as solitus or inversus is considered to be *situs ambiguous*. These may also be referred to as 'unknown' or 'complex' situs, isomerism, heterotaxy or cardio splenic syndromes. Cardio splenic syndrome was first used to describe *situs ambiguous* with an associated splenic abnormality [1]. However, since the spleen is not always abnormal in *in situs* ambiguous it cannot be reliably used for classification. The term 'heterotaxy' (Greek – *heteros* means different and *taxis* means arrangement) was then suggested to refer to these *situs* changes. Terms such as right and left isomerism - relating to the abnormal configuration of the heart and associated venous drainage pathways - have also found their place in the description of *situs ambiguous* abnormalities. These terms will be further addressed later in this chapter.

Heterotaxy syndrome is found in 2.2% - 4.2% of fetuses/infants with congenital heart disease [1]. Left isomerism is more common than right isomerism in fetuses while right isomerism is more common than left in infants. This phenomenon is attributed to the fact that *in-utero* demise is more likely in fetuses with left atrial isomerism, since complete heartblock and hydrops have an increased prevalence with this abnormality [1].

Heterotaxy syndrome has been linked to mutations of different genes during the establishment of left-right asymmetry within earliest embryonic stages. Mutations in at least 20 of the genes involved in this process have been identified in people with heterotaxy syndrome. There have been rare cases where genetic chromosomal changes such as deletions, insertions, duplications or other rearrangements have been associated with heterotaxy [10] (Fig. **9**).

To date, no single etiological factor responsible for the development of abnormal lateralization and isomerism has been reported. Evidence from human studies and animal models suggests causal heterogeneity. Interestingly however, Asian and Hispanic infants have shown a higher prevalence of heterotaxy syndrome when compared to Westerners [11, 12]. The reason for this has not been established.

Unlike with *situs solitus* or *situs inversus*, *situs ambiguous* is associated with various anomalies, both intra and extra cardiac. Associated extracardiac anomalies mainly involve organs within the abdominal cavity such as bowel atresia or bowel malrotation [1]. Persistent vomiting in the neonatal period should raise suspicion of an upper gastrointestinal obstruction owing to duodenal atresia or compression. Also, late intestinal obstruction might be caused by gastrointestinal malrotation or gastric volvulus [11].

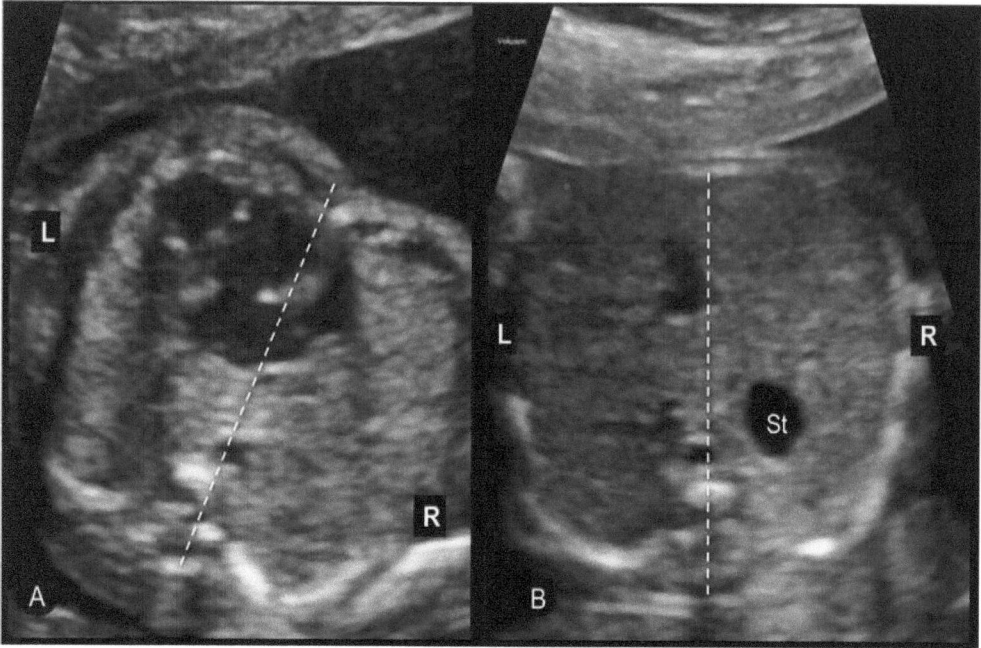

Fig. (9). Axial views of the fetal chest (**A**) and abdomen (**B**) in a fetus with heterotaxy syndrome. Heterotaxy was suspected on ultrasound examination by the presence of the heart in the left side of the chest (**A**) and the presence of the stomach (St) in the upper right abdomen (**B**). Note the presence of an abnormal four-chamber view suggesting a complex cardiac malformation. L: left; R: right.

There is also a high incidence of abnormalities of the biliary tree, especially biliary atresia, in isomerism. Routine abdominal ultrasound, with a focus on the biliary tree, is warranted even in the absence of jaundice in infants with left isomerism [11]. Anomalies of the spleen can present as asplenia (Ivemark syndrome) or polysplenia. The presence and/or state of the spleen should be established in all patients.

Features of *situs ambiguous* on prenatal ultrasound include polysplenia, non-immune hydrops fetalis, right-sided stomach, a mid-line liver, AVSD, heartblock and an interrupted IVC with azygous continuation.

HETEROTAXY

Heterotaxy is generally described as the deficiency of the natural left and right asymmetry of internal organs that have developed, usually, due to an underlying genetic condition. It is defined as the presence of a pattern of spatial organization of the thoracic and abdominal viscera that is neither that of *situs solitus* nor that of *situs inversus* [13]. Any arrangement other than *situs solitus* or inversus is known as *situs ambiguous*. Patients with heterotaxy syndrome can be further classified into cardio splenic syndromes; asplenia is generally associated with right atrial isomerism and polysplenia with left atrial isomerism which are the two most common forms [14]. Although right and left atrial isomerism are commonly used terms, it is important to note that actual atrial isomerism does not exist. It is only the appendages that are isomeric (symmetrical mirror images or each other) in the setting of Heterotaxy. Those having isomeric right atrial appendages frequently have bilaterally tri-lobed lungs, each with a short bronchus and absence of the spleen. Those having isomeric left atrial appendages frequently have bilaterally bi-lobed lungs, each with a long bronchus and multiple spleens [15]. Although it can be difficult to classify certain patients into a specific cardio splenic syndromes the majority of published studies estimate the incidence of heterotaxy at 10-14 per 100,000 live births [16, 17]. The relative frequency of heterotaxy syndrome is reported as 2.3-4.2% of congenital heart disease [18]. Whatever type of classification system is used, the imager should provide an accurate description of the thoraco-abdominal visceral *situs* and of all cardiovascular abnormalities though a detailed segmental approach. Noncardiac abnormalities associated with cardio splenic syndromes, aside from *situs* abnormalities, may include duodenal atresia, esophageal abnormalities, malrotation of the bowel and mesentery, absence of gall bladder and biliary atresia [14, 19].

Embryology/Etiology

Although it is still not known what causes each particular defect in conditions of Heterotaxy, an embryogenic insult occurring between the 28th and 35th days of gestation has been postulated to result in the spectrum of developmental abnormalities that is considered asplenia or polysplenia [14]. In normal development, growth of the endocardial cushions and septation of the conotruncus occur during the fifth week of gestation. Additionally, during this embryologic period, lobation of the lungs and rotation of the gut begin. The connection of the pulmonary veins occurs shortly after this, around 30-32 days, around the same time as the spleen develops from the mesogastrium. An insult during this period of development may give rise to certain malformations, including errors in symmetry or laterality. There may also be complex genetics that control different pathways that give rise to defects in left-right asymmetry. Studies in humans and mouse models suggest an autosomal recessive inheritance with variable penetrance, but polygenic or multifactorial causes have also been implicated [18, 20]. More recently, an X-linked recessive gene defect has been found in familial and sporadic forms of the laterality syndromes. Also, environmental factors can influence the incidence of the disease as studies have shown that diabetes and retinoic acid exposure *in utero* can be potential risk factors [18].

Left Atrial Isomerism

At first this condition may present itself to the obstetric sonographer as an arrhythmia or bradycardia. There is also a high incidence of complete heart block prenatally (68%) and may carry a differential diagnosis of a junctional escape rhythm. There may be identifiers that are curious due to associated defects that alter the initial presentation of the cardiac anatomy. The fetus may also present with fetal hydrops and the cardiac axis may be abnormal, with the apex either located more leftward or more centrally in the chest [21]. The most consistent indicators of polysplenia appear to be an interrupted inferior vena cava with azygous continuation which drains into the superior vena cava [14]. On cross-sectional scanning, two vessels are seen in the posterior mediastinum on long-axis or cross-sectional views of the thorax; the more posterior vessel is the azygous vein. There may be a partial or complete atrioventricular septal defect seen in the four-chamber view in common with an enlarged cardiac to thoracic circumference ratio (>50%) [21].

Sonographic Features

- Axis of the heart more leftward or more central than normal.
- Inferior vena cava not seen in the normal position in the upper abdomen.
- Hepatic veins drain directly to the atrial mass.
- Two vascular channels behind the heart.
- Atrioventricular septal defect.
- May be associated with complete heart block.
- Heart dilated and hypertrophied if complete heart block.
- Atrial septum may be abnormally aligned with anomalies of the pulmonary venous drainage.

Right Atrial Isomerism

Initially this condition may present itself to the obstetric sonographer due to the discrepancy between the stomach and sidedness of the heart. A common atrium with total anomalous pulmonary venous connection is synonymous with right atrial isomerism, because of this the pulmonary venous connection needs to be carefully examined. The most common connection is for a venous confluence to drain directly, with no obstruction, to the center of the atrial mass. Although the confluence may drain to an ascending or descending channel. The incidence of cardiac abnormalities associated with right atrial isomerism and asplenia is high. Atrioventricular septal defects are reported in approximately 85 to 95% of cases. Transposition of the great arteries, and pulmonary atresia or stenosis (80-90%) are also commonly associated with asplenia. A malpositioned inferior vena cava, which may be anterior or juxtaposed to the aorta, is frequently seen [14, 22].

Sonographic Features

- Discordant stomach and cardiac apex
- Inferior cava and aorta lie on the same side of spine
- Inferior vena cava lies directly anterior to the aorta in the upper abdomen
- Often associated with complex intracardiac anomalies and Pulmonary venous drainage

Prognosis

Long-term prognosis is frequently dependent on the occurrence of complications related to obstruction of the pulmonary veins, distortion of the pulmonary arteries, elevated pulmonary vascular resistance, atrioventricular valve regurgitation, or depressed ventricular function [18]. Many cases also have a more dominant ventricle due to unbalancing associated with certain lesions. The outlook for such cases has been poor for cases reported postnatally and this must be conveyed to the parents. If these conditions occur in combination with complete/third degree heart block, this sets the seen for an adverse prognostic indication with additional risk of intrauterine death. For both forms of isomerism associated with more complex cardiac abnormalities presenting before 24 weeks of gestation, termination of pregnancy is an option that the parents may want to consider [21]. Despite the improved success rate of corrective and palliative surgeries in recent years, mortality remains high with 5-year survival rates ranging from 30-74% for right atrial isomerism/asplenia and 65-84% for left isomerism/polysplenia [4].

CONSENT FOR PUBLICATION

Not applicable.

CONFLICT OF INTEREST

The authors confirm that the contents of this chapter have no conflict of interest.

ACKNOWLEDGEMENTS

Declare none.

REFERENCES

[1]   Abuhamad A, Chaoui R. A Practical Guide to Fetal Echocardiography. 3rd ed. Philadelphia: Wolters/Kluwer 2016; pp. 72-4.

[2]   Comstock CH. Normal fetal heart axis and position. Obstet Gynecol 1987; 70(2): 255-9. [PMID: 3299186]

[3]   Dobell AR, Williams HB, Long RW. Staged repair of ectopia cordis. J Pediatr Surg 1982; 17(4): 353-8. [http://dx.doi.org/10.1016/S0022-3468(82)80487-9] [PMID: 7120001]

[4]   Hagler DJ, O'Leary PW. Cardiac malposition and abnormalities of atrial and visceral situs.Heart Disease in Infants, Children, and Adolescents Including the Fetus and Young Adult. 5th ed. Baltimore, MD: Williams & Wilkins 1995; pp. 1307-36.

[5]   Oztunc F, Madazli R, Yuksel MA, Gökalp S, Oncul M. Diagnosis and outcome of pregnancies with prenatally diagnosed fetal dextrocardia. J Matern Fetal Neonatal Med 2015; 28(9): 1104-7. [http://dx.doi.org/10.3109/14767058.2014.943659] [PMID: 25007986]

[6]   Stamm ER, Drose JA. The Fetal Heart Rumack CM. 4th ed. Philadelphia, PA: Elsevier/Mosby 2011; p. 1297.

[7]   Lee MY, Won HS. Technique of fetal echocardiography. Obstet Gynecol Sci 2013; 56(4): 217-26. [http://dx.doi.org/10.5468/ogs.2013.56.4.217] [PMID: 24328006]

[8]   Drose J. Fetal Echocadiography. St. Louis, MS: Saunders Elsevier 2010.

[9]   Sharma S, Chaitanya KK, Suseelamma D. *Situs inversus* totalis (dextroversion) - an anatomical study. Anat Physiol 2012; 2: 112. [http://dx.doi.org/10.4172/2161-0940.1000112]

[10]   Reference GH. 2018.https://ghr.nlm.nih.gov/condition/heterotaxy-syndrome

[11]   Kim SJ. Heterotaxy syndrome. Korean Circ J 2011; 41(5): 227-32. [http://dx.doi.org/10.4070/kcj.2011.41.5.227] [PMID: 21731561]

[12]   Lopez KN, Marengo LK, Canfield MA, Belmont JW, Dickerson HA. Racial disparities in heterotaxy syndrome. Birth Defects Res A Clin Mol Teratol 2015; 103(11): 941-50. [http://dx.doi.org/10.1002/bdra.23416] [PMID: 26333177]

[13]   Jacobs JP, Anderson RH, Weinberg PM, *et al.* The nomenclature, definition and classification of cardiac structures in the setting of heterotaxy. Cardiol Young 2007; 17 (Suppl. 2): 1-28. [http://dx.doi.org/10.1017/S1047951107001138] [PMID: 18039396]

[14]   Derose JA. Cardio splenic Syndromes Fetal Echocardiograpy. 1st ed. Philidelphia, PA: WB Saunders Company 1998; pp. 253-62.

[15]   Van Praagh S, Kreutzer J, Alday L, Van Praagh R. Systemic and pulmonary venous connections in visceral heterotaxy, with emphasis on the diagnosis of atrial situs: a study of 109 postmortem cases.Developmental Cardiology: Morphogenesis and Function. Mount Kisko, NY: Futura Publishing Co 1990; pp. 671-727.

[16]   Gilljam T, McCrindle BW, Smallhorn JF, Williams WG, Freedom RM. Outcomes of left atrial isomerism over a 28-year period at a single institution. J Am Coll Cardiol 2000; 36(3): 908-16. [http://dx.doi.org/10.1016/S0735-1097(00)00812-3] [PMID: 10987619]

[17]   Lim JS, McCrindle BW, Smallhorn JF, *et al.* Clinical features, management, and outcome of children with fetal and postnatal diagnoses of isomerism syndromes. Circulation 2005; 112(16): 2454-61. [http://dx.doi.org/10.1161/CIRCULATIONAHA.105.552364] [PMID: 16216960]

[18]   Lai WW, Mertens LL, Cohen MS, Geva T. Cardiac Malpositions and Heterotaxy Syndrome Echocardiography in Pediatric and Congenital Heart Disease from fetus to adult. 2nd ed. West Sussex: John Wiley & Sons Ltd 2016; pp. 558-83. [http://dx.doi.org/10.1002/9781118742440]

[19]   Brown DL, Emerson DS, Shulman LP, Doubilet PM, Felker RE, Van Praagh S. Predicting aneuploidy in fetuses with cardiac anomalies: significance of visceral *situs* and noncardiac anomalies. J Ultrasound Med 1993; 12(3): 153-61. [http://dx.doi.org/10.7863/jum.1993.12.3.153] [PMID: 8492378]

[20]   Chin AJ, Saint-Jeannet JP, Lo CW. How insights from cardiovascular developmental biology have impacted the care of infants and children with congenital heart disease. Mech Dev 2012; 129(5-8): 75-97. [http://dx.doi.org/10.1016/j.mod.2012.05.005] [PMID: 22640994]

[21]   Allan L, Hornberger L, Sharland G. Heterotaxy syndromes/isomerism of the atrial appendages Textbook of Fetal Cardiology. 1ˢᵗ ed. London: Greenwich Medical Media Limited 2000; pp. 333-46.

[22]   Neil CA, Zukerberg AL. Syndromes and congenital heart defects.Critical Heart Disease in Infants and Children. St Louis, MS: Mosby-Year Book 1995; pp. 987-1012.

CHAPTER 9

Fetal Septal Defects

Darren Hutchinson[1,2] and **Ricardo Palma-Dias**[3,4,*]

[1] *Fetal Cardiology Unit, Royal Women's Hospital, Melbourne, Australia*

[2] *Department of Cardiology, Royal Children's Hospital Melbourne, Australia*

[3] *Ultrasound Department, Pauline Gandel Women's Imaging Centre, Royal Women's Hospital, Melbourne, Australia*

[4] *Department of Obstetrics and Gynaecology, University of Melbourne, Melbourne, Australia*

Abstract: The frequency of the different fetal septal defects and their presentation prenatally is described, including atrial septum defects (ASDs), ventricular septum defects (VSDs) and atrioventricular septum defects (AVSDs). Embryology of the defects and the association with underlying aneuploidy and genetic syndromes are discussed. Image findings in the fetal period are presented alongside diagrams to aide comprehension of the ultrasound views. A brief summary of prognosis and postnatal course of these conditions is also included.

Keywords: Atrial septum defect, Atrioventricular septum defect, Aneuploidy, Congenital anomalies, Fetal cardiology, Prenatal diagnosis, Ultrasound, Ventricular septum defect.

ATRIAL SEPTAL DEFECTS

Atrial septal defects (ASDs) postnatally are one of the commonest postnatal cardiac lesions [1], accounting for up to 10% of postnatal lesions. In the fetal circulation, the foramen ovale is essential in allowing streaming of highly oxygenated blood from the placental circulation through to the left atrium and then to the systemic fetal circulation. The foramen ovale is a normal fetal cardiac structure and not pathological. Persistence of a foramen ovale postnatally, termed a patent foramen ovale (PFO), is a very common finding and seen in up to 10% of the adult population [2]. Interventional closure of a PFO is rarely required.

Abnormal atrial septal defects are rarely diagnosed in the prenatal period, mostly due to the presence of the foramen ovale.

---

[*] **Corresponding author Ricardo Palma-Dias:** Department of Ultrasound , Pauline Gandel Women's Imaging Centre, Royal Women's Hospital, 20 Flemington Road, Parkville 3052, Melbourne, Victoria, Australia; E-mail: Ricardo.Palma-Dias@thewomens.org.au

Edward Araujo Júnior, Nathalie Jeanne M. Bravo-Valenzuela and Alberto Borges Peixoto (Eds.)

Atrial septal defects seen postnatally include:

1. Secundum atrial septal defects: these are the commonest subtype and occur in the area of the fossa ovalis. Many of these will become smaller over time with very few ultimately requiring intervention [3].
2. Sinus venosus defect: these occur as a defect in the superior or inferior atrial septum. These may be associated with partial anomalous pulmonary venous drainage and are rarely diagnosed prenatally.
3. Coronary sinus atrial septal defect: these are rare defects, associated with the roof of the coronary sinus, and generally not diagnosed in the prenatal or early postnatal period.
4. Primum atrial defect defects: these are generally associated with common atrioventricular (AV) valves and will be discussed further in this chapter.

Isolated atrial septal defects are not usually associated with chromosomal anomalies. One exception is Holt-Oram Syndrome, in which atrial septal defects are common along with upper limb skeletal anomalies.

Primum atrial septal defects are the most commonly prenatally diagnosed ASDs and, as mentioned, are usually part of the AV septal defect complex. On imaging it is important to distinguish these from dilation of the coronary sinus which can mimic a primum defect. A dilated coronary sinus is usually secondary to a persistent left superior vena cava (SVC) or, more rarely, in intracardiac total anomalous pulmonary venous drainage. The coronary sinus is a linear structure in the very back of the left atrium, behind the AV valves. Importantly with a dilated coronary sinus, the primum septum will still be present anterior to the coronary sinus, excluding a primum type ASD in this situation.

Postnatally, atrial septal defects rarely present in the newborn period and will often remain undiagnosed for many years even when large. A cardiac murmur is often not heard, and when it is, is related to increased flow across the pulmonary valve rather than flow across the atrial septal defect itself.

VENTRICULAR SEPTAL DEFECTS

Introduction

Ventricular septal defects (VSDs) are the most commonly diagnosed congenital heart defect postnatally [1]. However, prenatally this is not the case, with more complex congenital heart lesions predominating due to their severity and more obvious appearance on prenatal imaging.

Embryology

Ventricular septation occurs from days 38 through to 46. A muscular ridge forms in the floor of the early ventricle and propagates towards the base of the heart from its inferior aspect. Separately, the membranous septum fuses from both the endocardial cushions and the muscular septum [4].

Genetic Associations

Isolated VSDs are generally not associated with an increased risk of chromosomal anomalies [5], with Gomez *et al.* showing no clinically relevant chromosomal anomalies in 116 fetuses with isolated muscular VSDs. Perimembranous VSDs (pmVSD) have a slightly higher incidence of chromosomal anomalies, 3.1% in the same study. When additional cardiac anomalies are seen, or indeed any extra-cardiac malformations, then certainly the incidence of chromosomal abnormalities increases significantly [6].

Prenatal Detection

The majority of muscular and pmVSDs remain undiagnosed prenatally. Muscular VSDs are the commonest sub type diagnosed prenatally accounting for 85-90% of the VSDs found [5]. However, postnatally perimembranous defects predominate, likely due to the fact that they are less likely to spontaneously close and hence more likely to present with a cardiac murmur and clinical symptoms over time.

Classification

Ventricular septal defects can be divided into three main groups (Fig. **1**)

1. Inlet muscular VSDs: these are defects located immediately below the inlet valves and are usually associated with reduced offset of the AV valves and are in fact incomplete forms of AV septal defects.

2. Mid or apical muscular VSDs: these are the commonest types of ventricular septal defects seen prenatally. These may be seen on two-dimensional imaging and on colour flow, or in the smaller defects, on colour flow only. A common location for these defects is immediately below the moderator band of the right ventricle. These defects are the most likely to close in the prenatal or very early postnatal period.

3. Perimembranous and outlet VSDs: pmVSDs occur immediately below the aortic valve. They may be associated with a degree of aortic override but this is not always the case. If the aortic valve overrides the pmVSD by more than 50%, than this is termed double outlet right ventricle (DORV). A pmVSD which is

associated with aortic override (<50%) and pulmonary stenosis is then called tetralogy of Fallot.

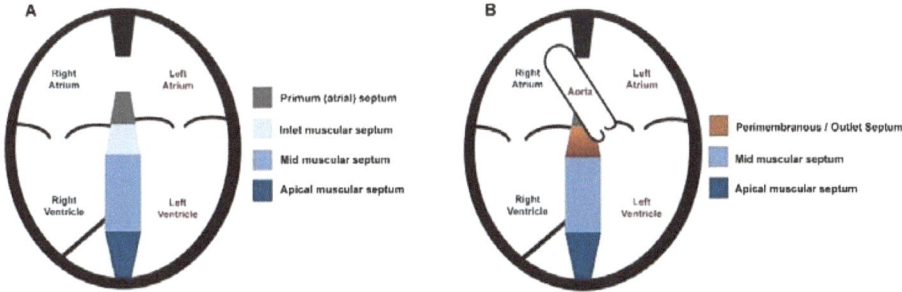

Fig. (1). A. Four chamber view showing different anatomical segments of the muscular ventricular septum. The moderator band is shown in the right ventricle. B. Left ventricular outflow tract view showing the mid-muscular and apical septum along with the perimembranous region with the aorta on view.

Fetal Imaging

The prenatal diagnosis of fetal VSDs relies on imaging the fetal ventricular septum in multiple imaging planes, using both two dimensional and colour flow imaging. The interventricular septum should be imaged perpendicular to the imaging beam wherever possible (Fig. 2). Multiple imaging planes should be utilised, including the four chamber view, the left ventricular outflow tract view and ideally short axis planes. The left ventricular outflow view (Fig. 3) is ideal for assessing pmVSDs, with lack of continuity between the ventricular septum and the aortic valve being seen with a pmVSD. A sweep through the ventricular septum in these multiple planes, one on two-dimensional (2D) and one with colour, allows complete assessment of the ventricular septum. Colour settings should be such to allow the diagnosis of smaller septal defects, whilst reducing false-positive findings. A Nyquist of 50 – 70cm/s is generally recommended.

Once the diagnosis of a fetal VSD is made a thorough assessment of the remainder of the fetal cardiac anatomy is needed. Muscular VSDs are often isolated. In comparison, a pmVSD may be associated with multiple additional intracardiac anomalies such as pulmonary stenosis, such as in tetralogy of Fallot. A subaortic ventricular septal defect with a sub aortic conus may display subaortic stenosis and consequently aortic valve stenosis and aortic arch coarctation or aortic interruption (Fig. 4).

Perinatal Management

Due to equalised left and right ventricular pressures in the fetal heart the presence of small or even large VSDs are generally of little haemodynamic consequence prenatally. Assuming no major extra cardiac lesions or fetal chromosomal anomalies, then timing of delivery should not be altered nor should mode of delivery. However, if there are any concerns regarding associated left or right ventricular outflow tract obstruction related to the VSD, then prenatal and early postnatal management may need to be appropriately modified.

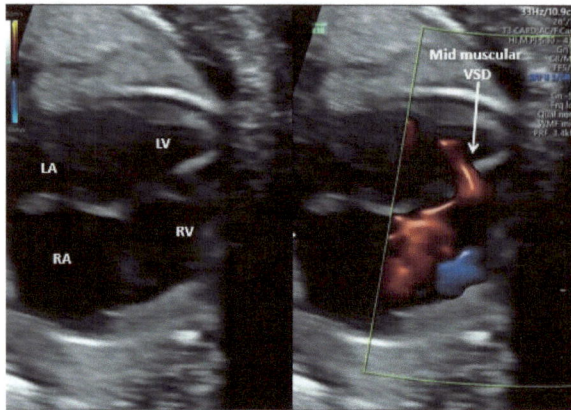

Fig. (2). Four-chamber view with ventricular septum perpendicular to ultrasound beam. Mid muscular ventricular septal defect (VSD) seen on 2D image and further defined with colour flow. RA: right atrium; LA: left atrium; RV: right ventricle; LV: left ventricle.

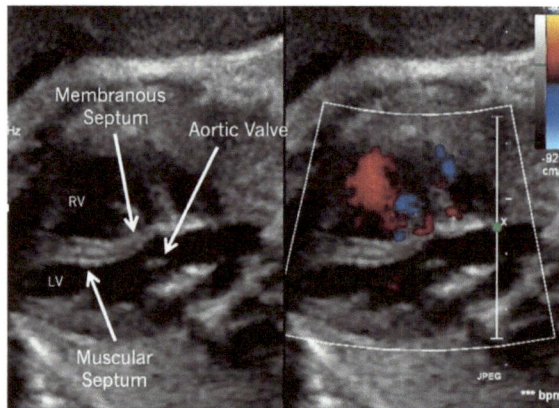

Fig. (3). Left ventricular outflow tract view showing location of the muscular and membranous septum. RV: right ventricle; LV: left ventricle.

Postnatally, the majority of isolated VSDs are asymptomatic in the first days and weeks after birth. It is not until the pulmonary pressure reduce that clinical symptoms may develop. Isolated mid or apical muscular ventricular septal defects have a very high chance of spontaneous closure over time: either in fetal life if diagnosed early in pregnancy or before school age over 90% of cases [7]. Perimembranous VSDs, due to their location, have a much lower rate of spontaneous closure, with only 50% closed by 7 years of age [6]. Postnatally, surveillance for additional complications of pmVSDs, such as aortic valve regurgitation is needed as it may indicate the need for surgery.

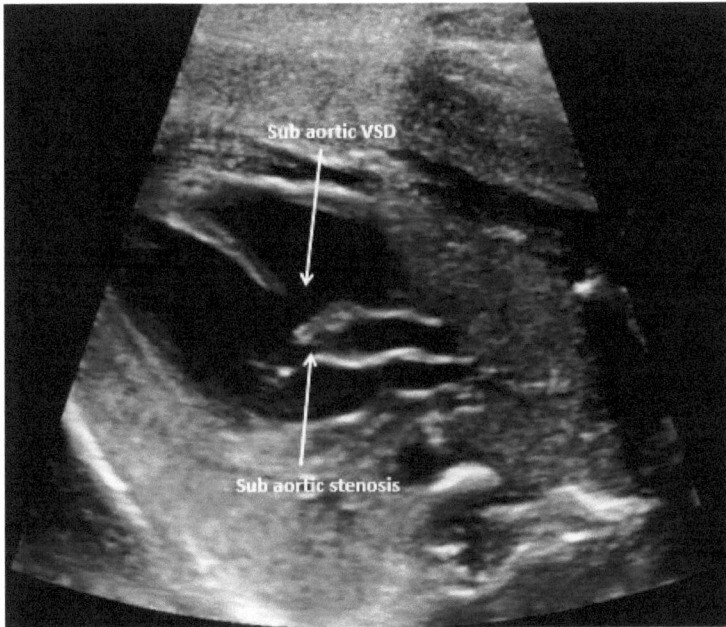

Fig. (4). Left ventricular outflow tract view showing subaortic ventricular septal defect (VSD) with subaortic muscular obstruction due to posterior deviation of the muscular conus. This fetus also had interrupted aortic arch.

ATRIOVENTRICULAR SEPTAL DEFECTS

Introduction

Atrioventricular septal defect (AVSD) is the fourth most common congenital heart lesion with an incidence of approximately 0.3 in 1,000 live births [1]. Due to the usually abnormal four-chamber view, and the frequently associated chromosomal anomalies, the prenatal incidence of AVSD is much higher than that seen postnatally.

Embryology

An AVSD arises due to the failure of fusion between the superior and inferior endocardial cushions. These endocardial cushions are formed from cellular proliferation with the transformation of epithelial to mesenchymal cells. This process is essential for the formation of not only the AV canal, but also the primum atrial septum and inlet ventricular septum. This normal process normally occurs early in the fifth week of gestation [4].

Genetic Associations

AVSD is strongly associated with chromosomal anomalies, especially trisomy 21. When an AVSD is found prenatally, trisomy 21 will be found in 40-50% of cases [8]. This is especially true for complete AVSDs or when an AVSD is associated with tetralogy of Fallot. The Down syndrome cell adhesion molecule (DSCAM) gene has been identified as the possible candidate gene for congenital heart disease associated with trisomy 21. An autosomal dominant inheritance pattern, not related to trisomy 21, has also been reported but remains uncommon [9].

Prenatal Detection

AVSD is prenatally diagnosed in 30 – 50% of cases [10, 11]. The highest prenatal detection is seen in the complete form of AVSD, those associated with additional cardiac malformations and those associated with trisomy 21. AVSDs, especially when complete, may be picked up as early as 10 – 12 weeks gestation. However, reduced offset of the AV valves in the first trimester is common and so caution should be taken with an early diagnosis.

Anatomy and Classification

An AVSD is most importantly characterised by a common atrioventricular (AV) valve, with complete loss of the normal mitral and aortic valves. However, depending on the subtype of AVSD, the common AV valve may be partitioned, giving the impression of two separate valves.

A number of classification systems have been used to describe the AVSD complex and the different subtypes. A system that is simple and descriptive, rather than using ambiguous names, is favoured by the authors of this chapter (Fig. 5).

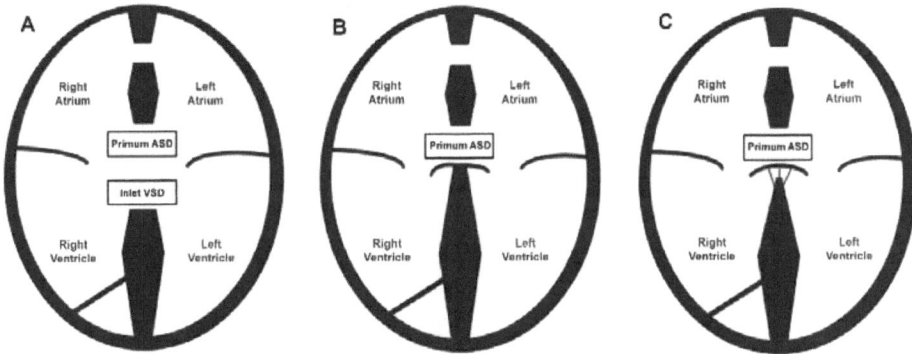

Fig. (5). Subtypes of atrial ventricular septal defect (AVSD). (**A**) Complete form with primum atrial septal defect (ASD) and inlet ventricular septal defect (VSD); (**B**) Incomplete AVSD with primum ASD and no VSD; (**C**) Incomplete form with primum ASD and a fenestrated VSD due to septal attachments of the chordae from the common valve. In B and C, there is no atrioventricular (AV) valve offset but separate left and right valve orifices.

Subtypes of AVSD include:

1. Complete AVSD: common AV valve. An atrial septal defect affecting the ostium primum septum, which is immediately below the normal fossa ovalis. An inlet type ventricular septal defect, positioned at the level of the AV valve (Fig. **6**). This VSD often extends into the membranous septum.

2. Incomplete or partial AVSD: despite no AV valve offset, the common AV valve is partitioned giving two separate orifices. The left and right AV valves are not morphologically normal mitral and tricuspid valves, and valvar incompetence is common.

a. In the first form of this subtype, there is only a defect in the ostium primum with no ventricular level shunt.

b. In the second form, often called a transitional AVSD, there is a primum level shunt and a small and restrictive ventricular level shunt. There remains to be partitioned left and right AV valve orifices despite some shunt at both the atrial and ventricular level.

In addition to the above classification, an AVSD may be either balanced or unbalanced. In an unbalanced defect, the common AV valve is generally more committed to one ventricle or the other, with possible progressive hypoplasia of one of the ventricles over time (Fig. **7**). If this leads to a single ventricle pathway postnatally, the outcomes are generally poorer, with an incompetent AV valve often being very problematic in a univentricular heart and conferring a significantly higher mortality than the usual single ventricle group.

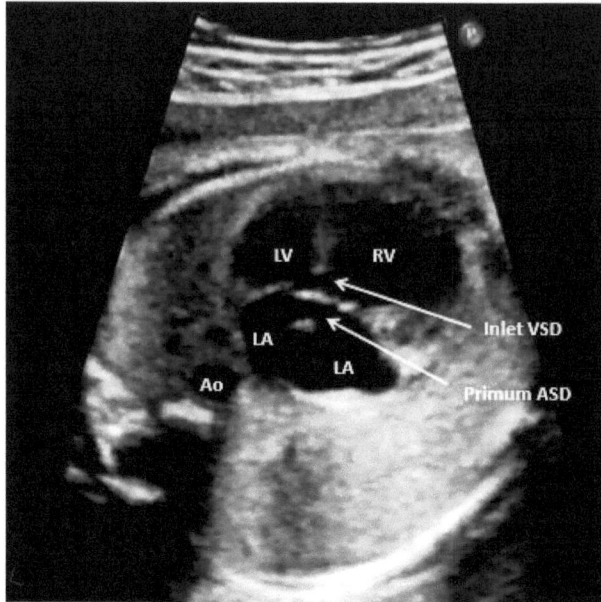

Fig. (6). Complete atrial ventricular septal defect (AVSD) with primum atrial septal defect (ASD) and inlet ventricular septal defect (VSD) shown. LA: left atrium; RA: right atrium; RV: right ventricle; LV: left ventricle; Ao: aorta.

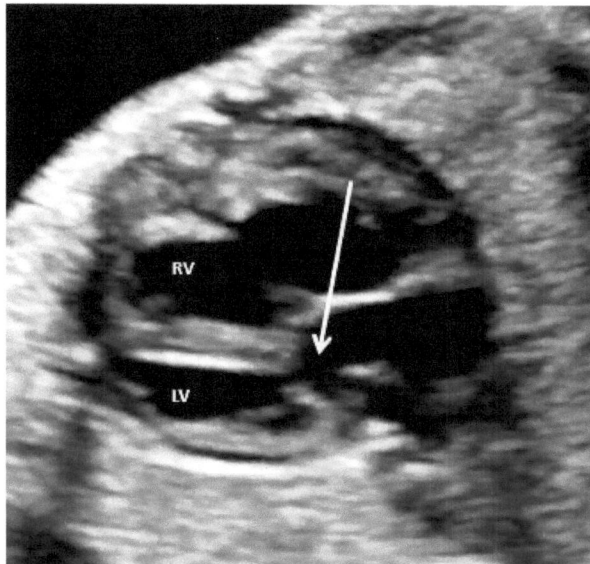

Fig. (7). Unbalanced atrial ventricular septal defect (AVSD) with primum atrial septal defect (ASD) shown (arrow). The right ventricle is dominant. RV: right ventricle; LV: left ventricle.

Additional cardiac malformations, outside of the AV valves, are commonly seen with an AVSD. Therefore, upon diagnosis of an AVSD a complete revaluation of the heart should be undertaken. Common associated malformations include tetralogy of Fallot in up to 9% (often related to trisomy 21) and also double outlet right ventricle in 12% - often related to heterotaxy syndromes [10, 12]. Up to two thirds of patients with heterotaxy will have an AVSD as part of their complex cardiac defect, often unbalanced.

Commonly in AVSD, the left ventricular (LV) outflow tract is displaced anteriorly and is elongated, the so called 'goose neck' deformity. This may lead to LV outflow tract obstruction in some and in the most severe cases lead to aortic coarctation or arch interruption.

Fetal Imaging

The diagnosis of an AVSD is generally made on the four chamber view. Particular attention is paid to the size of atrial and ventricular components of the defects. The size of the ventricular defect may determine how significant postnatal cardiac symptoms may be and how early surgical repair may be required. Using colour flow imaging, the atrial or ventricular level shunt may be further defined, although significant shunting is usually not seen given the equal left and right ventricular pressures. Increased shunting may be seen if outflow tract obstruction evolves, raising the pressure in one of the ventricles.

Atrioventricular valve regurgitation is commonly seen in AVSD and colour flow imaging is particularly important when assessing its severity. Left sided, right sided or biatrial enlargement may be seen with worsening AV valve regurgitation. Using colour flow, other concerning features for worsening AV valve regurgitation include: multiple jets of regurgitation, a broad-based jet or a jet that extends all the way to the superior or posterior atrial wall.

Short axis imaging of the common AV valve is achieved by 90-degree rotation on a four-chamber view that is perpendicular to the ultrasound beam. In this view there is loss of the normal mitral and aortic valve. In a complete AV septal defect, a single, common AV valve is seen with definition of the different leaflets of the common valve possible (superior bridging leaflet, inferior bridging leaflet, mural leaflet, lateral leaflet). The size and position of the papillary muscles can also be assessed in the short axis along with ventricular disproportion.

As mentioned previously, the left ventricular outflow tract is often elongated and displaced anteriorly. Assessment of the LV outflow tract for obstruction to flow on 2D, colour flow and PW Doppler is required. The aortic arch should be assessed for any obstruction in the three-vessel view and also sagittal plane.

The relative balance between the left and right heart size should be assessed at each review. If an unbalanced defect is seen, assessment for any reduction of outflow tract size or flow from the affected ventricle needs regular reassessment. In the most severe cases pulmonary or aortic stenosis or atresia may develop over time. Finally, again, detailed assessment for any additional cardiac lesions should be closely undertaken. This includes close review of systemic and pulmonary veins which may be abnormal in heterotaxy syndrome.

Perinatal Management

Generally, AVSDs are very well tolerated in the fetal circulation. This is due to the equalised pressures between left and right-sided circulation, and as such, the shunt through the ASD or VSD is minimal. Pulmonary over circulation is not possible in fetal life. Severe AV valve regurgitation may compromise fetal systemic output and needs to be assessed at each review. Equally, if heterotaxy is suspected, fetal cardiac rhythm may be affected and a more severe atrial bradycardia may lead to fetal hydrops.

Once the diagnosis of an AV septal defect is made, discussion and strong consideration of genetic testing needs to be offered. Even if termination of pregnancy is not being considered, the diagnosis of trisomy 21 prenatally will affect fetal surveillance, timing of delivery and early postnatal management.

In an ongoing pregnancy, serial fetal echocardiograms are required, especially to assess for progressive ventricular size disproportion or any outflow tract obstruction. We would generally repeat fetal echocardiograms monthly from 28 weeks gestation after a 20 weeks gestation diagnosis.

Assuming no significant outflow tract obstruction, early postnatal cardiac symptoms are not common. This is owing to the fact that pulmonary pressure remains high in the first few days or weeks after delivery, and so the left to right shunting remains small. However, with falling pulmonary pressures, symptoms related to increased pulmonary blood flow may evolve at 6 – 12 weeks postnatally. In children with trisomy 21 and complete AVSD surgical repair is generally undertaken at approximately 3 months of age, even in the absence of significant cardiac symptoms. This is to avoid the risk of ongoing and irreversible pulmonary hypertension for which they are at a greater risk. Repair of a complete AVSD, not related to trisomy 21, may be deferred to 6 – 9 months of age depending on clinical symptoms. Earlier surgery may be required in the setting of outflow tract obstruction. An incomplete AVSD with atrial defect only may avoid surgical repair for many years if asymptomatic and AV valve regurgitation is not significant. The aim of surgical repair is to close the septal defects whilst dividing the common AV valve into fairly equal portions. Attempt is made to minimise any residual AV valve regurgitation whilst not causing AV valve stenosis.

Long term outcomes after isolated AV repair are generally very good. The most common need for reoperation is left AV valve regurgitation, with reoperation seen in approximately 10% [13]. However, if there is more complex congenital heart defect associated with the AVSD or in patients with single ventricle anatomy, the outcomes are universally poorer.

CONSENT FOR PUBLICATION

Not applicable.

CONFLICT OF INTEREST

The authors confirm that the contents of this chapter have no conflict of interest.

ACKNOWLEDGEMENTS

Declare none.

REFERENCES

[1]   Hoffman JI, Kaplan S. The incidence of congenital heart disease. J Am Coll Cardiol 2002; 39(12): 1890-900.
       [http://dx.doi.org/10.1016/S0735-1097(02)01886-7] [PMID: 12084585]

[2]   Fisher DC, Fisher EA, Budd JH, Rosen SE, Goldman ME. The incidence of patent foramen ovale in 1,000 consecutive patients. A contrast transesophageal echocardiography study. Chest 1995; 107(6): 1504-9.
       [http://dx.doi.org/10.1378/chest.107.6.1504] [PMID: 7781337]

[3]   Radzik D, Davignon A, van Doesburg N, Fournier A, Marchand T, Ducharme G. Predictive factors for spontaneous closure of atrial septal defects diagnosed in the first 3 months of life. J Am Coll Cardiol 1993; 22(3): 851-3.
       [http://dx.doi.org/10.1016/0735-1097(93)90202-C] [PMID: 8354823]

[4]   Hill MA. Cardiac Embryology 2019. https://embryology.med.unsw.edu.au/embryology/index.php/Cardiac_Embryology

[5]   Gómez O, Martínez JM, Olivella A, et al. Isolated ventricular septal defects in the era of advanced fetal echocardiography: Risk of chromosomal anomalies and spontaneous closure rate from diagnosis to age of 1 year. Ultrasound Obstet Gynecol 2014; 43(1): 65-71.
       [http://dx.doi.org/10.1002/uog.12527] [PMID: 23733584]

[6]   Meberg A, Hals J, Thaulow E. Congenital heart defects--chromosomal anomalies, syndromes and extracardiac malformations. Acta Paediatr 2007; 96(8): 1142-5.
       [http://dx.doi.org/10.1111/j.1651-2227.2007.00381.x] [PMID: 17590185]

[7]   Zhao QM, Niu C, Liu F, Wu L, Ma XJ, Huang GY. Spontaneous closure rates of ventricular septal defects (6,750 consecutive neonates). Am J Cardiol 2019; 124(4): 613-7.
       [http://dx.doi.org/10.1016/j.amjcard.2019.05.022] [PMID: 31208700]

[8]   Paladini D, Tartaglione A, Agangi A, et al. The association between congenital heart disease and Down syndrome in prenatal life. Ultrasound Obstet Gynecol 2000; 15(2): 104-8.
       [http://dx.doi.org/10.1046/j.1469-0705.2000.00027.x] [PMID: 10775990]

[9]   Wilson L, Curtis A, Korenberg JR, *et al.* A large, dominant pedigree of atrioventricular septal defect (AVSD): Exclusion from the Down syndrome critical region on chromosome 21. Am J Hum Genet 1993; 53(6): 1262-8.
[PMID: 8250042]

[10]   Heide H, Thomson JD, Wharton GA, Gibbs JL. Poor sensitivity of routine fetal anomaly ultrasound screening for antenatal detection of atrioventricular septal defect. Heart 2004; 90(8): 916-7.
[http://dx.doi.org/10.1136/hrt.2003.018895] [PMID: 15253968]

[11]   Chew C, Halliday JL, Riley MM, Penny DJ. Population-based study of antenatal detection of congenital heart disease by ultrasound examination. Ultrasound Obstet Gynecol 2007; 29(6): 619-24.
[http://dx.doi.org/10.1002/uog.4023] [PMID: 17523161]

[12]   Yıldırım G, Gungorduk K, Yazıcıoğlu F, *et al.* Prenatal diagnosis of complete atrioventricular septal defect: Perinatal and neonatal outcomes. Obstet Gynecol Int 2009; 2009958496.
[http://dx.doi.org/10.1155/2009/958496] [PMID: 19960047]

[13]   Ten Harkel AD, Cromme-Dijkhuis AH, Heinerman BC, Hop WC, Bogers AJ. Development of left atrioventricular valve regurgitation after correction of atrioventricular septal defect. Ann Thorac Surg 2005; 79(2): 607-12.
[http://dx.doi.org/10.1016/j.athoracsur.2004.07.010] [PMID: 15680844]

CHAPTER 10

Fetal Right Heart Malformations

Jesus Rodríguez Calvo, Enery Gómez Montes, Ignacio Herraiz, Cecilia Villalaín and **Alberto Galindo**[*]

Department of Obstetrics and Gynaecology, Fetal Medicine Unit-Maternal and Child Health and Development Network (SAMID), Hospital Universitario 12 de Octubre, Instituto de Investigación Hospital 12 de Octubre (imas12), Faculty of Medicine, Universidad Complutense de Madrid, Madrid, Spain

Abstract: The fetal right heart malformations are a heterogeneous group of anomalies that basically involve the tricuspid and pulmonary valves. Ebstein´s anomaly usually consists of the existence of a downward displacement of the insertion of the septal and posterior leaflets of the tricuspid valve. Tricuspid dysplasia is an abnormality of the chordae tendinae and/or the leaflets, which are thickened, of a normally inserted tricuspid valve. Both conditions are characterized by an incomplete closure of the valve in systole, causing tricuspid regurgitation that may cause cardiomegaly, heart failure and hydrops. Chromosomal defects are rare and the mortality for prenatally detected forms is high, with survival rates at 5 years less than 25%. In tricuspid atresia there is a replacement of the valve by a fibromuscular tissue and is almost always associated with a ventricular septal defect. The right ventricle is invariably hypoplastic, and in up to 25% of cases there is ventriculo-arterial discordance. Chromosomal abnormalities are rare, and the outcome is usually good, with survival rates at 20 years of 61-75%. In mild to moderate forms of pulmonary stenosis, the pulmonary valve appears thickened and/or narrowed, and is visible continuously throughout the cardiac cycle. The four-chamber view is usually normal. On color Doppler, there is high-velocity turbulent flow across the pulmonary valve. The outcome is good in most cases. In severe forms of pulmonary stenosis or pulmonary atresia with intact ventricular septum there is an almost complete obstruction of the right ventricle outflow tract due to severe dysplasia or complete absence of the pulmonary valve, respectively. This can be assessed both in B-mode and with color Doppler. The only route for blood supply to the lungs is the ductus arteriosus. Depending on the tricuspid valve, the right ventricle can be severely small or normal sized, which has a paramount importance on the final outcome. Acquired forms of premature closure of the ductus arteriosus can be idiopathic or secondary to the administration to the mother of some medical treatments. It often appears abruptly, in the third trimester of pregnancy. The Doppler study shows an acceleration of the transductal flow, with a peak systolic velocity greater than 140 cm/s, a diastolic peak greater than 35 cm/s, and a pulsatility index lower than 1.9 m/s. When the closure is complete, there is an asymmetric cardiomegaly because of dilatation of the right chambers, right ventricle hypertrophy and dilatation of the pulmonary artery

[*] **Corresponding author Alberto Galindo:** Department of Obstetrics and Gynaecology, Hospital Universitario 12 de Octubre, Avda, Córdoba s/n, Madrid 28041, Spain; Tel: 034-1-3908376; E-mail: agalindo@salud.madrid.org

Edward Araujo Júnior, Nathalie Jeanne M. Bravo-Valenzuela and Alberto Borges Peixoto (Eds.)

and branches, while the duct is narrowed.

Keywords: Ebstein's anomaly, Premature closure of the ductus arteriosus, Pulmonary atresia with intact ventricular septum, Pulmonary stenosis, Tricuspid atresia, Tricuspid dysplasia.

TRICUSPID VALVE DISEASE

Ebstein's Anomaly, Tricuspid Dysplasia

Definition:

- Ebstein´s anomaly consists of the existence of an anomalous insertion of the septal and posterior leaflets of the tricuspid annulus in the right ventricle (RV), with an apical displacement of the leaflets which leads to a variable degree of valve dysplasia and of atrialization of the RV [1]. There is also a variable degree of adhesion of the leaflets to the ventricular wall, reducing significantly their mobility, causing incomplete closure and valvular regurgitation. The anterior leaflet can be relatively normal, although it is usually more elongated, redundant, and has multiple anchors to the RV walls that limit its movement. Therefore, the tricuspid valve (TV) in Ebstein's anomaly can be stenotic and regurgitant.

- Tricuspid dysplasia (TD) includes a wide spectrum of anomalies characterized by the existence of a malformation of the TV, at the level of the chordae tendinae and/or the leaflets, but in which the insertion of the TV is normal. However, their consequences are quite similar to those of Ebstein's anomaly. This is why TD is often called the "Ebstein´s-like" anomaly.

Incidence: Ebstein's anomaly is a rare condition, constituting 0.3-0.6% of all congenital heart defects (CHD), affecting 1 in 20,000 live births. It represents 3-7% of all CHD detected in fetal life. These data are similar for TD.

Recurrence: For Ebstein´s anomaly, it is 1% if there is one affected child, and 3% if there are 2 or more affected children.

Etiology: most cases are sporadic and their etiology is multifactorial because of the interaction between genetic and environmental factors. To date, the relationship between the appearance of this CHD and the maternal intake of lithium carbonate for the treatment of manic-depressive psychosis remains controversial.

Importance: the manifestations of both entities depend on the severity of the malformation of the TV, being of the few CHD that can cause intrauterine cardiac dysfunction and tachyarrhythmias, eventually leading to severe cardiomegaly, fetal hydrops, and perinatal death.

- The usually severe tricuspid regurgitation (TR) present in both entities together with the atrialization of the RV in Ebstein's anomaly causes the appearance of dilatation of the right atrium (RA), that also is dependent on the greater or fewer compliance of the foramen ovale. The increased pressure in the RA can be transmitted back and cause an increase in venous pressure, with alteration of the Doppler wave of the ductus venosus and, finally, get to the appearance of signs of right heart failure with effusions and fetal hydrops. In addition, the loss of forward flow through the pulmonary ring can cause a functional pulmonary stenosis or atresia, which is present in 30-50% of cases, with pulmonary filling from the ductus arteriosus (DA) (ductus-dependent pulmonary flow).

- In some cases, a "circular shunt" may even appear. In this situation, not only the filling of the pulmonary trunk is ductus-dependent but also the pulmonary valve is insufficient so that the blood re-enters the RV, creating a peculiar hemodynamic situation in which the blood flows in a permanent way. RV circuit → RA → left atrium → left ventricle → aorta → DA → pulmonary artery → RV → RA [2], which reduces cardiac output to the distal territory of the fetus and the placenta.

- Finally, the cardiomegaly due to massive RA enlargement causes a mass effect inside the thorax, with limited space for pulmonary development, conditioning a variable degree of pulmonary hypoplasia.

- However, there are also mild cases with better valve function and a higher degree of RV development that are usually well tolerated by the fetus.

Chromosome Abnormalities: very rare for both entities (<5%), although trisomy 13, 18 and 21 have been described.

Presentation: In 30% of cases of Ebstein's anomaly, there are associated anomalies, especially at the cardiac level, in the form of pulmonary stenosis or pulmonary atresia, septal defects, conotruncal anomalies, and aortic coarctation or interruption of the aortic arch. In approximately 20% of cases, there are extracardiac anomalies or genetic syndromes (Marfan, Cornelia de Lange). In TD, associated anomalies are very rare.

Prenatal Diagnosis:

• Ebstein's anomaly is characterized by the existence of a downwardly displacement of the septal and posterior leaflets of the TV, taking as reference the normal insertion of the anterior leaflet of the mitral valve (Fig. **1**). This difference in the insertions of the septal leaflets is usually greater than 8 mm although in the less severe forms it may be lower [3]. In the 4-chamber view, the increased size of the RA, the decreased size of the RV, the coarse, thickened and hyperechogenic aspect of the valve leaflets are observed as well as the limitation for their movement, especially the septal leaflet, which is hardly separated from the septal myocardium during the cardiac cycle (Fig. **2**).

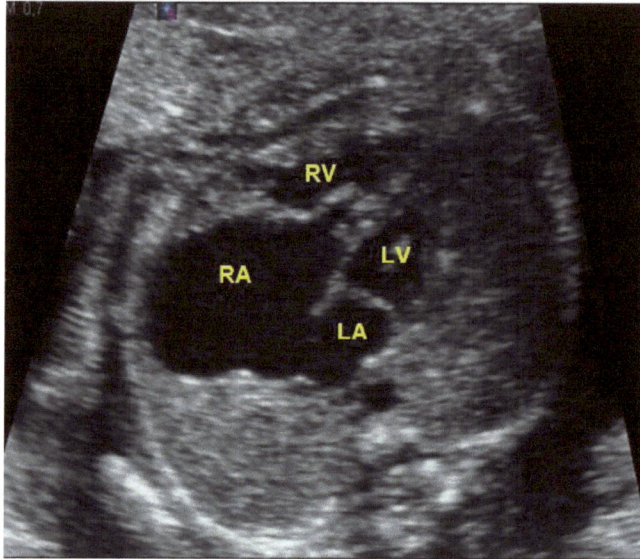

Fig. (1). Four chamber view of a fetus with Ebstein's anomaly. The apical displacement of the tricuspid valve is observed, especially of its septal leaflet (compare with the mitral valve insertion), and the atrialization of the right ventricle (RV). LV: left ventricle, RA: right atrium, LA: left atrium.

- TD is characterized in B mode by the existence of a thickened, coarse, hyperechoic, redundant TV leaflets, but with normal valve insertion. The movement of the leaflets may be limited, showing with an incomplete closure in systole. Usually, the degree of cardiomegaly is greater than in Ebstein's anomaly, and affects mainly the RA, which may show a massive enlargement, that usually increases as pregnancy advances (Figs. **3** and **4**).

In both conditions, color and pulsed Doppler allow to demonstrate the existence of TR, which, in the most severe cases, is holosystolic, of high speed and reaching the atrial roof. In TD, TR comes from the normal atrioventricular junction, while in Ebstein's anomaly the regurgitant flow appears more distally, at the level of the downwardly displaced valve (Figs. **5** and **6**). In both CHD, the RV outflow tract must be explored, to assess if there is forward flow through the pulmonary valve with antegrade filling of the pulmonary trunk and branches or, on the contrary, if there is retrograde flow coming from the DA with or without pulmonary insufficiency. In these last cases there may be a circular shunt (Fig. **7**). In the worst cases, the most severe and evolved signs of right heart failure and hydrops may appear (Fig. **8**).

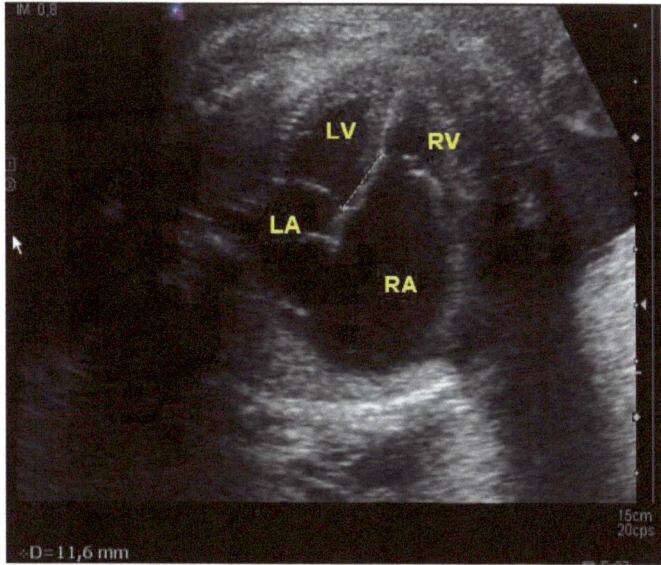

Fig. (2). Four chamber view of a fetus with Ebstein's anomaly. The apical displacement of the tricuspid valve is observed, with its septal valve being 11.6 mm from the insertion of the mitral valve, and the atrialization of the right ventricle (RV). LA: left atrium, LV: left ventricle, RA: right atrium.

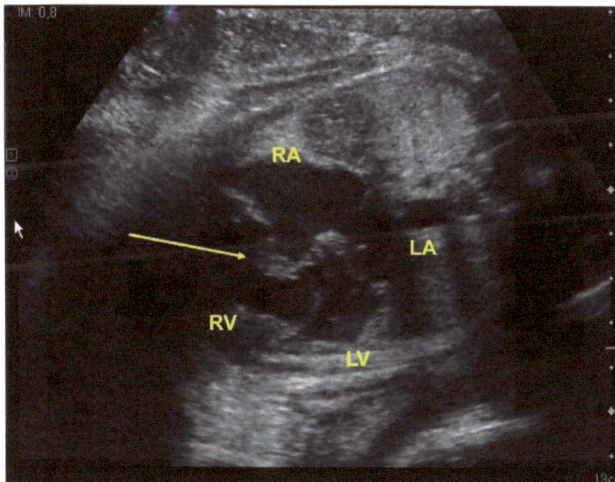

Fig. (3). Four chamber view of a fetus with tricuspid dysplasia. Dilatation of the right atrium (RA) and right ventricle (RV) is observed and the tricuspid valve is very thickened (arrow). LA: left atrium, LV: left ventricle.

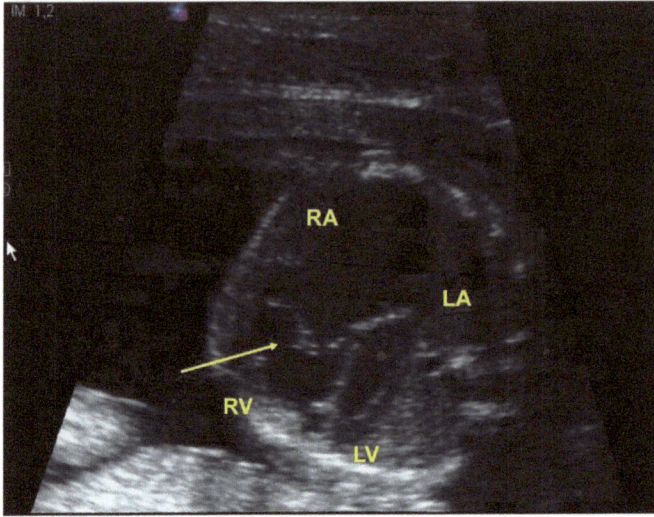

Fig. (4). Four chamber view of a fetus with tricuspid dysplasia. Severe asymmetric cardiomegaly is observed, mainly due to aneurysmal dilatation of the right atrium (RA) and right ventricle (RV), so that the heart practically occupies two thirds of the thorax. The tricuspid valve (arrow) is thickened. LA left atrium, LV: left ventricle.

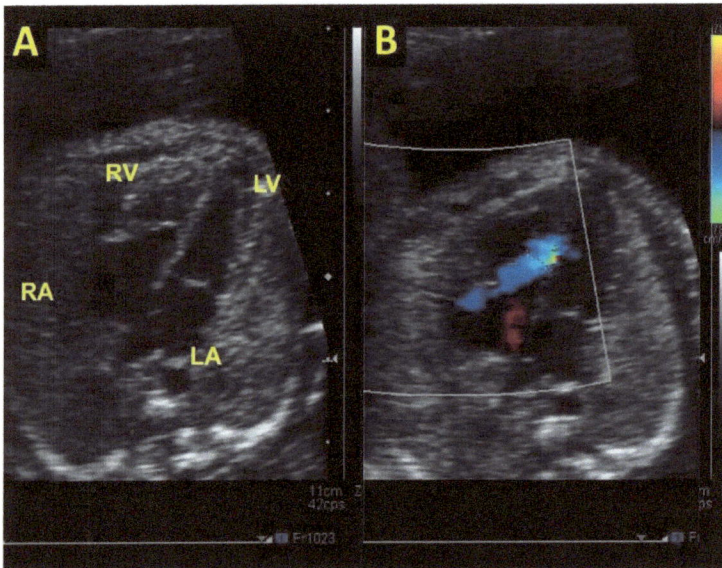

Fig. (5). (**A**) Four chamber view of a fetus with Ebstein's anomaly. The apical displacement of the tricuspid valve is observed, especially of its septal valve (compare with the insertion of the mitral valve), and the atrialization of the right ventricle (RV). (**B**) With color Doppler, with tricuspid regurgitation is confirmed through the septal valve, originating the regurgitation jet from the remaining RV cavity. RA: right atrium, LA: left atrium, LV: left ventricle.

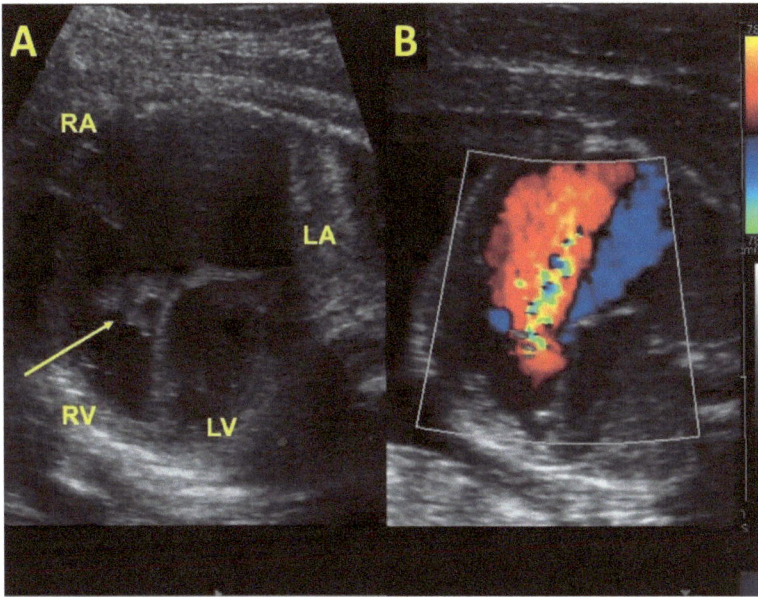

Fig. (6). (**A**) Four chamber view of a fetus with tricuspid dysplasia. Severe asymmetric cardiomegaly is observed, mainly because of an aneurysmal dilatation of the right atrium (RA), and the tricuspid valve (arrow) is irregular, echogenic and very thickened, but the insertion is normal. (**B**) With color Doppler, the massive tricuspid regurgitation of the right ventricle (RV) to the RA can be noted. LA: left atrium, LV: left ventricle.

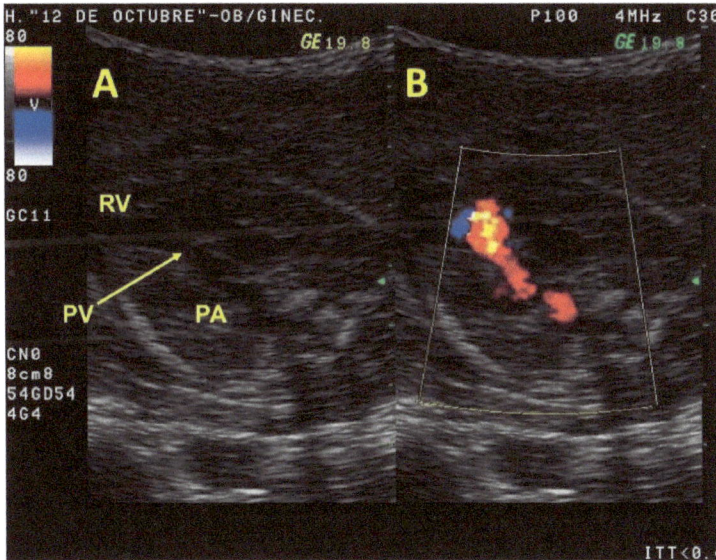

Fig. (7). Examination of the right ventricular (RV) outflow tract of a fetus with severe tricuspid dysplasia. (**A**) Anatomically it seems normal but (**B**) with color Doppler it is verified that the filling of the pulmonary artery (PA) is retrograde, coming from the ductus arteriosus, and the flow goes through the pulmonary valve (PV) that is insufficient and is introduced in the RV.

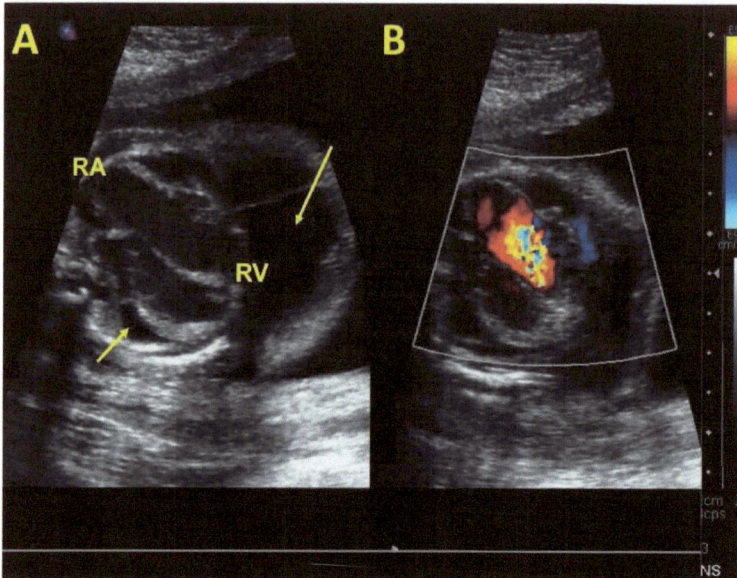

Fig. (8). (**A**) Oblique section of the thorax and abdomen of a hydropic fetus with severe Ebstein's anomaly, showing pericardial effusion and ascites (arrows). (**B**) With color Doppler, massive tricuspid regurgitation is observed. RA: right atrium, RV: right ventricle.

The milder forms of TD are characterized by the existence of a slight thickening of the valve leaflets, nodular and usually circumscribed to the free ends of the leaflets, and the TR is mild. In the most favorable forms of Ebstein's anomaly, the degree of atrialization of the RV is also minor and the competence of the TR is greater.

Differential Diagnosis: isolated cases of Ebstein's anomaly or TD should be differentiated of those conditions causing TR, especially critical pulmonary stenosis or pulmonary atresia with intact ventricular septum. The distinction is based on the features described for TD and Ebstein's anomaly as well as in the RV myocardial hypertrophy that is usually seen in obstructive diseases of the RV outflow tract. Similarly, it is important to differentiate these two conditions from premature closure of the DA: in this last situation, the TV is normal, there is almost no filling of the pulmonary trunk, and the flow in the DA is turbulent.

Natural History: the intrauterine mortality in these conditions is 20-30% and is usually associated with the onset of heart failure and hydrops. However, these figures may be, at least partially, explained by the fact that the more severe cases of TD and Ebstein's anomaly are those that are more often detected prenatally. Nevertheless, in fetal series the perinatal mortality for these CHD reaches 60-70%.

Perinatal Management: given the evolving nature of these conditions, once the diagnosis is made, follow up scans should be performed every 2-3 weeks.

- For both entities, signs of poor prognosis are severe cardiomegaly, severe TR, the presence of signs of right heart failure or tachyarrhythmia, and/or the absence of anterograde flow through the pulmonary valve. In all these cases, perinatal morbidity and mortality is very high, and perinatal assistance in a tertiary center with advanced cardiac and neonatal intensive care is mandatory.

- In favorable cases, parents should also be advised that perinatal care must ideally take place in a tertiary center, although in the neonatal period there may be some spontaneous improvement in the severity of the TR because of the physiological decline of pulmonary resistance.

Postnatal Treatment and Prognosis: depend largely on the severity of hemodynamic manifestations and the patient's situation.

- Children with milder forms may remain asymptomatic for a long time and surgical treatment can be delayed several years. This treatment usually consists of the reconstruction of the TV, the closure of the interatrial communication and the RA reduction plasty, if this is large. When it is not possible to perform the reconstruction of the TV, the only solution can be valve replacement, placing a biological or mechanical prosthesis. The prognosis of these more benign forms of Ebstein's anomaly is good, with a postoperative mortality of less than 5% and a survival at 20 years of over 90%.

- However, severe forms will require intensive inotropic and early ventilatory support, in addition to prostaglandin E1 to maintain pulmonary perfusion. In cases of Ebstein's anomaly, the surgical strategy is that of univentricular palliation. The prognosis of these more severe forms is poor and their mortality is very high, with survival rates at 5 years less than 25%. When there are signs of cardiac failure or cardiomegaly, early in gestation, mortality is very high.

Tricuspid Atresia

Definition: there is a complete absence of the TV, which is replaced by fibromuscular tissue. There is no communication between the RA and the RV, this being hypoplastic with absence of the entry portion, scarce development or absence of the trabecular portion and, usually, presence of the outflow tract. There is almost always a ventricular septal defect (VSD), whose size and number will modify the degree of development of the RV and the pulmonary artery (PA), since it is the only blood entry route to the RV [4].

Types: depending on the ventriculo-arterial junction, there are 3 types of tricuspid atresia (TA) [5]:

- Type I: concordant ventriculo-arterial connection (60-70%), with or without stenosis or pulmonary atresia.
- Type II: discordant ventriculo-arterial connection (D-transposition of the great arteries) (25-30%), with or without stenosis or pulmonary atresia or coarctation of the aorta.
- Type III: TA in the setting of L-transposition of the great arteries (1-2%).

Incidence: TA is a rare CHD that affects 1 in 15,000 live births. It constitutes 0.3-3.7% of all CHD, 4.5% in fetal series, and between 1 and 3% in pediatric series.

Recurrence: 1%

Etiology: most cases are sporadic and their etiology is multifactorial, as a result of the interaction between genetic and environmental factors.

Prognosis: note that there are three aspects affecting the severity of this condition:

a. The size of the foramen ovale. This is the natural way of escape of the blood flow coming to the RA from the systemic venous circulation. If the foramen is small, there will be an increase in pressure in the RA, which will be transmitted retrogradely, causing increased venous pressure and low cardiac output.
b. The presence or absence of ventricular septal defect (VSD) and its size: if there is no VSD or this is tiny, the RV is severely hypoplastic, and the degree of development of the PA will depend on the volume of blood that comes from the DA. The pulmonary valve is small and is often severely stenotic or atretic. On the contrary, if there is a larger VSD, this allows the filling of the RV and the pulmonary artery. Nevertheless, even in these cases, the RV is small but the size of the pulmonary artery and valve may be within normal limits. Regardless of the degree of prenatal development of the RV, all these patients will have univentricular circulation postnatally.
c. Ventriculo-arterial concordance or discordance: in cases of D-transposition of the great arteries, the situation of low flow from the RV may cause a subaortic stenosis (aortic atresia in the most severe cases) and underdevelopment of the aortic arch.

Presentation: in most cases (80%) TA presents isolated. In the rest there may be other anomalies, both cardiac (stenosis/pulmonary atresia, aortic stenosis, coarctation of the aorta or interruption of the arch) and extracardiac (musculoskeletal, neurological).

Chromosomal Abnormalities: they are present in 2-5% of cases.

Prenatal Diagnosis: in B mode, TA is characterized by the replacement of the TV by an immobile, thickened and hyperechoic structure corresponding to the fibromuscular tissue that replaces it. As said before, the degree of development of the RV depends on the size and number of the VSD, although in all cases the RV is small. Therefore, there is always a frank asymmetry in the size of both ventricles in the 4-chamber view. The RV loses its tripartite shape, lacking the inlet portion, having a small trabecular portion, to the point that it does not form apex, and a more developed infundibulum, in proportion with the size of the connection between both ventricles (Figs. **9** to **11**). The development of the pulmonary artery correlates with the development of the infundibulum and, therefore, it can be small and filled from the DA, at least partially, or it can be of practically normal size and filled antegrade from the RV. The VSD is usually located in the inlet portion and is, therefore, visible in the 4-chamber view, but sometimes there are also defects in the apical portion. It is important to explore the ventriculo-arterial junction and, when discordant, to analyze the integrity and size of the aortic arch. Color Doppler confirms the absence of tricuspid flow, the right-left interatrial shunt, the flow through the VSD, and the characteristics of the flow in the pulmonary trunk and valve (Fig. **12**) [6].

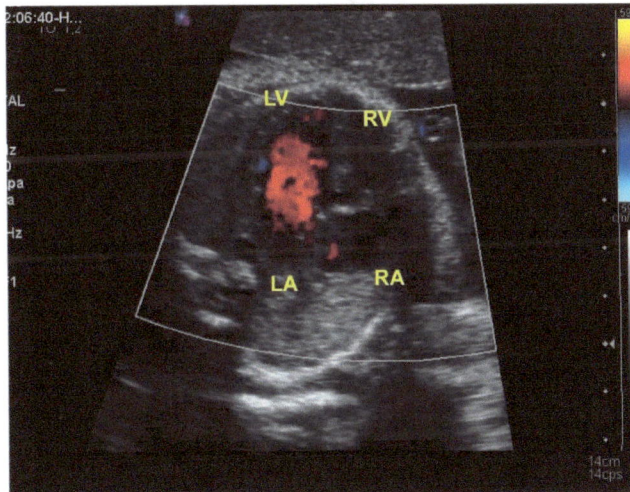

Fig. (9). Color Doppler examination of a fetus with tricuspid atresia showing a single atrioventricular (AV) flow jet corresponding to the mitral flow. LA: left atrium, RA: right atrium. LV: left ventricle, RV: right ventricle.

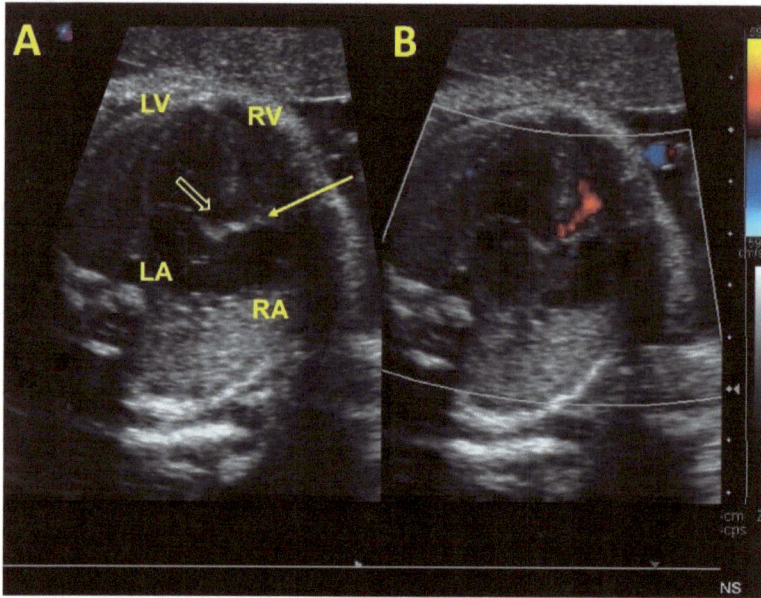

Fig. (10). (**A**) Four chamber view of a fetus with tricuspid atresia showing the closed, thickened and echogenic tricuspid valve (arrow), and an evident asymmetry between the size of the right ventricle (RV), extremely hypoplastic, and the left ventricle (LV). There is also a defect in the interventricular septum (hollow arrow). (**B**) With color Doppler, the passage of blood from the LV to the RV is verified through the defect of the interventricular septum. RA: right atrium, LA: left atrium.

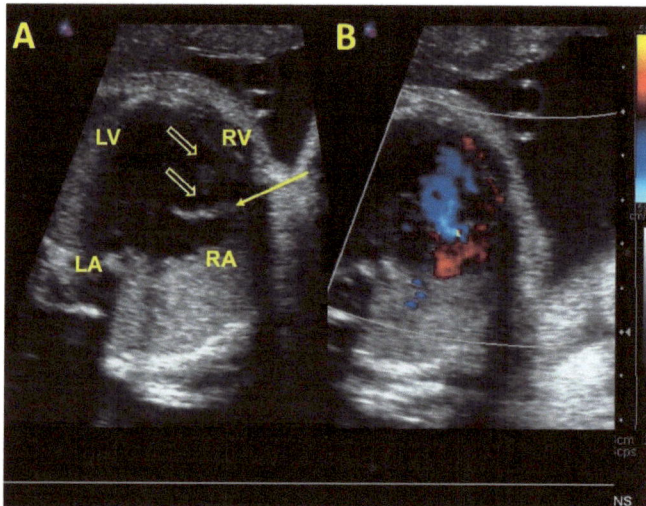

Fig. (11). (**A**) Four chamber view of a fetus with tricuspid atresia showing the closed, thickened and echogenic tricuspid valve (arrow), and an evident asymmetry between the size of the right ventricle (RV), extremely hypoplastic, and the left ventricle (LV). There are also two defects in the interventricular septum (hollow arrows). (**B**) With color Doppler, the passage of blood from the LV to the RV is verified through the defects of the interventricular septum. RA: right atrium, LA: left atrium.

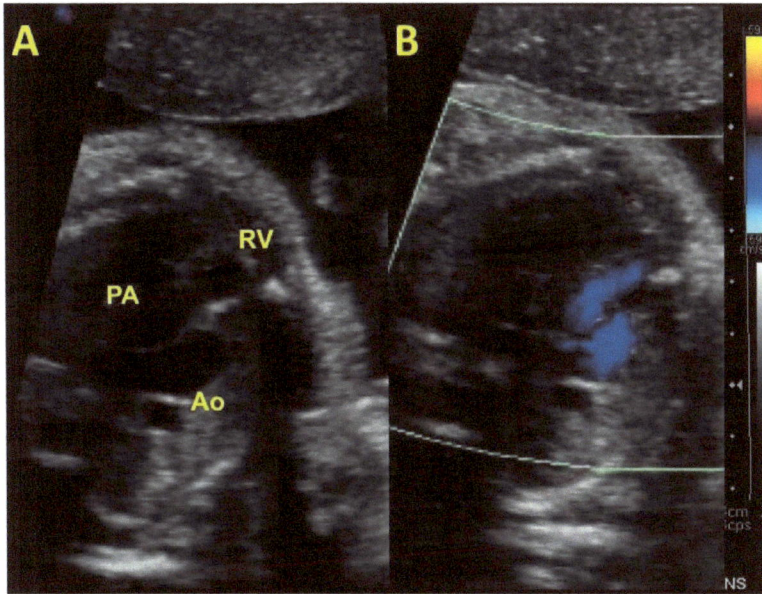

Fig. (12). (**A**) Image of the outflow tract of the right ventricle (RV) of a fetus with tricuspid atresia and several defects of the interventricular septum, observing the correct development of outflow tract, so that the size of the pulmonary artery (PA) and of the aorta (Ao) is similar. (**B**) With color Doppler, antegrade filling of the pulmonary trunk is observed.

Differential Diagnosis: mainly with pulmonary atresia with intact ventricular septum and restrictive TV, because in these cases the RV can also be hypoplastic. However, in this condition, the TV exists and shows the movement of opening and closing, although they may be very limited. With color and pulsed Doppler it is possible to demonstrate transtricuspid flow, even if it is minimal. Finally, there is no VSD, which is almost a constant finding in TA.

Natural History: TA usually remains stable prenatally, and the onset of signs of cardiac failure are rare.

Perinatal Management: all the factors that determine the severity of this condition need to be assessed. Therefore, the existence of associated congenital anomalies, including chromosome anomalies, should be ruled out. Similarly, the fetal biometry must be evaluated periodically since growth restriction is often present. Although the condition in itself usually remains stable throughout the pregnancy, follow-up scans every 4-6 weeks should be performed to monitor the evolution of the key findings, including the development of the aortic arch in cases of transposition of the great arteries. Perinatal care must take place always in a tertiary referral center with adequate cardiological and neonatal availability.

Postnatal Treatment and Prognosis:

- Initially, the essential point is to assure an adequate pulmonary flow, which is the rule when the VSD is large enough. However, when the VSD is restrictive it may be necessary to administer prostaglandin E1 in the neonatal period and even perform a provisional systemic-pulmonary shunt, either by communicating the right subclavian artery with the right pulmonary branch (the modified Blalock-Taussig fistula), or by placing a stent into the DA.

- The definitive treatment is surgical and palliative [7], creating a univentricular circulation by connecting both caval veins to the pulmonary arteries, and leaving the heart exclusively for the management of oxygenated blood. Firstly, at around 3-6 months, an anastomosis of the superior vena cava to the right pulmonary artery is performed (bidirectional Glenn). Then, between 18 months and 4 years, the connection between the inferior vena cava and the left pulmonary artery is made (Fontan surgery) with which the univentricular palliation is definitively established.

- The survival rates reported in the literature to the neonatal period, to the year of life, to 5 years and to 20 years are 89%, 82%, 72-80% and 61-75%, respectively.

PULMONARY VALVE DISEASE

Pulmonary Stenosis with Intact Ventricular Septum

Definition: it is a partial obstruction of the right ventricular (RV) outflow tract because of either an abnormal pulmonary valve (PV) or narrowing of the infundibulum.

Classification: according to the location of the obstruction, three forms are distinguished:

1. Supravalvular: the pulmonary artery just above the PV is narrowed. There is a fibrous ring or muscle thickening at the supravalvular level. It may appear isolated or associated with other CHD, such as tetralogy of Fallot, or in the context of congenital rubella, Williams, Noonan, or Alagille syndromes.
2. Valvular: is the most common type. The valve leaflets are thickened and/or narrowed, often with fusion of the leaflets, leaving a small hole in the middle. It is frequently associated with Noonan syndrome. Bicuspid pulmonary valve is found in 20% of cases.
3. Subvalvular: it is a rare form. There is a thickened fibrous ring or muscular thickening at the level of the RV infundibulum. It usually occurs in VSD and

tetralogy of Fallot.

In addition, depending on the severity of the obstruction, two types of pulmonary stenosis are differentiated [7], which will have different ultrasound expression, clinical presentation and prognosis:

1. Mild-moderate forms: with subtle sonographic expressiveness and, therefore, difficult prenatal diagnosis.
2. Severe forms (critical pulmonary stenosis - CPS): it has a pathophysiology similar to that of pulmonary atresia with intact ventricular septum (PAIVS). Therefore, in the same way that occurs with this condition, its behavior and echocardiographic manifestations depend on the status of the tricuspid valve (TV):

- Stenotic-competent TV: the only way out of the blood that enters the RV will be the severely obstructed PV. Consequently, the RV pressure will increase, which will hinder its filling and, therefore, its development, leading to a hypoplastic RV. The great pressure existing within the RV will favor the escape of blood through a thick-walled, distended intertrabecular myocardial spaces between a capillary bed and the subepicardial coronary arteries, leading to the formation of ventriculo-coronary connections (VCC) or fistulas (connections of the coronary system with the RV cavity).

- Incompetent or insufficient TV: this insufficiency can be functional, due to the increase in pressure in the RV, or because of a tricuspid valve dysplasia. In these cases, the alternating flow of entry and exit of the RV will allow some development of it and, therefore, the RV may be of normal size or even be dilated. In addition, the incompetence of the TV will make the pressure existing in the RV to be lower than in the previous situation and, therefore, the existence of VCC is unlikely.

Frequency: it represents 7.8% of all CHD, but only represents 1% of the CHD detected in fetal life.

Recurrence: incidence of 2% when a brother is affected and 6% when two siblings are affected. The risk of recurrence when the affected is the father is 2%, being 4-6.5% when is the mother.

Presentation: most cases detected prenatally are part of other more complex CHD such as conotruncal anomalies (tetralogy of Fallot, double outlet RV, transposition of the great arteries), tricuspid anomalies (atresia, dysplasia, Ebstein's anomaly), heterotaxy syndromes, aortic or mitral stenosis, or atrioventricular septal defects, or also in the context of monochorionic twin gestations complicated with twin-twin transfusion syndrome.

Chromosome Abnormality: present in 15-20% of cases (partial trisomy of chromosome 22, monosomy XO, trisomy 18). It can also be part of genetic syndromes.

Prenatal Diagnosis: its echocardiographic manifestation will depend on the severity of the obstruction:

1. Mild-moderate forms: they have subtle sonographic features. The morphology and development of the RV can be normal or have minimal changes. In B mode, the "four-chamber" view may show an almost completely normal appearance. In moderate forms, myocardial hypertrophy may appear, mainly in the third trimester. The RA can be dilated if there is tricuspid insufficiency (Fig. **13**). It is the study of the PV what allows the diagnosis: in B mode a dysplastic, thickened, hyperechoic and hypokinetic PV is observed, and is visible continuously throughout the cardiac cycle, with decreased pulmonary diameter in relation to the aortic valve (Fig. **14**). Along with this, a post-stenotic dilatation of the main pulmonary artery (MPA) can be seen. With Doppler, the turbulence of the flow at the level of the PV and the acceleration of the pulmonary systolic peak are observed (Figs. **15** and **16**). The perfusion of the MPA is usually antegrade.

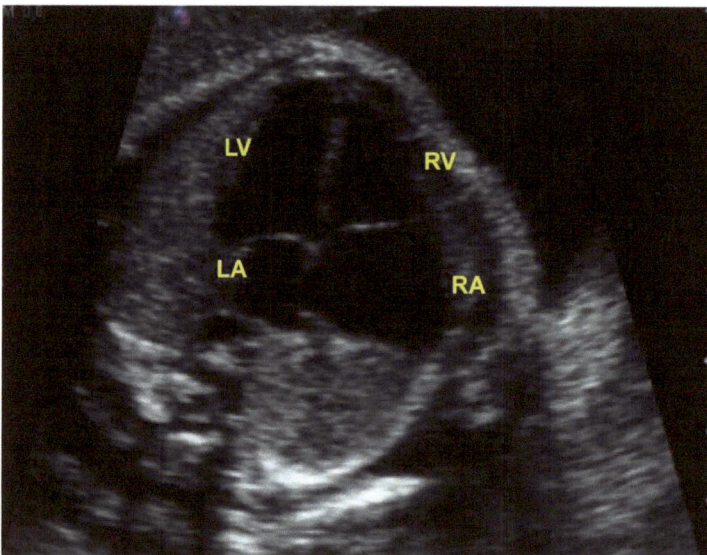

Fig. (13). Four chamber view of a fetus with mild-moderate pulmonary stenosis, in which only a discrete dilation of the right atrium (RA) is observed. LA: left atrium, LV: left ventricle, RV: right ventricle.

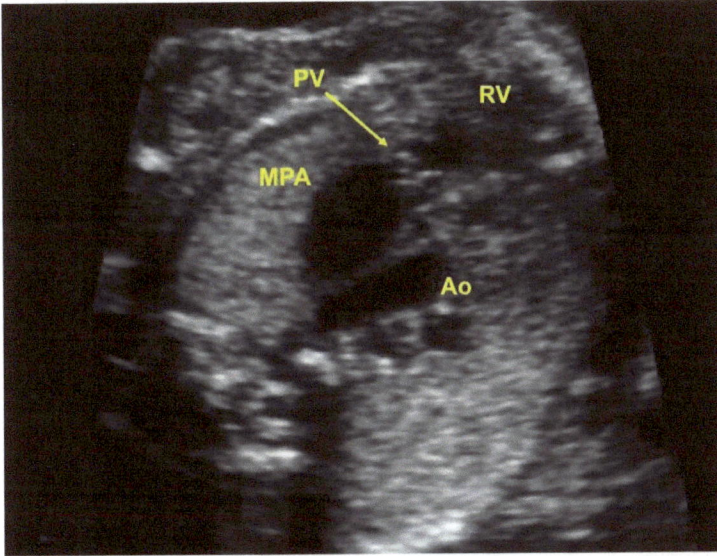

Fig. (14). Image of the right ventricle (RV) outflow tract of a fetus with pulmonary stenosis showing a thickened, irregular and hyperechogenic pulmonary valve (PV), as well as a post-stenotic dilatation of the main pulmonary artery (MPA). Compare with the size of the aorta (Ao).

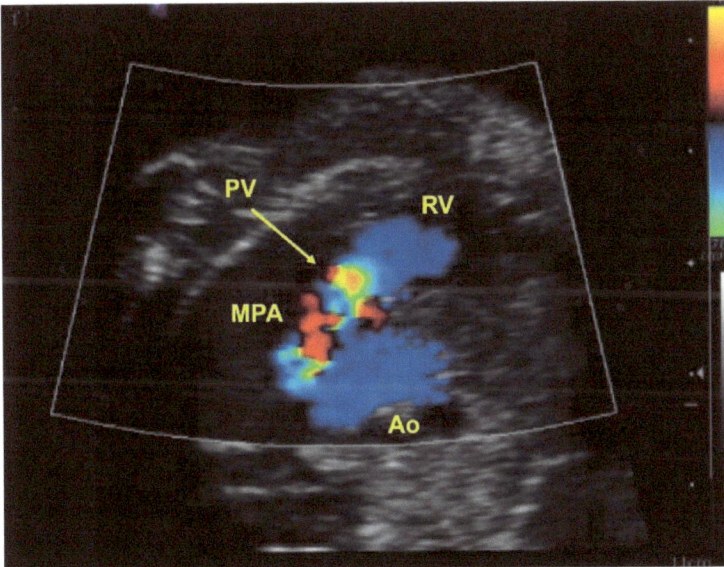

Fig. (15). Color Doppler assessment of the right ventricular (RV) outflow tract of a fetus with moderate pulmonary stenosis in which the turbulent flow of blood through the pulmonary valve (PV) is observed. Ao: aorta, MPA: main pulmonary artery.

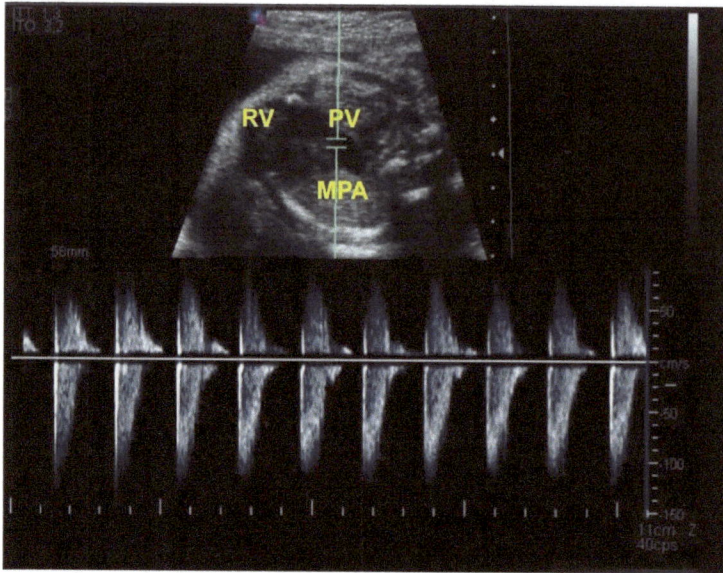

Fig. (16). Pulsed Doppler evaluation of the right ventricular (RV) outflow tract of a fetus with moderate pulmonary stenosis showing an acceleration of the pulmonary systolic peak (close to 1.5 m/s). MPA: main pulmonary artery, PV: pulmonary valve.

1. Severe forms (CPS): the pulmonary valve also is dysplastic, thickened, hyperechoic and hypokinetic. Its leaflets have a dome movement to leave a small exit orifice in systole, central or eccentric, but the leaflets are visible at all times during the cardiac cycle (Fig. **17**). The diameter of the MPA is usually lower than expected for gestational age (GA), but occasionally a post-stenotic dilatation may be found. Doppler demonstrates the presence of anterograde and turbulent flow, with acceleration of the systolic peak in the PV. This makes it possible to distinguish this entity from the PAIVS in which there is no flow through the PV (Fig. **18**). The filling of the MPA is mixed, there being a large component of reversed flow from the DA (Fig. **19**). It is not uncommon in dysplastic PV that behave mainly as stenotic to observe also a small jet of diastolic pulmonary insufficiency.

As has already been pointed out, the CPS has many similarities with PAIVS, so that in both cases the findings will be conditioned by the status of the TV. In cases in which the TV is severely stenotic the RV may eventually become hypoplastic (Fig. **20**). In these cases, the CPS may even evolve to pulmonary atresia (PA). On the contrary, RV growth is usually preserved when the TV is insufficient (Fig. **21**). Both situations, stenosis and tricuspid insufficiency, can be assessed with Doppler: in the case of stenosis, a small jet of transtricuspid anterograde flow will be observed, often monophasic, followed in systole by also a small jet of regurgitation that does not reach the roof of the RA (Fig. **22**). On the other hand, in the case of insufficient TV, a holosystolic regurgitation jet, with a velocity of more than 2-3 m/s and reaching the RA roof, will be observed. In these cases, the diastolic transtricuspid antegrade flow is often normal (Fig. **23**). In the most severe forms of TR, signs of congestive heart failure may appear, even leading to fetal hydrops.

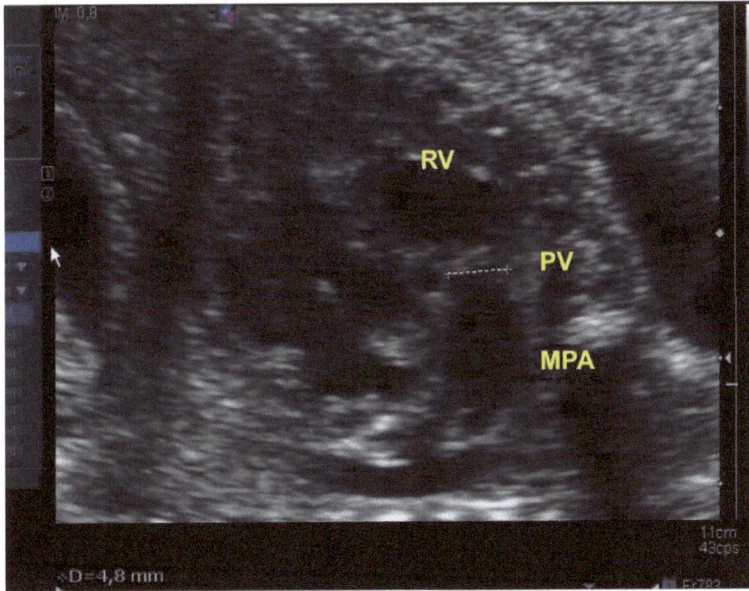

Fig. (17). Image of the right ventricular (RV) outflow tract of a fetus with critical pulmonary stenosis in systole in which it is observed a thickened and hyperechoic pulmonary valve (PV) and whose leaflets do not separate. MPA: main pulmonary artery.

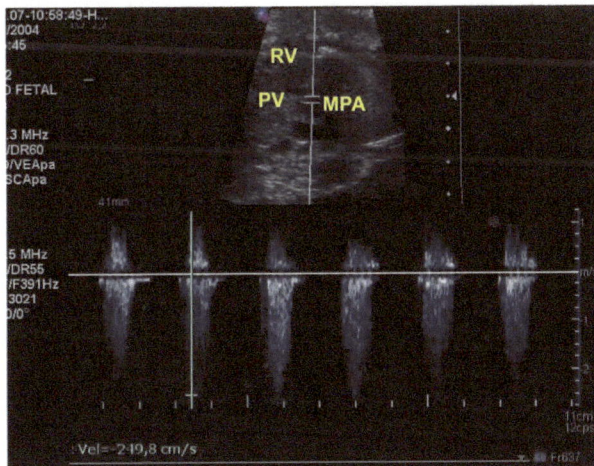

Fig. (18). Pulsed Doppler assessment of the right ventricular (RV) outflow tract of a fetus with severe pulmonary stenosis showing an acceleration of the pulmonary systolic peak (2.5 m/s). MPA: pulmonary artery, PV: pulmonary valve.

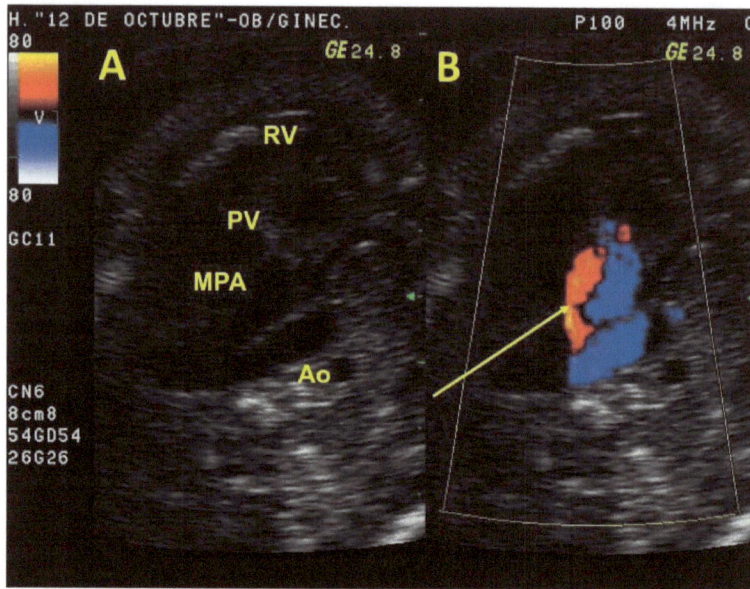

Fig. (19). (A) Image of the right ventricular (RV) outflow tract of a fetus with severe pulmonary stenosis showing a thickened pulmonary valve (PV). (B) Color Doppler examination of the same patient in which mixed perfusion of the main pulmonary artery (MPA) with anterograde component (blue) and another of similar size from the ductus (red, arrow) is observed. Ao: aorta.

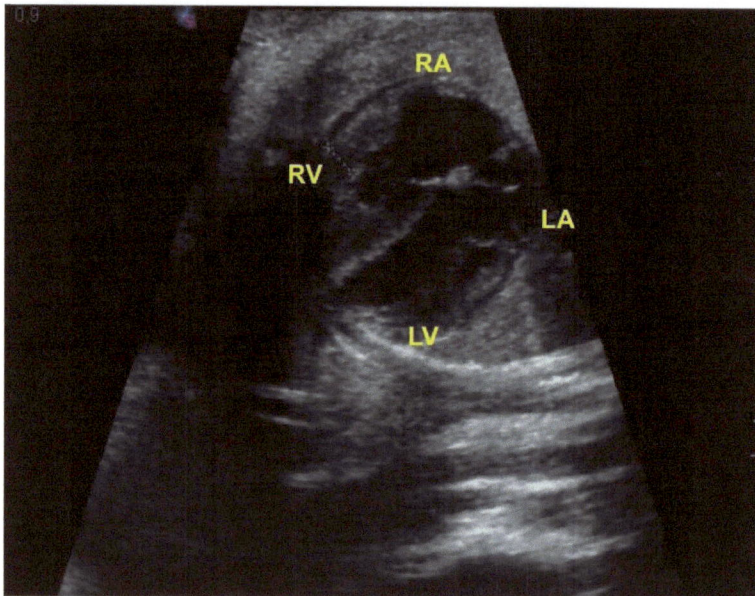

Fig. (20). Four chamber view of a fetus with critical pulmonary stenosis in which a significant asymmetry between the size of the left (LV) and right ventricle (RV) is observed. The RV is underdeveloped and only the inlet portion is seen. The trabecular portion is obliterated and the and the RV does not form the cardiac apex. LA: left atrium, RA: right atrium.

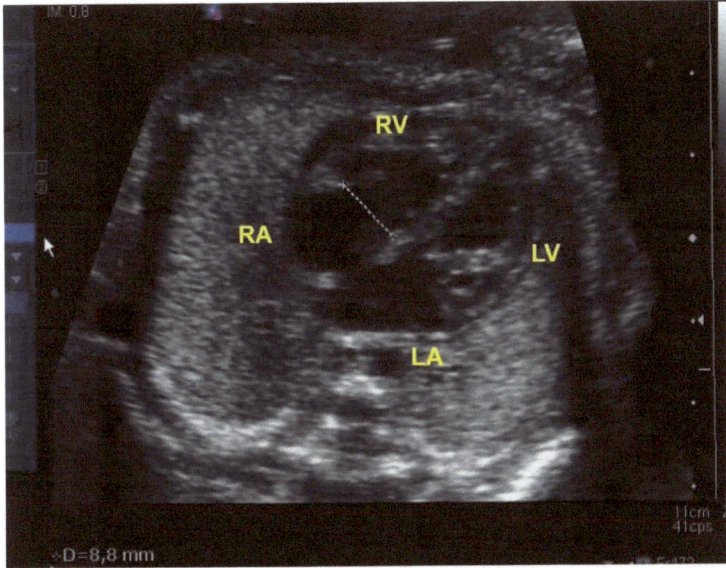

Fig. (21). Four chamber view of a fetus with critical pulmonary stenosis with an adequate development of the right ventricle (RV), which preserves the inlet and trabecular portions. RA: right atrium; LA: left atrium; LV: left ventricle.

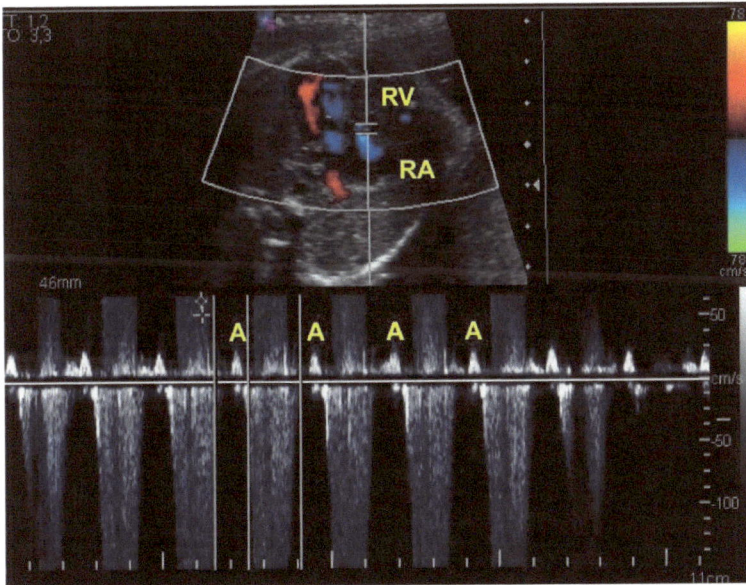

Fig. (22). Color and pulsed Doppler evaluation of the tricuspid flow in a fetus with severe pulmonary stenosis, stenotic tricuspid valve and small right ventricle (RV). In diastole, the antegrade flow is low speed, of short duration and monophasic, only A wave being identified, which is followed by a flow of holosystolic regurgitation that does not reach the atrial roof. RA: right atrium.

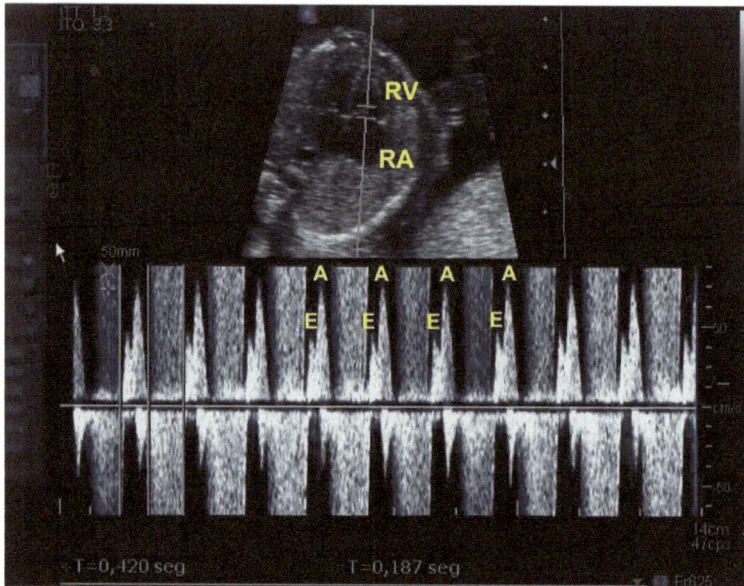

Fig. (23). Color and pulsed Doppler assessment of the tricuspid flow in a fetus with severe pulmonary stenosis, insufficient tricuspid valve and normally developed right ventricle (RV). In diastole, the anterograde flow is biphasic, identifying both the E and A waves, which is followed by a flow of holosystolic regurgitation. RA: right atrium.

In all cases, the existence of other CHD and associated extracardiac malformations should be ruled out, and a study of the fetal karyotype should be offered.

Evolution and Perinatal Management: this condition may remain stable throughout gestation but also may evolve to a more severe disease [8]. Therefore, it is important to perform follow up scans every 3-4 weeks, assessing the growth of the MPA and the PV, as well as the presence of forward flow through the valve, since it can progress to PA. The severity of the TR, the flow through the foramen ovale, the appearance of signs of right heart failure and the growth of the RV should also be assessed. These last two aspects are the most important from a prognostic point of view so that when there are signs of right heart failure or a tendency towards RV underdevelopment, a fetal pulmonary valvuloplasty trying to modify the natural history of this condition may be offered. In cases of CPS, perinatal care must be made in a tertiary care referral center since it is a ductus-dependent CHD. However, neonates with mild forms of PS do not require immediate postnatal cardiological care.

Postnatal Treatment and Prognosis: patients with mild forms may be completely asymptomatic and do not need any type of early treatment. In symptomatic patients, with moderate or severe forms of PS, the treatment of choice is balloon pulmonary valvuloplasty, which has excellent results. Refractory cases or those with a dysplastic valve are candidates to surgical valvulotomy. The treatment of cases of CPS and severe RV hypoplasia is discussed in the PAIVS section.

Pulmonary Atresia with Intact Ventricular Septum

Definition: total obstruction of the RV outflow tract due to the absence of development of the PV. The only route of blood supply to the lungs is the DA.

Classification: depending on the location of the obstruction, there are two types of pulmonary atresia with intact ventricular septum (PAIVS):

- PAIVS with valvular or membranous obstruction: 80% of cases.

- PAIVS with subvalvular, infundibular or muscular obstruction: 20% of cases.

In addition to this, according to the behavior of the TV there are two forms of PAIVS [9]:

- Type I (75%): TV is competent or restrictive. In the same way that it occurred with CPS, this form is usually associated with an underdeveloped RV (80%), or even frankly hypoplastic RV, and it can be associated with VCC in 40% of these cases.

- Type II (25%): TV is incompetent or insufficient. As for CPS, in most cases the RV can have a normal size (80-85%) and maintain its tripartite morphology (80-85%). The VCC are not common. The more severe the TR, the more likely it is that there is dysplasia of the TV or that it is even an Ebstein's anomaly (10% of cases). In these cases of severe TR, there can be an asymmetric cardiomegaly because of enlargement of the RA. It can cause right heart failure and fetal hydrops.

Frequency: it constitutes 1-5% of all CHD, and 2.5-4% of the CHD detected prenatally.

Recurrence: 1% if there is an affected child and 3% if there are two affected children.

Presentation: most cases are isolated, but in 20% of cases there are associated other cardiac anomalies (Ebstein, right aortic arch, aortic stenosis) or extracardiac (musculoskeletal, central nervous system).

Chromosome Abnormality: present in 10% of cases (trisomy 21, trisomy 18 and deletion 4p).

Prenatal Diagnosis:

- Type I: the echocardiographic findings are dependent on the stage of evolution of the condition. In B mode, the four-chamber view is abnormal due to the presence of a hypertrophic, hypokinetic RV with a variable degree of underdevelopment. According to the tripartite aspect that the RV has in normal conditions, three different morphologies of the RV can be observed in this CHD:

- Tripartite (59%): none of the three portions is lost.
- Bipartite (34%): the apical portion is obliterated, and only the inlet and outlet portions are seen.
- Unipartite (<8%): presence of the inlet portion only.

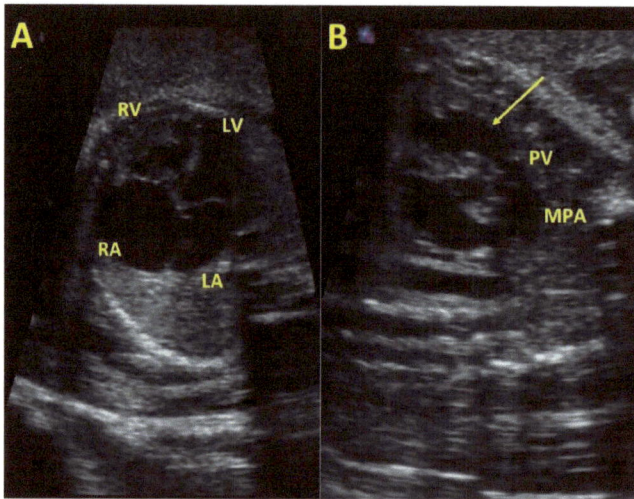

Fig. (24). (**A**) Four chamber view of a fetus with pulmonary atresia and intact ventricular septum with an adequate development of the right ventricle (RV), which preserves the inlet and trabecular portions. (**B**) Image of the RV outflow tract of the same fetus in which the normal development of the infundibulum is observed (arrow). LA: left atrium, LV: left ventricle, MPA: main pulmonary artery, PV: pulmonary valve, RA: right atrium.

The importance of this classification relies in the association with the postnatal prognosis [10], since the type of surgery depends on the morphology and size of the RV (Figs. **24-26**). Unlike what happens in the left ventricle (LV), when there is a severe obstruction in the RV outflow tract, it is uncommon for the RV to show fibroelastosis. There may be an increase in the size of the left atrium (LA) and LV due to the volume overload. The size of the TV is generally proportional to that of the RV, and it presents a low mobility, with frank limitation to its opening, due to its stenotic character and to the high pressure in the RV (Fig. **27**). The PV is dysplastic, showing a thickened and hyperechogenic appearance, and although it can show movement during the cardiac cycle, no separation of its leaflets is identified (Fig. **28**). The diameter of the main pulmonary artery (MPA) and its branches is usually lower than expected for GA (Figs. **29** and **30**).

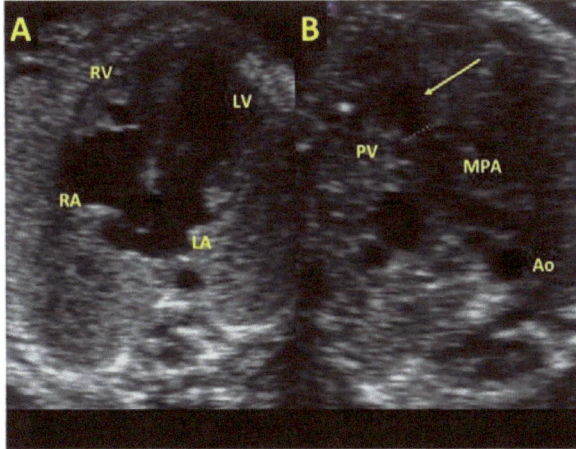

Fig. (25). (**A**) Four chamber view of a fetus with pulmonary atresia and intact ventricular septum, in which only the inlet portion is observed in the right ventricle (RV). (**B**) Image of the RV outflow tract of the same fetus in which the infundibulum is very small (arrow). Ao: aorta, LA: left atrium, LV: left ventricle, MPA: main pulmonary artery, PV: pulmonary valve, RA: right atrium.

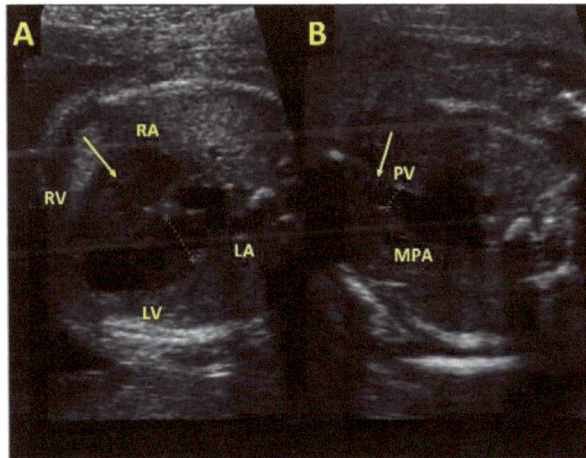

Fig. (26). (**A**) Four chamber view of a fetus with pulmonary atresia and intact ventricular septum with a hypoplastic right ventricle (RV), in which only a minimal development of the inlet portion is identified. The arrow points to the tricuspid valve. (**B**) Image of the RV outflow tract of the same fetus where there is also no development of the infundibulum (arrow). LA: left atrium, LV: left ventricle, MPA: main pulmonary artery, PV: pulmonary valve, RA: right atrium.

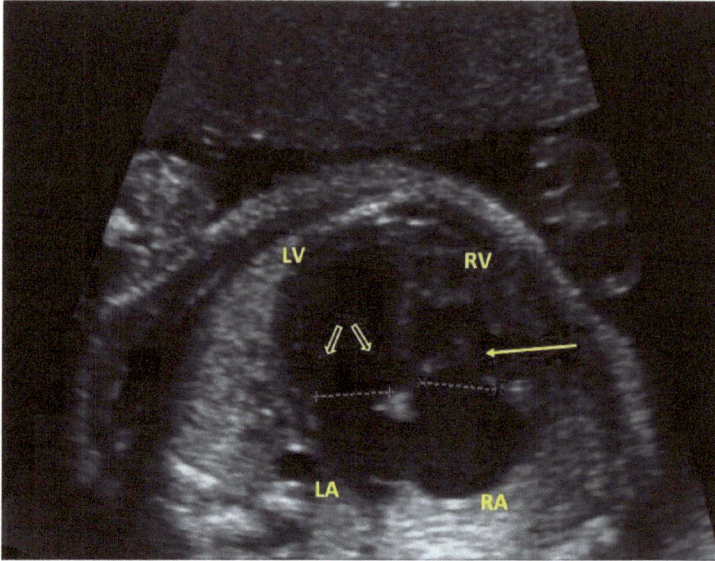

Fig. (27). Four chamber view of a fetus with pulmonary atresia and intact ventricular septum, in which there is a limitation for the opening of the tricuspid valve (arrow) in diastole because of the increased pressure in the right ventricle (RV). Compare with the separate leaflets of the mitral valve (empty arrows). LA: left atrium, LV: left ventricle, RA: right atrium.

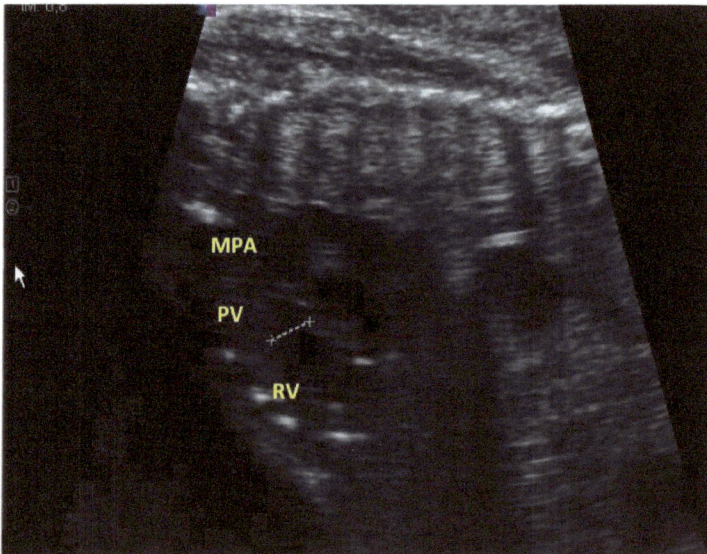

Fig. (28). Image of the right ventricular (RV) outflow tract of a fetus with pulmonary atresia and intact ventricular septum in which the pulmonary valve (PV) is closed, thickened and hyperechoic. MPA: main pulmonary artery.

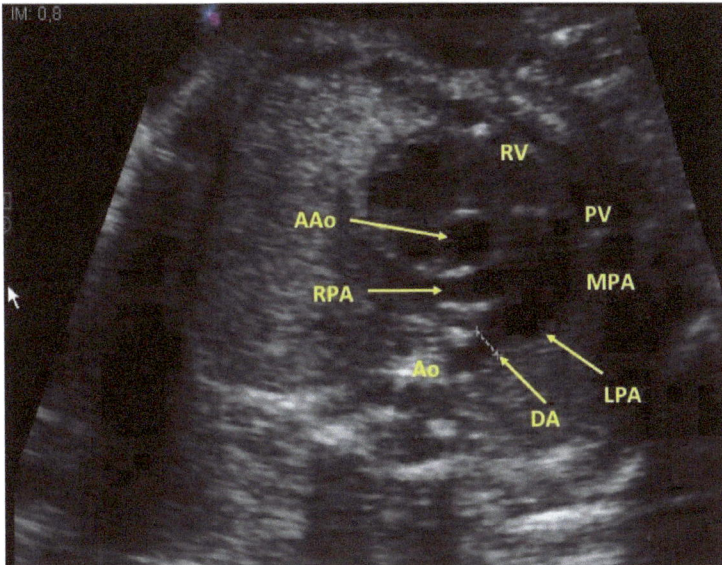

Fig. (29). Short axis view of the great vessels of a fetus with pulmonary atresia and intact ventricular septum in which it is observed that, despite the valvular atresia, the anatomy is conserved. Ao: descending aorta, AAo: ascending aorta, DA: ductus arteriosus, LPA: left pulmonary artery, MPA: main pulmonary artery, PV: pulmonary valve, RPA: right pulmonary artery, RV: right ventricle.

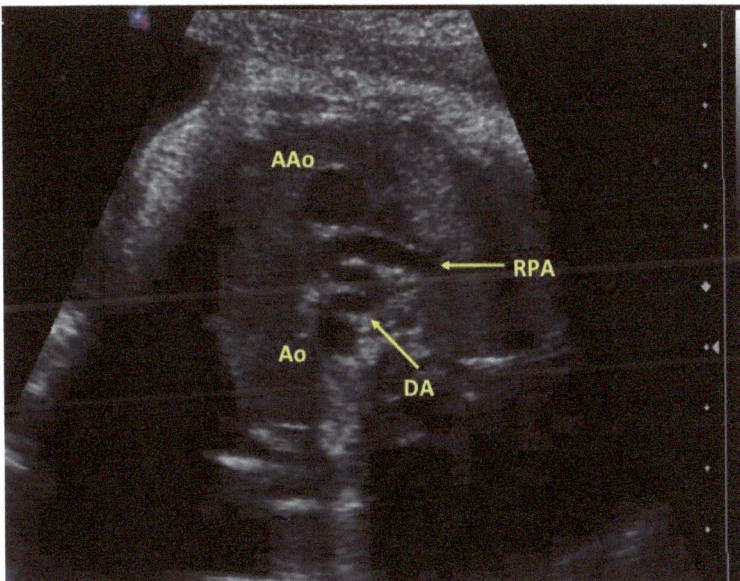

Fig. (30). Examination of the central pulmonary arteries of a fetus with muscular atresia of the pulmonary valve and intact ventricular septum, in which it is observed that the right pulmonary artery (RPA) is connected to a tortuous and sinusoidal ductus arteriosus (DA) that originates from the lower side of the aorta (Ao). AAo: ascending aorta.

With color and pulsed Doppler, there is an absence of transvalvular flow through the PV, with retrograde flow in the MPA from the DA (Fig. **31**). The tricuspid flow is antegrade, although monophasic, followed by a mild TR that usually does not reach the atrial roof (Fig. **32**).

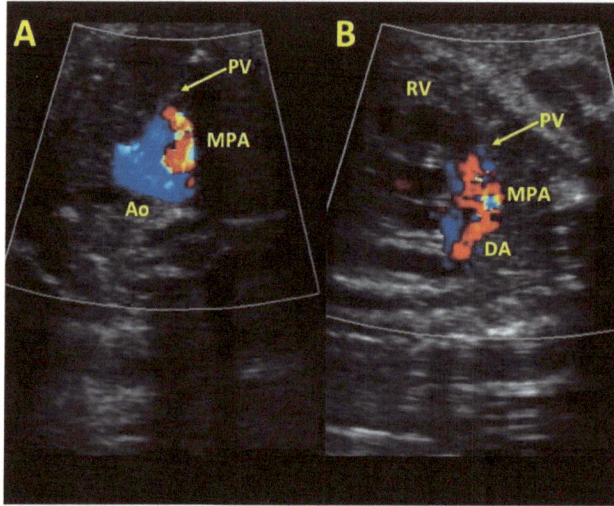

Fig. (31). (**A**) Three vessels and trachea view of a fetus with pulmonary atresia and intact ventricular septum, in which the ductus-dependent retrograde filling of the main pulmonary artery (MPA) is observed in red. (**B**) Image of the ductal arch of the same fetus showing the same phenomenon. Ao: aorta, DA: ductus arteriosus, PV: pulmonary valve, RV: right ventricle.

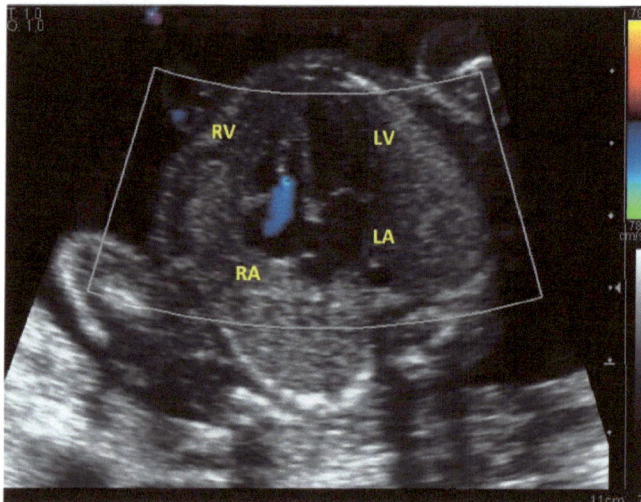

Fig. (32). Four chamber view of a fetus with pulmonary atresia and intact ventricular septum type I, with a mild tricuspid regurgitation that does not reach the atrial roof. LA: left atrium, LV: left ventricle, RA: right atrium, RV: right ventricle.

In approximately 40% of PAIVS type I, the presence of VCC is observed in the lateral wall or in the apex of the RV. The probability that there are VCC is inversely proportional to the size of the TV and RV: the smaller these are, the more likely it is to find them. It is more common to observe it in the five-chamber view, in which a vessel arising in the aortic root and following the path of the coronary artery, generally right, is noted. A bidirectional flow (antegrade and low speed in diastole, and retrograde and high velocity in systole) will be observed and that can also be demonstrated with pulsed Doppler (Figs. **33** and **34**).

- Type II: RV has a normal or dilated appearance, with a dysplastic TV and/or an anomalous insertion with high velocity pansystolic TR that causes a dilatation of the RA. With Doppler the severity of the TR is demonstrated and quantified (Figs. **35** and **36**), and it is even possible to detect reverse flow in the ductus venosus, coinciding with atrial contraction, and even pulsatile flow in the inferior vena cava. The VCC are rarely seen in this form.

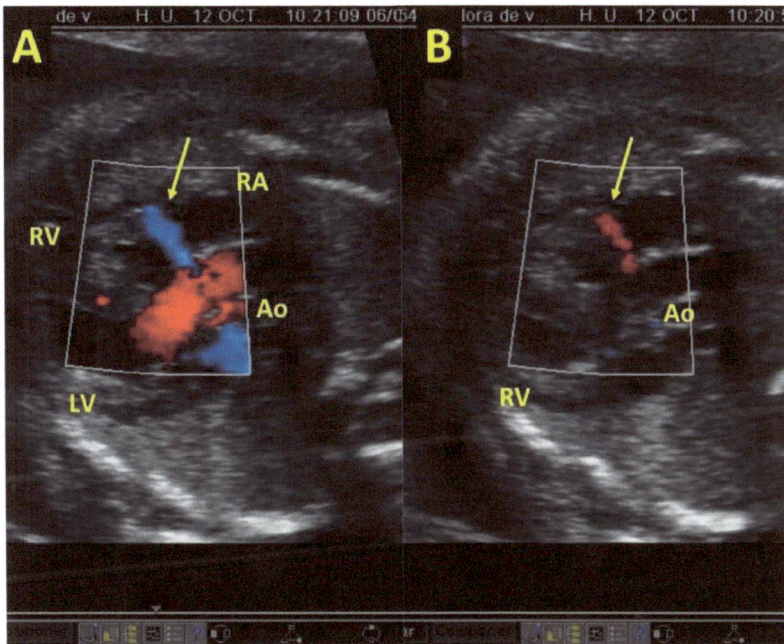

Fig. (33). Five chamber view of a fetus with pulmonary atresia and intact ventricular septum and ventriculo-coronary connections. (**A**) In systole, the flow through the coronary artery is retrograde (arrow), towards the aorta (Ao). (**B**) In diastole, the flow through the coronary artery is antegrade (arrow). LV: left ventricle, RA: right atrium, RV: right ventricle.

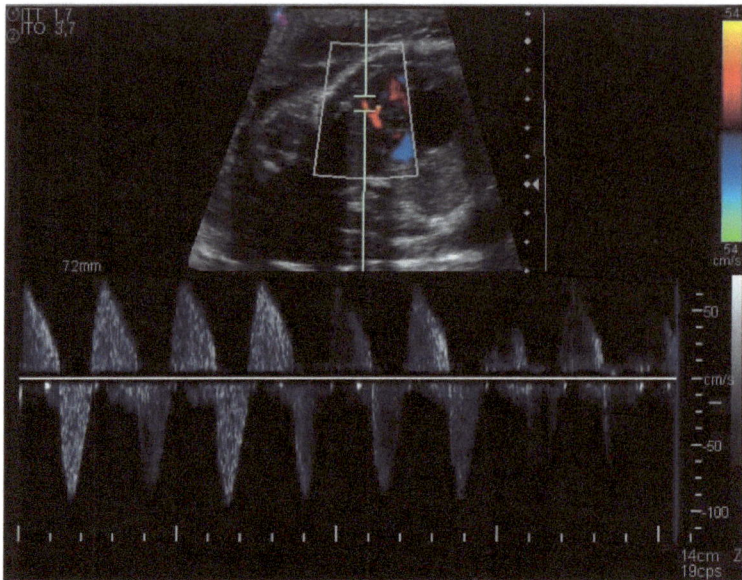

Fig. (34). Pulsed Doppler examination of a fetus with pulmonary atresia and intact ventricular septum and ventriculo-coronary connections, in which the characteristic alternating antegrade-retrograde (diastole-systole) pattern is seen.

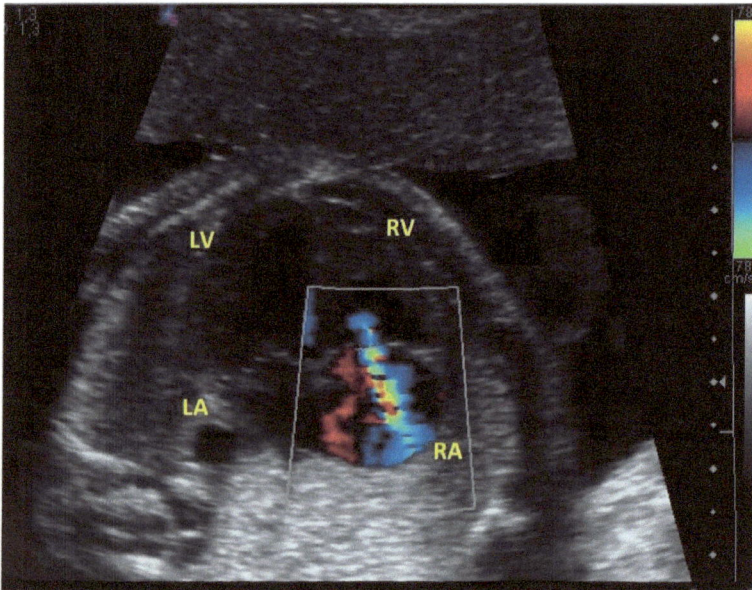

Fig. (35). Four chamber view of a fetus with pulmonary atresia and intact ventricular septum type II, with a severe tricuspid insufficiency that reaches the atrial roof, and returns to the right ventricle (RV). LA: left atrium, LV: left ventricle, RA: right atrium.

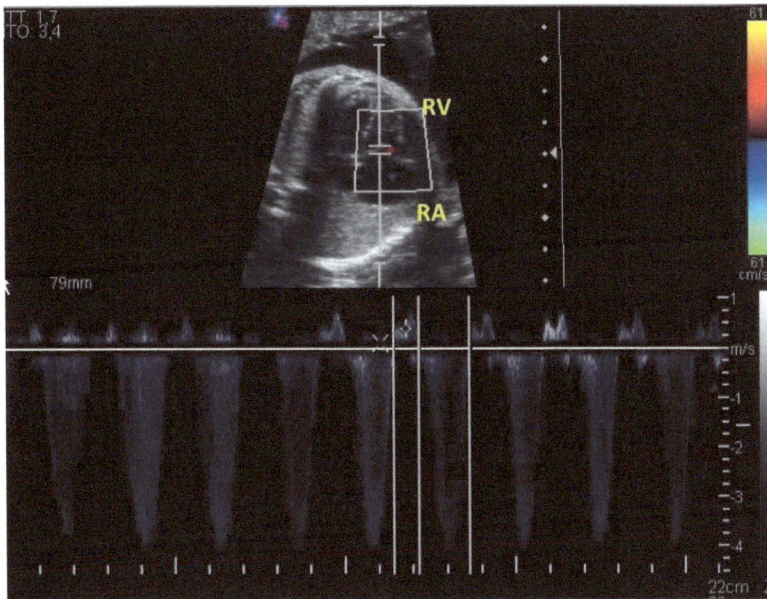

Fig. (36). Pulsed Doppler evaluation of transtricuspid flow in a fetus with pulmonary atresia and intact ventricular septum type II, showing a severe high velocity holosystolic insufficiency (4 m/s). RA: right atrium, RV: right ventricle.

Perinatal Management: the prognosis depends primarily on, first, the degree of RV development and whether it is possible to maintain a biventricular circulation or not, and second, the appearance of signs of cardiac failure. Therefore, the sonographic assessment will also include the analysis of the viability of the RV and of the hemodynamic situation. It is also important a close surveillance, in order to propose, in selected cases, intrauterine cardiac intervention. These controls will be performed every 2-4 weeks, depending on the characteristics of each case, and they will assess the growth of the affected structures, the severity of the TR, interatrial flow, cardiac function and the global hemodynamic situation. All patients diagnosed prenatally with PAIVS must be born in a tertiary care center.

Postnatal Treatment and Prognosis: the factors that will influence the type of treatment are the degree of development of the RV, which will determine the type of postnatal circulation (uni or biventricular), and the presence of VCC with RV-dependent coronary circulation. Based on this, there are three situations:

- Hypoplastic RV (uni- or bipartite, absence of infundibulum, z-score of the TV <-5) and/or RV-dependent coronary circulation: univentricular palliation is chosen, for which three serial surgical interventions are necessary.

- RV adequately developed (tripartite, z-score of the TV >-2): biventricular circulation is usually possible. Commonly the treatment consists of radiofrequency perforation followed by balloon dilation, although surgical valve opening can also be chosen.

- Borderline RV (bipartite, z-score of the TV between -2 and -5) and with a compromise of diastolic function and a variable cardiac output reduction. In these cases, the initial therapy is similar to the previous point, but it may be necessary to add the placement of a systemic-pulmonary fistula or a stent in the DA to assure an adequate pulmonary flow. The subsequent re-evaluation of the RV size and function, approximately at 6 months, allows to decide if the RV is able to assume all the RV output, in which case the systemic-pulmonary connection is closed, or not. In the latter case, a bidirectional Glenn procedure is usually chosen, reassessing the situation between the 1st and 3rd year of life to decide whether to opt for univentricular palliation or for an intermediate situation of "1 and a half ventricle repair".

Finally, a biventricular circulation is achieved in 30-50% of all PAIVS cases, with a child survival rate at around 90%. At 10-15 years the survival is 80-86%.

EARLY CLOSURE OF DUCTUS ARTERIOSUS

Definition: partial or complete obstruction to the flow between the MPA and the descending aorta through the DA in fetal life.

Etiology: it may be a congenital absence of DA or a total or partial closure of a DA previously normal. In the first case, it is usually associated with CHD (tetralogy of Fallot with absence of PV, truncus arteriosus). Acquired forms can be idiopathic, which are the most common, or secondary to the administration to the mother of some medical treatments [non-steroidal anti-inflammatory drugs such as indoleacetic acid derivatives (indomethacin), arylacetic acid derivatives (diclofenac), and the arylpropionic acid derivatives (ibuprofen), or corticosteroids, such as dexamethasone] [11]. We will focus in acquired forms.

Presentation: it often appears abruptly, in the third trimester of pregnancy, and is usually reversible after discontinuation of the medication. The pharmacological forms usually appear beyond 32-34 weeks, since this period is when DA becomes more sensitive to constricting factors. However, the response to these drugs is often fetus-dependent and not always dose-dependent.

Prenatal Diagnosis: the Doppler study shows an acceleration of the transductal flow, with a peak systolic velocity greater than 140 cm/s, a diastolic peak greater than 35 cm/s, and a pulsatility index (PI) lower than 1.9 m/s (Fig. **37**). This PI is smaller the more marked the constriction to the ductal flow is. In addition, there may be signs of volume overload in the RV. When the closure of the DA is complete, in B-mode there is an asymmetric cardiomegaly because of dilatation of the RA and RV, RV hypertrophy (Fig. **38**) and dilatation of the MPA and its branches, while the DA is narrowed showing an hourglass appearance. With Doppler, the poor antegrade filling of the MPA is noted, usually accompanied by pulmonary insufficiency, moderate-severe TR, absent or reverse flow in the ductus venosus, and a dilated MPA (Fig. **39**). In more advanced cases signs of right heart failure may even appear, eventually leading in undiagnosed cases to fetal hydrops and intrauterine death.

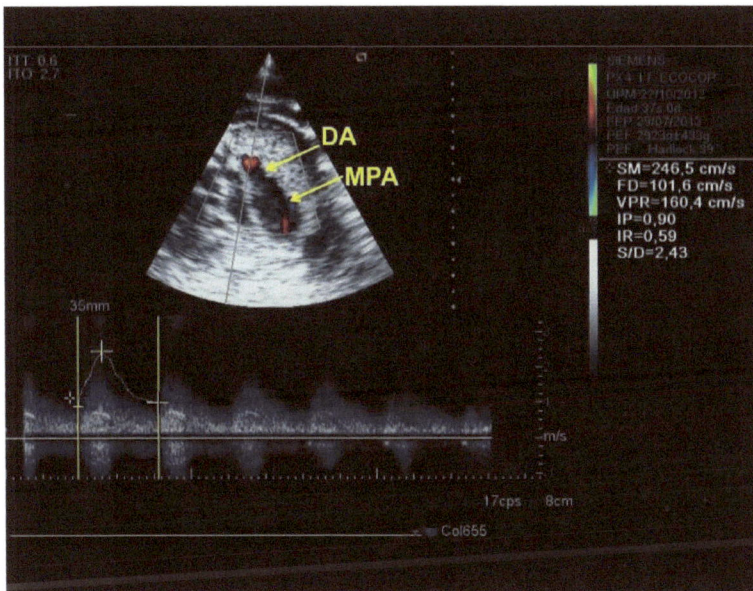

Fig. (37). Doppler waveform of the ductus arteriosus (DA) of a fetus with premature closure of the DA. There is a high velocity systolic peak (246.5 cm/s), a high end-diastolic velocity (101.6 cm/s) with a pulsatility index (PI) of 0.9. MPA: main pulmonary artery.

Evolution and prenatal management: the first step is to interrogate the mother about the use of drugs that can cause an early closure of the DA. If so, the immediate cessation of such consumption must be recommended, which can lead to a progressive reopening of the DA.

The attitude will depend on the degree of hemodynamic repercussion:

- If the etiological agent has been identified, the fetal situation is adequate, and the GA is < 34-36 weeks: expectant management with monitoring every 24-48h and if it progresses, delivery is recommended.

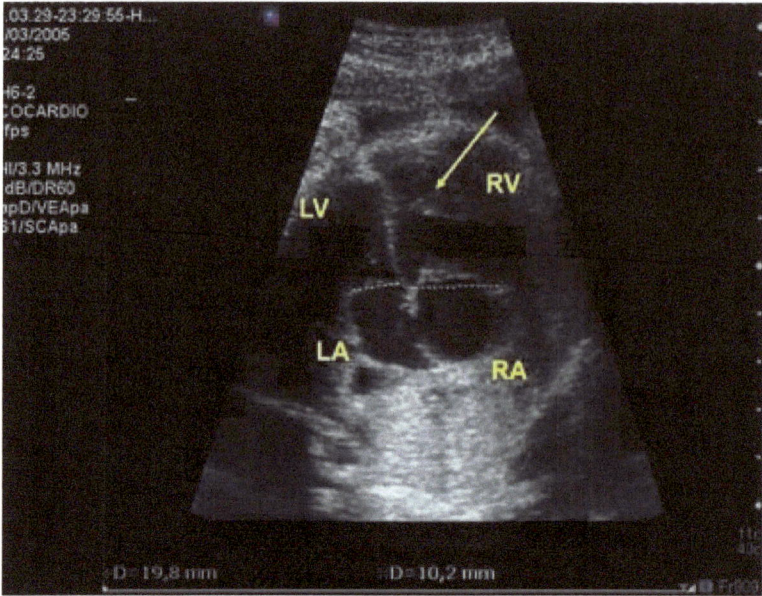

Fig. (38). Four chamber view of a fetus with premature closure of the ductus arteriosus in the third trimester of gestation. There is a cardiac asymmetry, with dilatation of the right atrium (RA) and right ventricle (RV) as well as hypertrophy of the latter (arrow). LA: left atrium, LV: left ventricle.

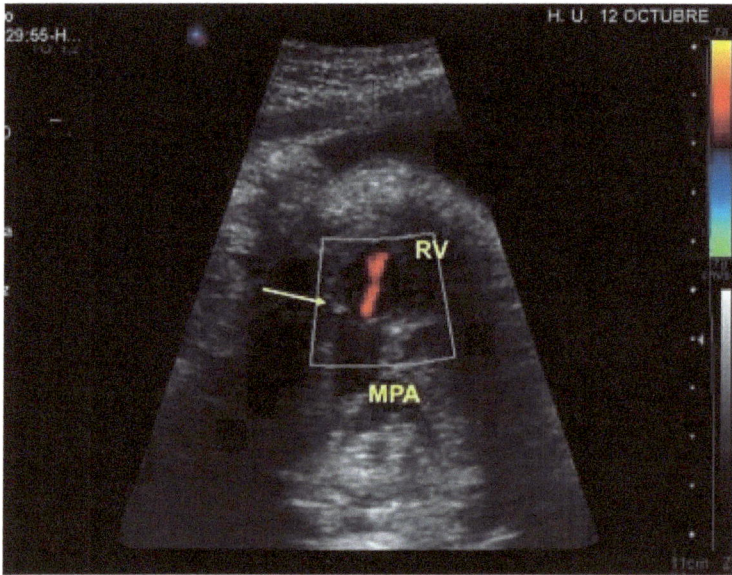

Fig. (39). Color Doppler assessment of the right ventricular (RV) outflow tract of a fetus with premature closure of the ductus arteriosus in which a jet of pulmonary insufficiency (arrow) is observed during diastole. MPA: main pulmonary artery.

- If the etiological agent has been identified, the fetal situation is adequate and the GA is > 34-36 weeks: delivery is recommended.

- If the etiological agent has been identified, and there is a severe fetal repercussion (hydrops): delivery is recommended. If the GA is < 32 weeks, a close surveillance for 24-48h to assess if the DA reopens and the fetal situation improves after cessation of the administration of the etiological agent can be chosen.

- If the etiological agent has not been identified: delivery is recommended, unless the fetal situation is adequate and the GA is < 32-34 weeks, in which case expectant management with close fetal monitoring can be elected.

Most of the prenatal echocardiographic findings disappear at three weeks of birth although the changes produced at the RV (hypertrophy) take longer to normalize. However, fetuses with long-term ductal constriction during pregnancy can develop pulmonary hypertension in the neonatal period, and occasionally respond poorly to medical treatment with nitric oxide. Survival is around 75-80%.

CONSENT FOR PUBLICATION

Not applicable.

CONFLICT OF INTEREST

The authors confirm that the contents of this chapter have no conflict of interest.

ACKNOWLEDGEMENTS

Declare none.

REFERENCES

[1]   Paladini D, Volpe P. Ultrasound of congenital fetal anomalies Differential diagnosis and prognostic indicators. 2nd ed., Boca Raton, FL: CRC Press, Taylor & Francis Group 2014.
        [http://dx.doi.org/10.1201/b16779]

[2]   Torigoe T, Mawad W, Seed M, *et al.* Treatment of fetal circular shunt with non-steroidal anti-inflammatory drugs. Ultrasound Obstet Gynecol 2019; 53(6): 841-6.
        [http://dx.doi.org/10.1002/uog.20169] [PMID: 30381862]

[3]   Aly S, Bokowski J, Diab K, Muller BA. Fetal and postnatal echocardiographic diagnosis of ebstein anomaly of the mitral valve. Pediatr Cardiol 2018; 39(6): 1276-9.
        [http://dx.doi.org/10.1007/s00246-018-1903-y] [PMID: 29756160]

[4]   Allen HD, Driscoll DJ, Shaddy RE, Feltes TF. Moss and Adams' Heart disease in infants, children, and adolescents Including the fetus and young adult. 7th ed., Philadelphia, PA: Lippincott Williams and Wilkins 2008.

[5]   Rao PS. A unified classification for tricuspid atresia. Am Heart J 1980; 99(6): 799-804.

[http://dx.doi.org/10.1016/0002-8703(80)90632-8] [PMID: 6990738]

[6]   Berg C, Lachmann R, Kaiser C, *et al.* Prenatal diagnosis of tricuspid atresia: intrauterine course and outcome. Ultrasound Obstet Gynecol 2010; 35(2): 183-90.
[http://dx.doi.org/10.1002/uog.7499] [PMID: 20101636]

[7]   Yagel S, Silverman NH, Gembruch U. Fetal Cardiology: Embryology, Genetics, Physiology, Echocardiographic Evaluation, Diagnosis and Perinatal Management of Cardiac Disease. 2nd ed., Boca Raton, FL: CRC Press, Taylor & Francis Group 2009.

[8]   Redington AN, Van Arsdell GS, Anderson RH. Congenital diseases in the right heart. London: Springer-Verlag 2009.
[http://dx.doi.org/10.1007/978-1-84800-378-1]

[9]   Drose J. Fetal echocardiography. 2nd ed., St Louis, MO: Saunders Elsevier 2010.

[10]   Galindo A, Gratacós E, Martínez JM. Cardiología Fetal. Madrid: Marbán 2015.

[11]   Ishida H, Kawazu Y, Kayatani F, Inamura N. Prognostic factors of premature closure of the ductus arteriosus *in utero*: a systematic literature review. Cardiol Young 2017; 27(4): 634-8.
[http://dx.doi.org/10.1017/S1047951116000871] [PMID: 27322829]

CHAPTER 11

Fetal Left Cardiac Malformations

Gabriele Tonni[1,*] and **Gianpaolo Grisolia**[2]

[1] *Department of Obstetrics and Gynecology, Prenatal Diagnostic Service, Guastalla Civil Hospital, Istituto di Ricerca a Carattere Clinico Scientifico (IRCCS), AUSL di Reggio Emilia, Reggio Emilia, Italy*

[2] *Maternal Fetal Unit, Department of Obstetrics and Gynecology, "Carlo Poma" Hospital, Mantua, Italy*

Abstract: Congenital heart defects (CHDs) represent the most common congenital malformations, especially those affecting the left side of the fetal heart. During fetal life, the presence of the ductus arteriosus is responsible for the low intrauterine mortality rate if compared with the postnatal life. Prenatal diagnosis of CHDs has improved over the past 20 years and diagnostic enhancement has been obtained with the introduction of standardized examination of the fetal heart together with the technological advancement of the ultrasound equipment, particularly with the introduction of the four-dimensional (4D) ultrasound technique based on spatio-temporal-image correlation (STIC) or the application of the three-vessels and trachea view (3VT). The chapter describes and reports the evolution of the antenatal detection of left cardiac malformations, with emphasis regarding the echocardiographic characteristics that need to be evaluated in order to assess the hemodynamic state of the fetus. An extending search and analysis of the medical literature has been sought and describe in relation to the prenatal ultrasound diagnosis of aortic coarctation (CoA), aortic stenosis (AS), interrupted aortic arch (IAA), hypoplastic left heart syndrome (HLHS), aortic arch abnormalities and aorto-pulmonary window (APW). Understanding the cardiac performance of the fertus is of vital and critical importance to plan appropriate management and prognosis. Cardiac defect as critical aortic stenosis (CAS), IAA and HLHS are described as a potential emerging pathogenetic *continuum*. Attention has been paid to the latest improvement of *in utero* surgery and technique such as fetal aortic valvuloplasty in case of CAS or severe CoA and the use of multiple scoring system to predict postnatal biventricular circulation are described in great details. Notewithstanding, the chapter is enriched by a series of 2D- as well as 3D/4D ultrasound imaging and videos for each type of left cardiac malformation.

Keywords: 3 Vessel and Trachea view, Aortic arch abnormalities, Aortic coarctation, Aortic stenosis, Congenital heart defects, Doppler ultrasound,

* **Corresponding author Gabriele Tonni:** Department of Obstetrics and Gynecology, Guastalla Civil Hospital, Istituto di Ricerca a Carattere Clinico Scientifico Associate Professorship in Obstetrics & Gynecology, Department (IRCCS), AUSL di Reggio Emilia, Reggio Emilia, Italy;
E-mail: Tonni.Gabriele@ausl.re.it

Edward Araujo Júnior, Nathalie Jeanne M. Bravo-Valenzuela and Alberto Borges Peixoto (Eds.)

Echocardiography, Fetal surgery, Hypoplastic left heart syndrome, Interrupted aortic arch, Prenatal diagnosis, Spatio-temporal image correlation.

INTRODUCTION

Malformations involving the left myocardium as well the aorta are of critical importance, especially when postnatal outcome is considered. Congenital heart defects (CHDs) are the most common congenital anomalies with an estimated incidence of 8 per 1,000 births [1].

During fetal life, the right-to-left shift due to the presence of the ductus arteriosus usually prevents cardiovascular complications and heart failure that become apparent sooner or later after birth.

EMBRYOLOGIC DEVELOPMENT OF THE AORTA

At approximately 27 days post-fertilization, the bulbous cordis is divided into the conus cordis and the truncus arteriosus. The conotruncal cushions consisting of cells derived from the endothelium, fuse to form the aortic-pulmonary septum that later undergo to a process of dextral looping of the septum itself and of both the aorta and pulmonary artery. These events occur at around 6 weeks of gestation. Once the fusion of the outflow tract cushions is completed at 8 weeks, the separation of the blood flow between the left and the right ventricle occur.

The aortic vessels, which extend from the aortic sac to the paired dorsal aortae, develop and obliterate asymmetrically. The vessels deriving from the left 4th arch and the left 6th arch give origin to the aortic arch and the pulmonary artery and ductus arteriosus, respectively.

AORTIC COARCTATION

A standardized definition of aortic coarctation (CoA) is still to be assessed, which may contribute to a challenging antenatal ultrasound diagnosis. In general, CoA may be defined as a narrowing of the aorta at the level of the aortic arch or the isthmus to different degrees and may affect 5 to 8% of newborns with CHDs [2, 3]. Disproportion between the right and left ventricle is one of the prenatal echocardiographic clusters of CoA but it may also imply false positive diagnosis *in utero* [4, 5]. Hayett *et al.* [6] described how a high proportion of fetuses with increased nuchal translucency during the first trimester had narrowing of the aortic arch as an associated ultrasound finding.

However, such disproportion may develop during the third trimester of gestation where the vast majority of the international guidelines do not foresee screening for cardiac malformations unless suspected CHDs elicited a thorough fetal echocardiogram late in gestation. Fetuses affected by CoA have several cardiac parameters that may aid the antenatal diagnosis and prenatal diagnosis of the condition, which is important as it is associated with a better postnatal outcome [7].

A systematic metanalysis of medical literature showed that antecedents with pulmonary valve / aortic valve (PV/AoV) ratio >1.6 statistically increased the risk of CoA with an OR of 15.11 (95% CI, 6.80–33.6), good sensitivity (86.2%; 95% CI, 77.5–92.4), but low specificity (51.8%; 95% CI, 46.1–57.4) [8]. Several echocardiographic parameters can be used to assess cardiac outflow tract of the great arteries in cases of CoA such as aortic valve Z-score, ascending aorta Z-score, aortic isthmus Z-score, pulmonary valve Z-score or ratios such as right ventricle/left ventricle (diameters, mm), right ventricle/left ventricle (areas, mm^2), pulmonary artery/ascending aorta (diameters, mm), aortic isthmus/arterial duct (diameters, mm) and arterial duct/aortic isthmus (diameters, mm). Z-score was calculated using the formula Z-score = (f (x) − E(x))/SD(x), where f(x) is the transformation function to which the variable was subjected to generate a distribution that was closer to normal (square root or logarithmic), E(x) is the expected value generated through regression (when the variable depends on gestational age (GA) and calculated as E(x)= α+β x GA) or through the mean (when the variable is independent of gestational age, R2 ~ 0), and SD(x) is the standard deviation estimated by the data sample [9].

However, hypoplastic aortic arch showed a sensitivity (SEN) of 90.0%, a specificity (SPE) of 87.1%, a positive likelihood ratio (LR+) of 6.99 and a negative likelihood ratio (LR−) of 0.12 [8]. Unfortunately, a standardized definition of hypoplastic arch has not yet been established and this may hinder accurate diagnosis. In addition, persistent left superior vena cava (PLSVC) may represent an independent associated antecedent to CoA [10, 11].

Durand *et al.* [12] confirmed hypoplastic aortic arch and a PV/AoV > 1.6 as echocardiographic parameters with good SEN for CoA but also considered aortic arch angulation, ventricular septal defects (VSD) and AoV < 5 mm as additional diagnostic clusters at 36 weeks of gestation with an overall OR > 1 in a multiple logistic regression model. In this series, the prenatal diagnostic accuracy for isolated CoA was 45%. In addition, this study showed that the true positive rate (TPR) for CoA considering the associated presence of VSD or not was 74% and 65% for isolated CoA, respectively. Importantly, Durand *et al.* [12] identified with ROC (receiver operator characteristics) analysis that an AoV Z-score of -1.2, an AoV Z-score of -1.72 and an AoV diameter of 4.9 mm were the best cutoff points of these three qualitative predictors for diagnosing CoA. Nevertheless, the use of such predictors, especially the measurement of AoV, was more feasible and predictable than the measurement of the isthmus [13, 14].

Unfortunately, the detection rate of prenatally diagnosed CoA at the time of the routine anomaly scan in low-risk obstetric complications has shown low performance levels [15, 16] and other ultrasound markers such as anatomical abnormalities within the aortic arch and the ductus arteriosus or the use of predictive models based on multiple risk factors should potentially enhance diagnostic accuracy [14, 17, 18]. But why is it so important to diagnose CoA antenatally? This type of congenital heart malformation may be associated with poor prognosis after birth if undetected prenatally and antenatal management in tertiary care centers and *in utero* treatment are not provided [7, 19]. By doing this, Jowett *et al.* [20] have obtained enhanced diagnostic accuracy for CoA from 62.5% [21] to 86% by including four echocardiographic parameters, namely isthmal Z score, isthmus to duct ratio, shelf and flow.

In addition, the inclusion in clinical practice of reference ranges of fetal aortic arch may contribute to the standardized echocardiographic examination of the aortic arch thus reducing both false-positive or false-negative diagnosis of CoA [22]. These authors reported that the transverse arch diameter in millimeters (TAD) as a function of gestational age (GA) in weeks was expressed by the regression equation TAD= - 1.17 + 0.169 x GA while distal aortic arch isthmus diameter (DAID)= - 1.39 + 0.189 x GA. Both diameters showed a statistically significant correlation of r= 0.924 and r= 0.938, respectively.

However, caution may be exercised in the use of these charts because the width of the reference range remains constant across the gestational age range studied as although this model was mathematically based, it did not take into account the gestation-specific standard deviation value. This issue should be considered as it may contribute to the false-negative or false-positive diagnosis of CoA when screening in early or late gestation [23].

Furthermore, Pasquini *et al.* [24] constructed a Z score reference range for aortic isthmus and ductal arch assessment using the three vessel and trachea (3VT) view, with the advantage that a hypoplastic aortic arch can also be directly compared with the ductal arch [25, 26].

On the other hand, the use of advanced ultrasound technology based on four-dimensional (4D) ultrasound may also contribute to distinguishing diagnostic artefacts and pitfalls in the prenatal diagnosis of CoA [27, 28].

AORTIC STENOSIS

The disease has a prevalence of 3% of overall CHDs [29]. According to the level of the stenosis, aortic stenosis can be classified as being valvular, supravalvular or subvalvular. While the latter may be associated with monosomy X, the supravalvular type may be associated with peripheral pulmonary stenosis in Williams syndrome and/or trisomy 13. The valvular type can jeopardize the fetus and be a cause of congestive heart failure [30]. Usually, the left ventricle appears dilated with hyperechogenic lining of the myocardium representing endocardial fibroelastosis (Fig. **1**).

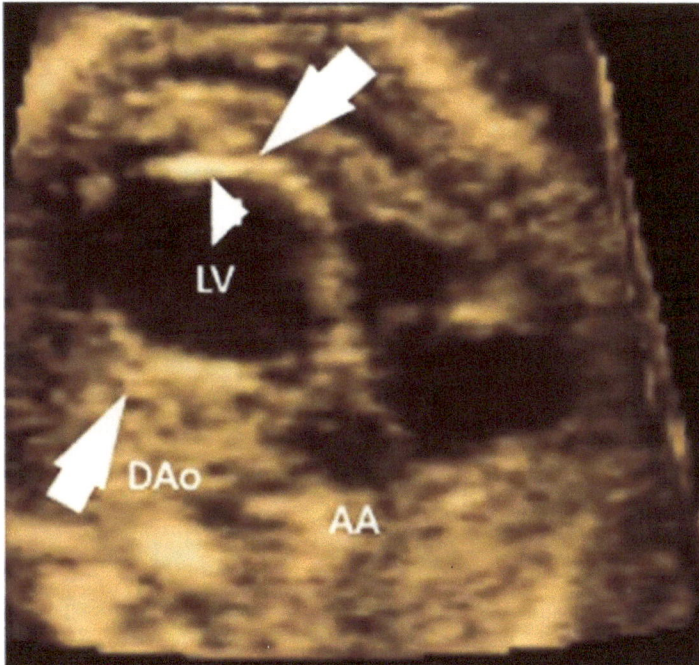

Fig. (1). Three-dimensional (3D) ultrasound showing enlarged left ventricle in critical aortic stenosis (CAS). Also note hyperechogenic endocardial cushion lining secondary to endocardial fibroelastosis (EFE) (arrows). LV: left ventricle; DAo: descending aorta; AA: ascending aorta.

In critical aortic stenosis, the aortic valve can demonstrate hypertrophy and the ascending aorta may be enlarged with turbulent flow and reversed with high velocity flow across the arch and ascending aorta using color Doppler ultrasound (Figs. **2** and **3**).

This cardiac defect may be characterized also by subaortic membranous or muscular stenosis, supravalvular mitral membrane (SVMM), parachute-like mitral valve and CoA, all diagnostic clusters of the syndrome described by Shone in the late 1963 [31] (Fig. **4**).

In a study conducted over 7 years, 107 fetuses with aortic stenosis (AS) have been followed up, representing one of the largest clinical series considering that a prenatal diagnosis of aortic stenosis has occurred in no more than 10% of cases

[32]. This study showed that 42% of newborns that satisfied the Boston criteria for emerging hypoplastic left heart syndrome (eHLHS) had had biventricular circulation (BV) without undergoing fetal intervention. Fetal aortic valvuloplasty (fAVP) at mid-gestation is intended to prevent, where possible, a progression from aortic valve stenosis to HLHS and to establish a BV circulation, either *in utero* or postnatally. This is highly important as critical aortic valve stenosis is complicated by intrauterine fetal demise (IUFD) of around 7.5% and procedure-related demise of 10% [33].

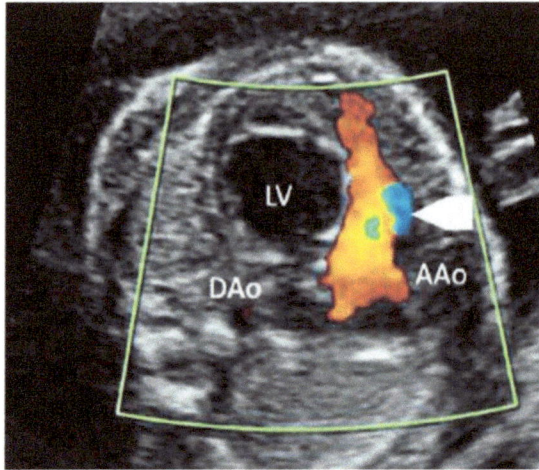

Fig. (2). Color Doppler ultrasound showing turbulent jet flow across the ascending aorta in critical aortic stenosis (CAS). LV: left ventricle; DAo: descending aorta; AAo: ascending aorta.

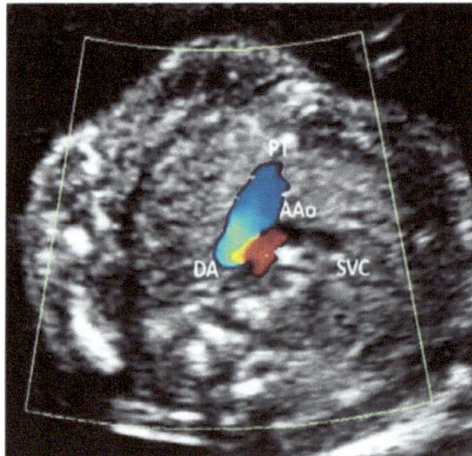

Fig. (3). Three-vessel view (3VV) showing reverse blood flow at the level of the descending aorta (DA) in critical aortic stenosis (CAS). AAo: ascending aorta; PT: pulmonary trunk; SVC: superior vena cava.

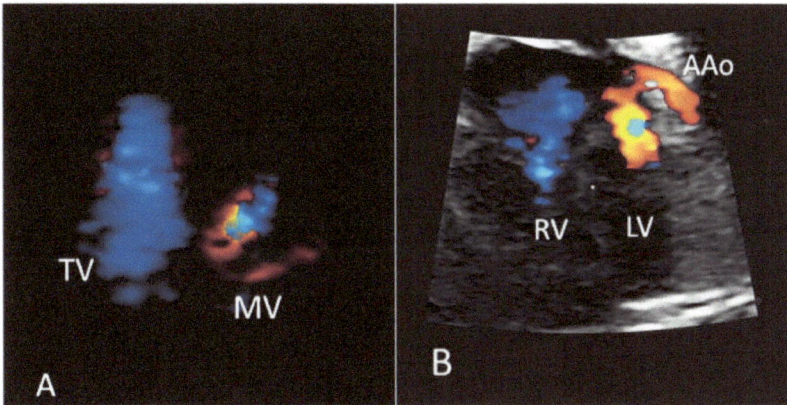

Fig. (4). Four-dimensional (4D) ultrasound performed at 33+2 weeks of gestation using color Doppler ultrasound with spatio-temporal image correlation (STIC) demonstrating mitral stenosis (**A**) and subaortic stenosis (**B**) in a fetus with Shone syndrome (Courtesy of Dr. Nathalie Bravo-Valenzuela). TV: tricuspid valve; MV: mitral valve; RV: right ventricle; LV: left ventricle; AAo: ascending aorta.

Following adequate fetus selection for *in utero* therapy with fAVP, an improvement in the growth of the left myocardium as well as the mitral valve and hemodynamic functions have been demonstrated [34 - 39]. Cardiovascular perfor-mance can be assessed by means of pulsed wave tissue Doppler imaging (TDI), an echocardiographic technique capable of measuring the contraction and relaxation velocities of the myocardium [40, 41]. TDI has been shown to be feasible and reproducible, to have low level intra- and inter-observer variability and reference charts have also been developed for clinical purposes [42 - 49].

TDI can be used to assess myocardium performance both before and after fAVP treatment in case of critical aortic stenosis (CAS) [50]. Wohlmuth *et al.* [51] have documented that pulsed wave TDI-derived parameters correlate well with newborns with BV circulation who have undergone successful fAVP surgery. However, criteria to select which fetuses with CAS will further develop HLHS and thus may benefit from fAVP may vary between physicians and institutions. These criteria usually reflect echocardiographic hemodynamic characteristics including the direction of flow across the ostium primum and the transverse aortic arch as well as the mitral valve (MV) inflow pattern [52]. In a series by McElhinney *et al.* [37] on 70 fetuses with CAS that were predicted to develop HLHS, a multiple regression scoring system to predict which ones would lead to BV circulation after birth following fAVP at a median gestational age of 23 weeks showed that a higher LV long-axis Z score (odds ratio, 2.6; 95% confidence interval, 1.4 to 4.9) and "high" LV pressure (odds ratio, 17.0; 95% confidence interval, 2.5 to 117) were independently associated with a high probability of BV at birth. "High" LV pressure was defined as a maximum instantaneous MR (mitral regurgitation) jet predicting a gradient of ≥20 mm Hg or, if there was no MR, as a maximum instantaneous AS gradient ≥16 mm Hg. A multivariate model was developed based on threshold Z scores of the left heart function and expressed in the range of 0 to 5. Interestingly, fetuses scoring ≥4 had 100% SEN, 53% SPE, 38% positive predictive value (PPV) and 100% negative predictive value (NPV) in identifying fetuses with BV circulation at the time of birth. This study demonstrated that fAVP can be successfully be performed in 74% of cases at mid-gestation, producing an improved cardiac output with aortic growth although the left ventricle dimension did not differ from controls [37] Table **1**.

Table 1. Fetal echocardiographic characteristic and multiple regression scoring system to predict postnatal biventricular circulation in fetuses undergoing fetal aortic valvuloplasty at mid-gestation.

Critical AS with Emerging HLHS	Scoring System: Definition and Diagnostic Criteria	BV Circulation Score (O-5)
↑ LV long-axis Z score	Odds ratio: 2.6 (1.4-4.9, 95% CI)	If score ≥4, 100% SEN, 53% SPE, 38% PPV, 100% NPV
↑ LV pressure	Odds ratio: 17.0 (2.5-117, 95% CI)	
High level pressure	Max. instantaneous MR jet with a gradient ≥ 20 mmHg OR No MR, max. instantaneous AS gradient ≥ 16 mmHg	

AS: aortic stenosis; BV: biventricular circulation; HLHS: hypoplastic left heart syndrome; CI: confidence interval; LV: left ventricle; MR: mitral regurgitation; NPV: negative predictive value; PPV: positive predictive value; SEN: sensibility; SPE: specificity

INTERRUPTED AORTIC ARCH

Coarctation of the aorta, interrupted aortic arch (IAA) and HLHS can represent an etiopathogenetic *continuum* [53]. It is usually classified into three types according to the level of interruption in relation to the brachiocephalic vessels [54]: type A, where the aorta supplies the head and neck vessels and the pulmonary artery, the descending aorta *via*the ductus arteriosus; type B, where the interruption burdens the left subclavian artery and type C where the interruption is located between the right innonimate artery and the left common carotid artery. In types B and C, the head and neck vessels are supplied *via*the ductus arteriosus. Type B is the most frequent subtype (65%) and frequently associated with 22q11.2 of (Di George) syndrome in almost 60-70% of cases [55 - 59] while type A may be seen in 30% of cases [60] with type C as the rarest form of IAA although associated with the worse prognosis [29].

Prenatally, ultrasound diagnosis between IAA type A and CoA may be very challenging and a vertical course of the ascending aorta giving rise to a single brachiocephalic vessel may aid echocardiographic diagnosis [29]. The low Ao/main pulmonary artery (MPA) ratio as seen in CoA may help the differential diagnosis between the two conditions [25 - 28]. In the case series of Hirano *et al.* [55] ventricular septal defect (VSD) was seen in 100% of cases of IAA type A and type B using the three-vessel view (3VV) compared with a cumulative association of 85.7% in IAA of type A from previous observations [61 - 63] (Figs. **5** and **6**).

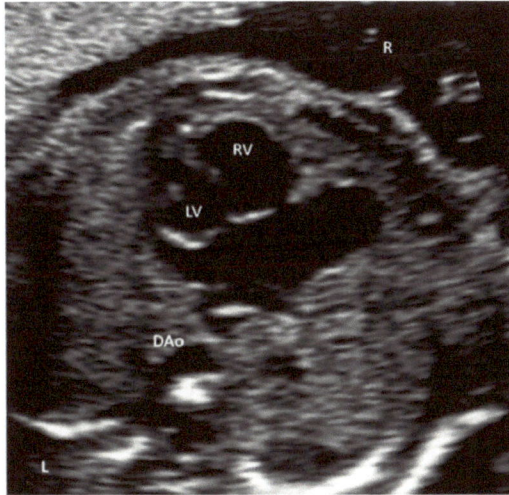

Fig. (5). Second trimester scan at 20 weeks showing right atrial and ventricular prevalence in a case of interrupted aortic arch (IAA) in a trisomy 13 fetus with cerebral and renal lesions and single umbilical artery (SUA). LV: left ventricle; RV: right ventricle; DAo: descending aorta; L: left; R: right.

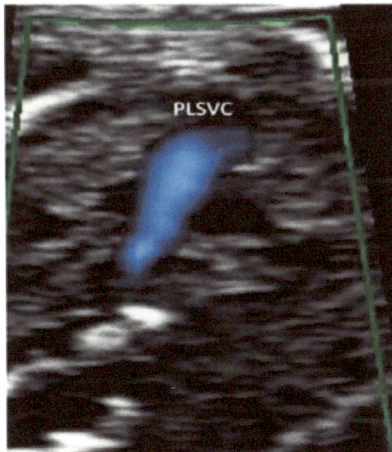

Fig. (6). Persistent left superior vena cava (PLSVC) by color Doppler in the same fetus affected by trisomy 13.

HYPOPLASTIC LEFT HEART SYNDROME

Hypoplastic left heart syndrome (HLHS) may represent the end stage of a disease causing an underdevelopment of the left ventricular inlet (mitral valve stenosis/foramen ovale restriction) [64 - 66] and left ventricular outflow tract (LVOT) obstruction and hypoplasia, accounting for 7-9% of all CHDs [29]. The term was first used by Noonan and Nadas in 1958 [67].

LVOT with associated mitral and aortic atresia prevents communication between the left atrium and ventricle whereas aortic atresia leads to left ventricle hypoplasia. In these conditions, the systemic circulation in the fetus is almost maintained by the ductus arteriosus [29]. Consequently, the end-diastolic length and the diameter of the left ventricle (LV) decreased as compared with normal controls while the right ventricle (RV) diameter increased leading to a higher RV:LV ratio (median value=2.44, range 1.33-6.25) and a decreased ratio of Ao/PA artery diameter (median value=0.49, range 0.24-0.69) [68] (Figs. **7** to **9**).

Alterations in myocardial growth signaling pathways at cellular level and failed or absent cardiomyocytes mitosis may explain why myocardial remodeling when LV has developed is limited to LV hypertrophy only and not to hyperplasia [69].

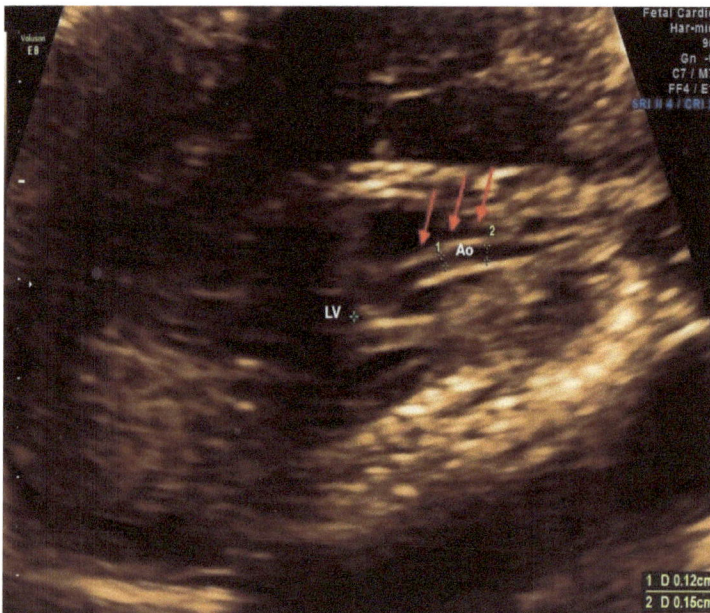

Fig. (7). Two-dimensional (2D) ultrasound performed at 21 weeks of gestation showing hypoplastic left heart syndrome (HLHS) with severe aortic hypoplasia (red arrows). LV: left ventricle; Ao: aorta. (Courtesy of Dr. Nathalie Bravo-Valenzuela).

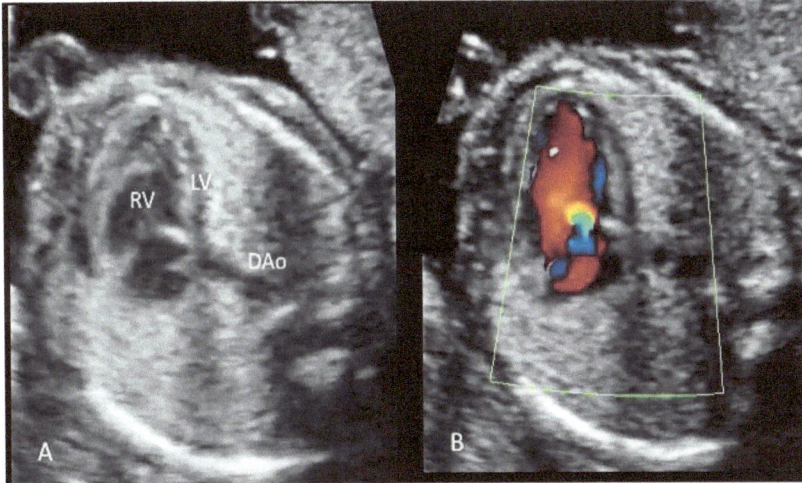

Fig. (8). Two-dimensional (2D) ultrasound in apical four-chamber view (4CV) (**A**): severe hypoplasia of the left ventricle is clearly seen; (**B**) Doppler ultrasound showing almost absent transmitral flow. DAo: descending aorta; LV: left ventricle; RV: right ventricle. (Courtesy of Dr. Nathalie Bravo-Valenzuela).

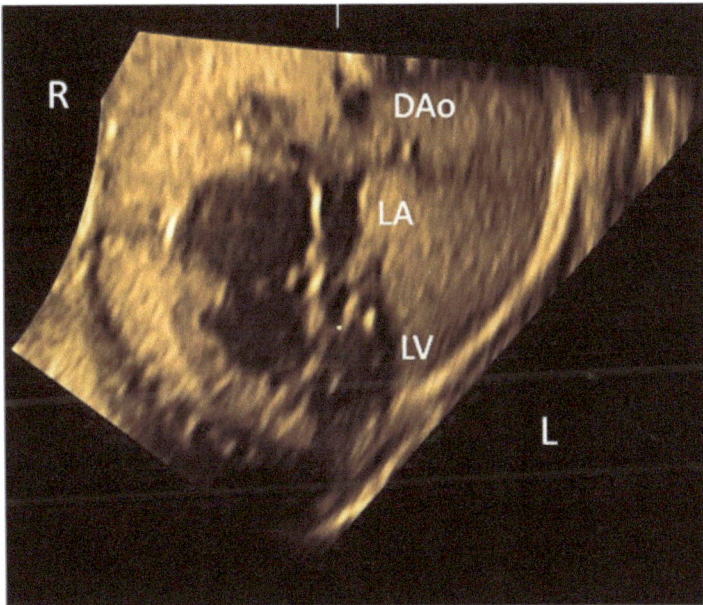

Fig. (9). Four-dimensional (4D) ultrasound in the same case using spatio-temporal image correlation (STIC). DAo: descending aorta; L: left; LA: left atrium; LV: left ventricle; R: right. (Cortesy of Dr. Nathalie Bravo-Valenzuela).

Furthermore, necropsy findings in HLHS showed histologic signs of LV myocardial fibrosis, aortic elastic fragmentation and grade 3 fibrosis [68]. HLHS may be a *continuum* of cardiac malformations evolving from critical aortic stenosis and interrupted aortic arch [70].

When critical aortic valve stenosis is present, a decreased flow or a reversal of flow through the ostium primum is observed, contributing to left ventricular dilation and hypoplasia. Additional risk factors for developing HLHS have been recognized as reversed transverse aortic arch (TAA), monophasic mitral inlet flow and varying degrees of abnormal left ventricle cardiac performance. These findings may be also predictors of CAS evolving into HLHS [34, 71, 72].

The disease is associated with poor postnatal outcome unless staged palliative surgery and transplantation are available [37, 73] and is associated with increased multisystem organ failure [74, 75]. The pathogenesis of HLHS may comprise developmental as well as genetic factors. Genetic factors may be present in 15-30% of cases and include common trisomy and monosomy X, Kabuki syndrome, Noonan and Jacobsen syndrome [76, 77].

Association with fetal growth restriction has been described [78, 79] with up to 40% suggesting placental dysfunction [80]. These authors demonstrated that fetuses with HLHS have a disturbed regulation of angiogenetic factors acting at the level of the syncitium and fetal endothelium characterized by reduced placental growth factor (PlGF) RNA expression and a compensatory increase in leptin RNA expression and leptin and leptin-receptor staining both in the syncytium and in the endothelium of the villus vasculature compared with controls. Leptin is a trophic and angiogenetic factor that is important for the physiological function of the placenta. In addition, this study showed subchorionic fibrin deposition with reduced placental weight in 40% of placentas from fetuses affected by HLHS [80].

The rationale for *in utero* fetal cardiac intervention (FCI) is to establish BV circulation where possible. Selection criteria of fetuses that would benefit from FCI are severe aortic stenosis with HLHS with intact or severely restrictive atrial septum. HLHS with mitral and aortic stenosis represents the most severe type of restrictive left-sided cardiac defect and is associated with increased mortality [81, 82].

In HLHS with intact or severely restrictive atrial septum (IAS), the cardiac functions are based on pulmonary vein flow that is directed towards the atrial septum. The hemodynamic changes that occur postnatally cause left atrial hypertension, pulmonary edema and decreased systemic perfusion resulting in congestive heart failure and high risk of neonatal mortality [82 - 85].

Criteria for FCI in fetuses with HLHS/IAS should consider the following echocardiographic parameters: IAS or ≤1 mm atrial septal defect, prominent pulmonary vein flow reversal and forward-to-reverse pulmonary vein velocity time integral ratio <5 [86]. Data from the International Fetal Cardiac Intervention

Registry (IFCIR) obtained from 13 centers in 72 fetuses with HLHS/IAS demonstrated a septoplasty success rate of 77% although procedure-related intrauterine fetal demise was seen in 13% of fetuses. In addition, a patent foramen ovale was only seen in 45% of all FCI neonates and overall survival rate at discharge was only 35%, with no statistical difference between fetuses who underwent FCI and those who did not [87 - 92].

A recent publication [93] evaluating the results of fAVP in 123 fetuses with eHLHS showed that fetuses with LV pressure > 47 mmHg and AAo Z-score≥0.57 had a 92% probability of BV circulation. This study compared the Boston experience in two periods (2000-2008) and (2009-2015) during which successful fAVP procedure increased from 73% from inception to 94% in recent time, with BV circulation achieved in 59% of cases and procedure-related IUFD of 4%. The authors also propose the use of a classification and regression tree (CART) analysis based on pre-fAV echocardiographic parameters to better advise the couple regarding the risks and benefits of undergoing *in utero* FCI. This study demonstrated that LV long-axis dimension Z-score, higher LV pressure, longer MV inflow duration and larger ascending aorta dimension Z-score were independent antecedents predicting a BV outcome after birth. Furthermore, it also demonstrated for the first time how postnatal outcome is dependent on myocardium remodeling in terms of lower LV long-axis Z-score and higher sphericity.

In utero balloon fAVP dramatically improved from the first series in the 1990s [94 - 96] and again during the last 6 years if we consider that in the series by Galindo *et al.* [97] the overall survival rate of the intention-to-treat cohort was 50% and that 22.2% of surviving infants had neurologic sequelae. Moreover, newborns with HLHS with IAS (6%) or restrictive atrial septum (RAS, 22%) [83, 97, 98] still represent the subset of infants with the highest mortality rate (almost 70%) [82, 99] secondary to hemodynamic dysfunction causing acidosis and tissue hypoxia [100, 101]. Table **2** reports clinical risk factors and predictors of evolving in HLHS in 43 fetuses with fetal aortic valve stenosis and normal left ventricle length in mid-gestation.

AORTIC ARCH ANOMALIES

The anatomical variant of the normal aortic arch can be found in approximately 0.1% of low-risk pregnancies [102 - 104]. These abnormalities can be detected together with CHDs and aneuploidy, mainly 22q11.2 microdeletion syndrome [105 - 109]. They are classified according to the anatomical relationship established between the aortic arch and ductus arteriosus with the trachea [110] as left aortic arch with an aberrant right subclavian artery (ARSA), right aortic arch anomaly with an aberrant left subclavian artery (ALSA), right aortic arch anomaly with mirror image branching and double aortic arch (DAA) anomaly [106, 110 - 112].

Table 2. Fetal aortic valve stenosis: clinical risk factors and predictors of evolving in hypoplastic left heart syndrome in 43 fetuses with critical aortic stenosis and normal left ventricle length in mid-gestation.

Clinical Risk Factors for Developing HLHS	Predictors (%) of Evolving in HLHS
Reversed transverse aortic arch flow	100%
Left-to-right flow across the foramen ovale	88%
Monophasic mitral inlet flow	91%
Abnormal left ventricle cardiac dysfunction	94%

HLHS: hypoplastic left heart syndrome.

Aortic arch maldevelopment is not usually important per se but when it is found associated with anomalies of the brachiocephalic vessels such as either the right or left aberrant subclavian artery and high association with DiGeorge syndrome [113] or when it forms a vascular sling around the trachea and esophagus, that may cause airway obstruction and dysphagia postnatally until late complications consisting of tracheomalacia [114 - 117].

Accordingly, when a prenatal diagnosis of abnormal aortic arch is posed, thorough evaluation of the "thy-box" with two-dimensional (2D) ultrasound measurement or three-dimensional (3D) ultrasound calculation of the thymus volume should be performed [118, 119].

The RAA derived from an embryologic maldevelopment affecting the fourth branchial arch [120] and would form a vascular ring around the trachea when associated with an ALSA or with a DAA [105]. Peng *et al.* [105] have reported that RAA was associated with a left DA in 73.2% of cases (causing a U-shape vascular ring at the 3VT view) and with intracardiac malformation such as tetralogy of Fallot (TOF) and 22q11.21 microdeletion in 5% of RAA fetuses and right isomerism in a 16p11.2 microdeletion, a finding also confirmed by Miranda *et al.* [106].

When a vascular sling is detected prenatally, it is important to advise parents to monitor possible signs of airway obstruction postnatally or signs of left arm ischemia such as brachial palsy in case of ALSA [115]. Rarely, DAA with vascular ring may cause intrauterine airway compression, mirroring a congenital high airway obstruction syndrome (pseudo-CHAOS). In such cases, the prenatal detection is of critical importance in order to plan appropriate perinatal management that would be based on *ex-utero* intrapartum treatment (EXIT) procedure and/or operation on placental support (OOPS) in a tertiary care center with a multidisciplinary team [121,122].

Prenatal diagnosis of aortic arch abnormalities can be performed using the 3VT view although an upward insonating plane of the mediastinum, cephalad to the classic 3VT view, is required in order to detect the relationship between the great arteries and brachiocephalic vessels [104, 123, 124] whose course is like a bike handlebar [102]. In addition, 3D ultrasound with spatio-temporal image correlation (STIC) has been shown to improve the antenatal diagnosis of aortic arch abnormalities in the 3VT view in a way that resembles that of postnatal imaging [125].

At the time of routine anomaly scan in the second trimester in an unselected pregnant population, the prevalence of RAA has been reported to be 0.05% and 83% of cases presented with a left-sided ductus arteriosus. In this situation, correct prenatal diagnosis is facilitated by a change of the 3VT view from a V-shape to a U-shape [126] (Figs. **10** to **12**).

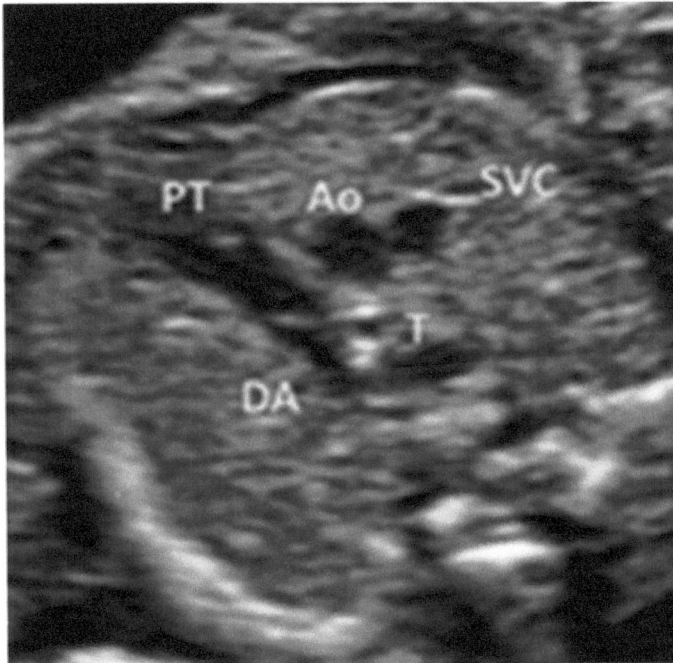

Fig. (10). Two-dimensional (2D) ultrasound at 20+5 weeks of gestation of a fetus showing a right aortic arch (RAA) on the 3 vessel view and trachea (3VT). PT, pulmonary trunk; DA; ductus arteriosus; Ao: ascending aorta; SVC: superior vena cava; T: trachea.

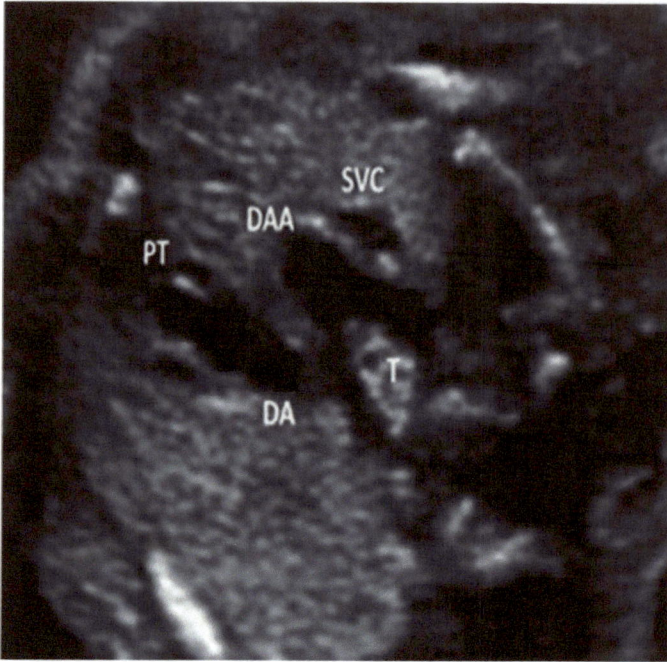

Fig. (11). Two-dimensional (2D) ultrasound in the axial plane performed at 20+5 of gestation in a fetus diagnosed with a double aortic arch (DAA): note that the trachea lies in the center of the two aortic branches. DA: ductus arteriosus; PT: main pulmonary trunk; SVC: superior vena cava; T: trachea.

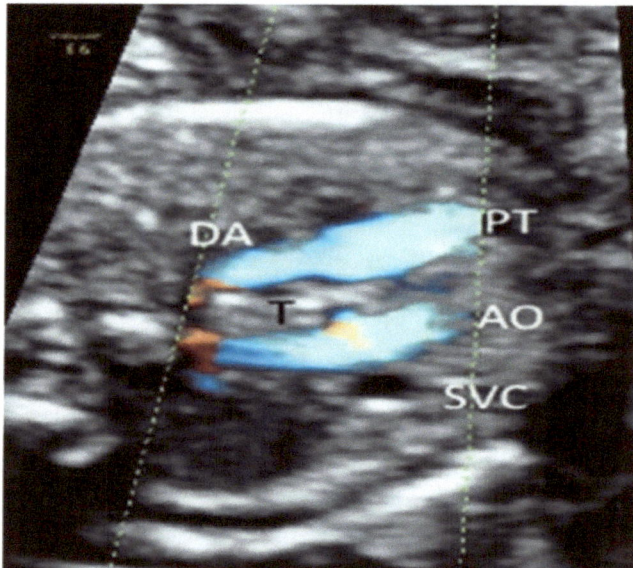

Fig. (12). Three-vessel view and trachea (3VT) using color Doppler: a typical U-shaped vascular ring surrounding the trachea (T) is seen. AO: ascending aorta; PT: pulmonary trunk; SVC: superior vena cava; DA: ductus arteriosus.

Isolated aortic arch abnormalities are usually asymptomatic whereas DAA and RAA especially if associated with ALSA or with mirror-image branching, left descending aorta and left ductus arteriosus are the subtypes most commonly associated with upper airway obstruction [112]. The series by Galindo *et al.* [112] conducted over 48 fetuses diagnosed with RAA showed that 30 fetuses with mirror-image branching without vascular sling had associated CHDs in 97% of cases, extracardiac malformations in 37% and chromosomal abnormalities in 20% of cases. In this subset of fetuses (RAA with mirror-image branching) these authors have calculated a 300-fold increase in associated CHDs. When either the aorta and the DA are to the right of the trachea without a vascular ring, a strong association with CHDs has been described [127].

When RAA is associated with ALSA, the ALSA is perfused dorsally from the descending aorta by a vascular retrotracheal remnant vessel called the Kommerell's diverticulum whereas ventrally, the ALSA is connected to the DA arising from the left pulmonary artery [128].

Discrepancy in medical literature still exists between a favorable prognosis in fetuses diagnosed in the prenatal series compared with a high percentage of symptomatic neonates as reported in the pediatric series [117, 129, 130]. In the series by Evans *et al.* [131] in 204 fetuses with RAA and situs solitus a prevalence of RAA in the order of 5.8 per 10,000 live births was seen. Isolated RAA was detected in 47% of cases while the rest had intracardiac malformations; fetuses with isolated RAA showed a vascular ring around the trachea and esophagus in 94% of fetuses, in agreement with previous observations [112].

Vascular rings can be accurately detected by prenatal echocardiography especially using the so-called "supra-aortic branch view" [111]. RAA with normal intracardiac anatomy was seen in 0.35% of cases among 16,450 fetuses screened with echocardiography over a 12-year period. The detection of RAA at routine fetal echocardiogram warrants karyotyping as well as a differential diagnosis with the double aortic arch (DAA), as the differentiation between these two entities is sometimes challenging antenatally [113].

A uncommon type of RAA is represented by cervical aortic arch that has been described very recently in a fetus with tetralogy of Fallot (TOF) and associated 22q11.2 microdeletion syndrome [132] or other rarer anatomical variants such as RAA with bilateral DA with origin of the left subclavian artery from the left pulmonary artery [133] or RAA with bilateral DA associated with nonconfluent pulmonary arteries [134] or associated with trisomy 9 with variant phenotype including Dandy-Walker syndrome and cleft lip and cleft palate [135].

DOUBLE AORTIC ARCH

This type of aortic arch anomaly is characterized, in the vast majority of cases, by the formation of an incomplete or complete vascular sling encircling the trachea and esophagus. The vascular ring is caused by the association of double aortic arch (DAA) with an aberrant right or left subclavian artery. Tracheal compression by DAA with the vascular ring is a rare finding during fetal life; however, if pulmonary distension and hydrops fetalis ensue, it should be suspected [136].

DAA has been reported to occur from 5.2% [110] to 13% reaching 19% in the clinical series by Mogra *et al.* [126] and Razon *et al.* [113], respectively and is also seen associated with 22q11.2 microdeletion in almost 4-5% of fetuses [126].

DAA derives according to the model proposed by Edwards *at al* [137]. a consequence of the formation and regression of the pharyngeal arches between the 35- to 40-day embryonic period ending in the remnant of both fourth pharyngeal arches and both dorsal aortas encircling the trachea and the esophagus. In the vast majority of cases, the right aortic arch is dominant and atresia of the contralateral branch of the DAA may occur at a different level, usually distal to the left subclavian artery [138] (Figs. **13** to **15**).

In the review of 35 cases by Trobo *et al.* [138] postnatal signs of tracheoesophageal compression were present in 72.4% of cases whereas 22q11.2 microdeletion was only seen in one case.

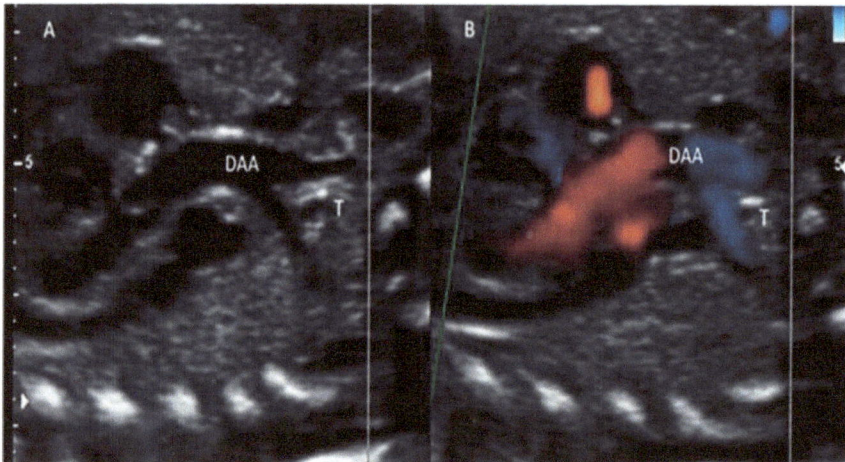

Fig. (13). Two-dimensional ultrasound (2DUS) in the sagittal plane using B-mode (**A**) and color flow mapping (**B**): the branching of the ascending aorta in two arms (DAA) is clearly visible with the trachea (T) lying in between.

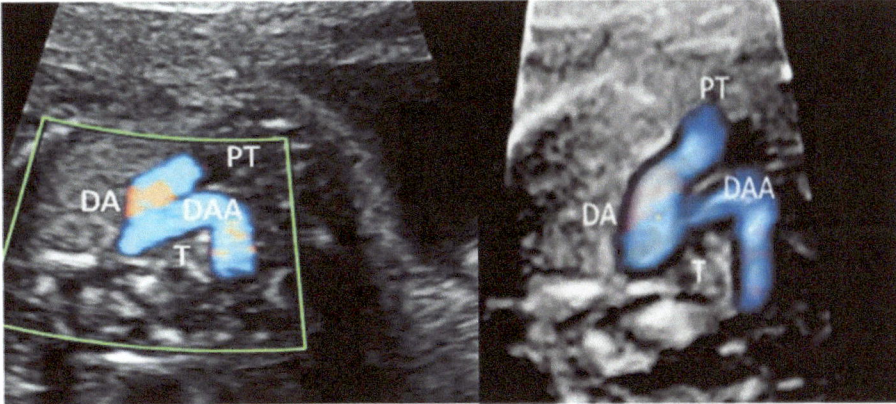

Fig. (14). Three vessels and trachea (3VT) view in the axial plane of the mediastinum with color Doppler (**A**) clearly shows the two aortic branches (DAA) encircling the trachea (T) (**B**). PT: pulmonary trunk; DA: ductus arteriosus.

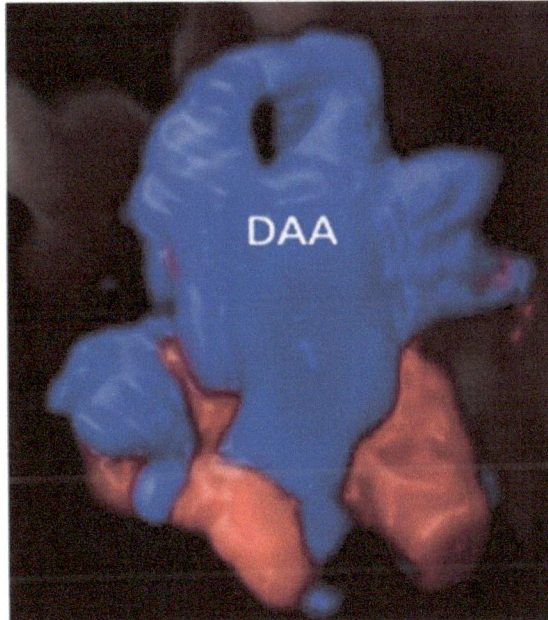

Fig. (15). Four-dimensional (4D) ultrasound using SonoVCAD™ rendering in the same case with DAA (double aortic arch).

The prenatal diagnosis is feasible using the 3VT view [124] giving rise to an image of a trident or a number 6 or 9 [138]. When DAA with vascular rings are detected prenatally it is clinically useful to control the correctness of the antenatal echocardiographic diagnosis during the neonatal period not only using ultrasound but also computed tomography (CT) scan and/or magnetic resonance (MR) imaging [139].

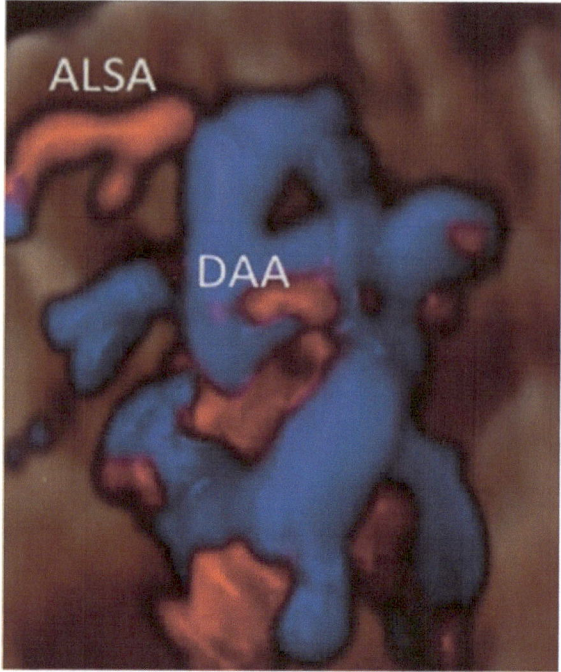

Fig. (16). Four-dimensional (4D) ultrasound using SonoVCAD™ rendering in a case of DAA (double aortic arch) with aberrant left subclavian artery (ALSA).

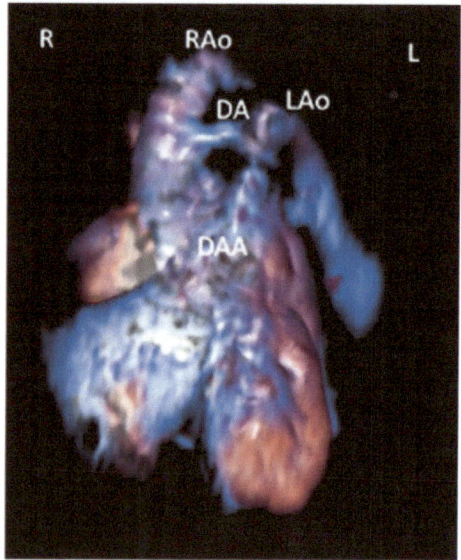

Fig. (17). Four-dimensional (4D) ultrasound using Realistic Vue™ showing a DAA (double aortic arch) with a prevalent right aortic branch compared with a hypoplastic/atretic left aortic branch. DA: ductus arteriosus; RAo: right aorta; LAo: left aorta; L: left side; R: right side.

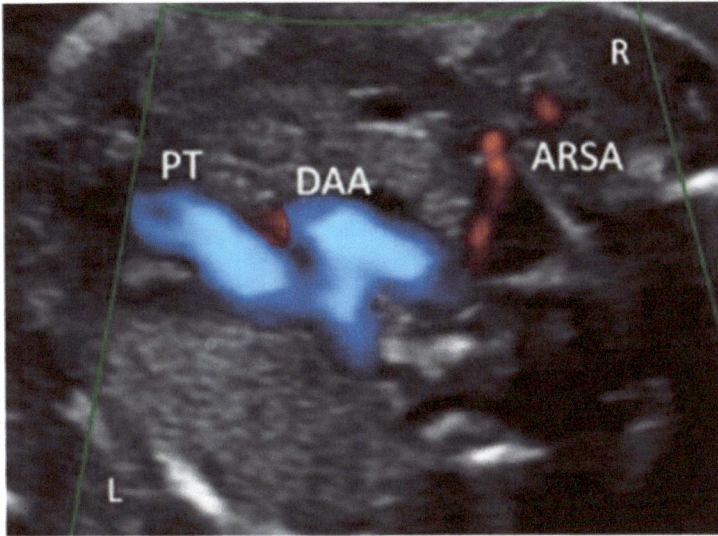

Fig. (18). Three vessels and trachea (3VT) view in a second trimester fetus with DAA (double aortic arch) and associated aberrant right subclavian artery (ARSA). PT: pulmonary trunk; R: right side.

Xiong *et al.* [140] have proposed Live xPlane as a novel echocardiographic ultrasound approach to the diagnosis of the aortic and ductal arches Live xPlane is an ultrasound technique that provides two insonation planes in real time allowing 3VT rendering on the axial plane on one side and a sagittal plane of the ductal and aortic arches on the other side [140, 141].

DAA can be seen associated with intracardiac malformations such as d-transposition of the great arteries [142, 143] or associated with a concurrent RAA and an aberrant artery arising from the ascending aorta [144]. Table **3** describes different type of left heart malformations with associated congenital anomalies and ultrasound diagnostic clusters of left CHDs.

AORTO-PULMONARY WINDOW

Aorto-pulmonary window (APW) is uncommonly seen in association with tricuspid atresia and truncus arteriosus [145]. Autopsy finding documented an APW in a fetus with fetal growth restriction and multiple congenital malformations where a severe pulmonary regurgitation was an indirect sign of the disease during the intrauterine period [146] (Fig. **19**).

Table 3. Type of left heart malformations, congenital associated anomalies and diagnostic ultrasound clusters.

Cardiac Malformations	Associated Anomalies	Diagnostic US Clusters
Aortic stenosis (AS)	Shone syndrome, Williams syndrome, trisomy 13, monosomy X	Thickened AoV, enlarged AAo, enlarged LV, endocardial fibroelastosis, ↑ velocity turbulent flow across the AA and AAo at color Doppler
Interrupted aortic arch (IAA) Type A (30%) Type B (65%) Type C (5%)	VSD in 89% Type A and 100% Type B cases on 4CV, 22q11.2 (in 60-70% of Type B), CDH, bilateral renal agenesis, esophageal atresia and duplicated stomach	Average Ao/MPA ratio: 0.47±0.10, Average AoV/PV ratio: 0.49±0.09, RV prevalence with RV/LV ratio: 0.8±0.23, Ductal arch ↑ in size Vertical course of the AAo with only one H&N vessel
Aortic coarctation (CoA)	PLSVC, ↑ NT	PV/AoV ratio >1.6 RV predominance, hypoplastic aortic arch, turbulent flow in DAo at color Doppler
Hypoplastic left heart syndrome (HLHS)	Trisomy 18, trisomy 13, monosomy X, Kabuki syndrome, Noonan syndrome, Jacobsen syndrome	↑ RV:LV ratio (median value=2.44, range 1.33-6.25); ↓Ao/PA artery diameter (median value=0.49, range 0.24-0.69);
Right aortic arch (RAA)	Aberrant subclavian artery, absent ductus arteriosus, TOF, 22q11.2 microdeletion, 16p11.2 microdeletion, extracardiac malformations	Aortic arch to the right of the trachea in the 3VT view U-shaped vascular sling around the trachea at color Doppler at 3VT view Evaluate the presence of aberrant subclavian artery at color Doppler Evaluate the presence of the thymus ("Thy box")
Double aortic arch (DAA)	Prevalence 13-19%, association with vascular sling and clinical signs of tracheal and esophageal compression postnatally; 22q11.2 microdeletion (4-5%)	Two aortic branching with a horseshoe appearance with the trachea lying in between at 3VT view Evaluate incomplete or complete vascular sling at 3VT view Evaluate the presence of the thymus ("Thy box")

AA: aortic arch; AAo: ascending aorta; AoV: aortic valve; CDH: congenital diaphragmatic hernia; DAo: descending aorta; H&N: head and neck vessels; LV: left ventricle; MPA: main pulmonary artery; NT: nuchal translucency; PV: pulmonary valve; PLSVC: persistent left superior vena cava; RV: right ventricle; TOF: tetralogy of Fallot; 3VT: three vessel and trachea view; 4CV: four chamber view.

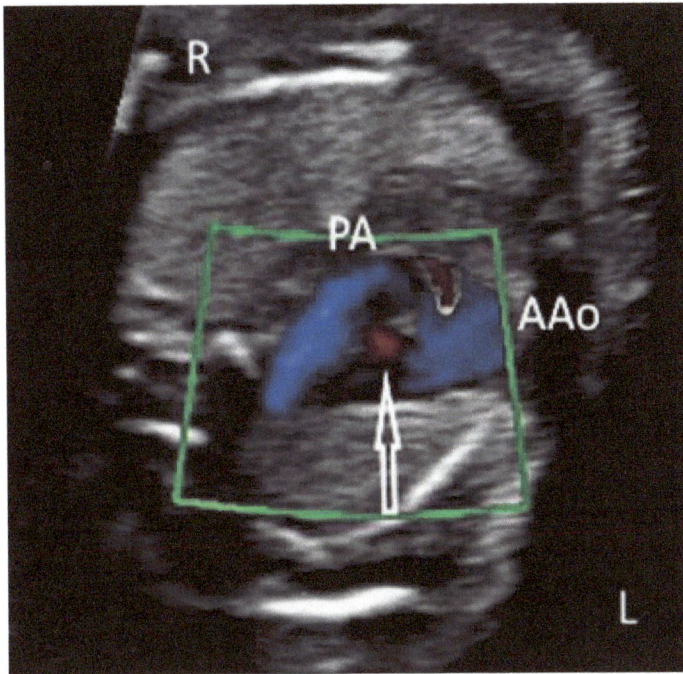

Fig. (19). Three-vessel and trachea (3VT) view performed at 21+2 weeks of gestation using color Doppler ultrasound: an aorto-pulmonary window (arrow) is demonstrated in a trisomy 21 fetus. AAo: ascending aorta; L: left; PA: pulmonary artery; R: right.

CONSENT FOR PUBLICATION

Not applicable.

CONFLICT OF INTEREST

The authors confirm that the contents of this chapter have no conflict of interest.

ACKNOWLEDGEMENTS

Declare none.

REFERENCES

[1]   Mitchell SC, Korones SB, Berendes HW. Congenital heart disease in 56,109 births. Incidence and natural history. Circulation 1971; 43(3): 323-32.
       [http://dx.doi.org/10.1161/01.CIR.43.3.323] [PMID: 5102136]

[2]   Rosenthal E. Coarctation of the aorta from fetus to adult: curable condition or life long disease process? Heart 2005; 91(11): 1495-502.
       [http://dx.doi.org/10.1136/hrt.2004.057182] [PMID: 16230458]

[3]   Reifenstein GH, Levine SA, Gross RE. Coarctation of the aorta; a review of 104 autopsied cases of the adult type, 2 years of age or older. Am Heart J 1947; 33(2): 146-68.
       [http://dx.doi.org/10.1016/0002-8703(47)90002-1] [PMID: 20283558]

[4]   Tegnander E, Williams W, Johansen OJ, Blaas HG, Eik-Nes SH. Prenatal detection of heart defects in a non-selected population of 30,149 fetuses--detection rates and outcome. Ultrasound Obstet Gynecol 2006; 27(3): 252-65.
[http://dx.doi.org/10.1002/uog.2710] [PMID: 16456842]

[5]   Hornberger LK, Sahn DJ, Kleinman CS, Copel J, Silverman NH. Antenatal diagnosis of coarctation of the aorta: a multicenter experience. J Am Coll Cardiol 1994; 23(2): 417-23.
[http://dx.doi.org/10.1016/0735-1097(94)90429-4] [PMID: 8294696]

[6]   Hyett J, Moscoso G, Nicolaides K. Increased nuchal translucency in trisomy 21 fetuses: relationship to narrowing of the aortic isthmus. Hum Reprod 1995; 10(11): 3049-51.
[http://dx.doi.org/10.1093/oxfordjournals.humrep.a135845] [PMID: 8747070]

[7]   Franklin O, Burch M, Manning N, Sleeman K, Gould S, Archer N. Prenatal diagnosis of coarctation of the aorta improves survival and reduces morbidity. Heart 2002; 87(1): 67-9.
[http://dx.doi.org/10.1136/heart.87.1.67] [PMID: 11751670]

[8]   Familiari A, Morlando M, Khalil A, *et al.* Risk factors for coarctation of the aorta on prenatal ultrasound: a systematic review and meta-analysis. Circulation 2017; 135(8): 772-85.
[http://dx.doi.org/10.1161/CIRCULATIONAHA.116.024068] [PMID: 28034902]

[9]   Rocha LA, Rolo LC, Nardozza LMM, Tonni G, Araujo Júnior E. Z-score reference ranges for fetal heart functional measurements in a large brazilian pregnant women sample. Pediatr Cardiol 2019; 40(3): 554-62.
[http://dx.doi.org/10.1007/s00246-018-2026-1] [PMID: 30415382]

[10]   Berg C, Knüppel M, Geipel A, *et al.* Prenatal diagnosis of persistent left superior vena cava and its associated congenital anomalies. Ultrasound Obstet Gynecol 2006; 27(3): 274-80.
[http://dx.doi.org/10.1002/uog.2704] [PMID: 16456841]

[11]   Gustapane S, Leombroni M, Khalil A, *et al.* Systematic review and meta-analysis of persistent left superior vena cava on prenatal ultrasound: associated anomalies, diagnostic accuracy and postnatal outcome. Ultrasound Obstet Gynecol 2016; 48(6): 701-8.
[http://dx.doi.org/10.1002/uog.15914] [PMID: 26970258]

[12]   Durand I, Deverriere G, Thill C, *et al.* Prenatal detection of coarctation of the aorta in a non-selected population: a prospective analysis of 10 years of experience. Pediatr Cardiol 2015; 36(6): 1248-54.
[http://dx.doi.org/10.1007/s00246-015-1153-1] [PMID: 25845939]

[13]   Gómez-Montes E, Herraiz I, Mendoza A, Escribano D, Galindo A. Prediction of coarctation of the aorta in the second half of pregnancy. Ultrasound Obstet Gynecol 2013; 41(3): 298-305.
[http://dx.doi.org/10.1002/uog.11228] [PMID: 22744957]

[14]   Gómez-Montes E, Herraiz I, Gómez-Arriaga PI, Escribano D, Mendoza A, Galindo A. Gestational age-specific scoring systems for the prediction of coarctation of the aorta. Prenat Diagn 2014; 34(12): 1198-206.
[http://dx.doi.org/10.1002/pd.4452] [PMID: 25042904]

[15]   Sharland GK, Chan KY, Allan LD. Coarctation of the aorta: difficulties in prenatal diagnosis. Br Heart J 1994; 71(1): 70-5.
[http://dx.doi.org/10.1136/hrt.71.1.70] [PMID: 8297700]

[16]   Quarello E, Trabbia A. High-definition flow combined with spatiotemporal image correlation in the diagnosis of fetal coarctation of the aorta. Ultrasound Obstet Gynecol 2009; 33(3): 365-7.
[http://dx.doi.org/10.1002/uog.6270] [PMID: 19194864]

[17]   Arya B, Bhat A, Vernon M, Conwell J, Lewin M. Utility of novel fetal echocardiographic morphometric measures of the aortic arch in the diagnosis of neonatal coarctation of the aorta. Prenat Diagn 2016; 36(2): 127-34.
[http://dx.doi.org/10.1002/pd.4753] [PMID: 26630206]

[18]   Toole BJ, Schlosser B, McCracken CE, Stauffer N, Border WL, Sachdeva R. Importance of

relationship between ductus and isthmus in fetal diagnosis of coarctation of aorta. Echocardiography 2016; 33(5): 771-7.
[http://dx.doi.org/10.1111/echo.13140] [PMID: 26667892]

[19]   Gómez-Montes E, Herraiz I, Mendoza A, Escribano D, Martínez-Moratalla Valcárcel JM, Galindo A. Prenatal prediction of surgical approach for coarctation of the aorta repair. Fetal Diagn Ther 2014; 35(1): 27-35.
[http://dx.doi.org/10.1159/000356077] [PMID: 24356526]

[20]   Jowett V, Aparicio P, Santhakumaran S, Seale A, Jicinska H, Gardiner HM. Sonographic predictors of surgery in fetal coarctation of the aorta. Ultrasound Obstet Gynecol 2012; 40(1): 47-54.
[http://dx.doi.org/10.1002/uog.11161] [PMID: 22461316]

[21]   Matsui H, Mellander M, Roughton M, Jicinska H, Gardiner HM. Morphological and physiological predictors of fetal aortic coarctation. Circulation 2008; 118(18): 1793-801.
[http://dx.doi.org/10.1161/CIRCULATIONAHA.108.787598] [PMID: 18852365]

[22]   Achiron R, Zimand S, Hegesh J, Lipitz S, Zalel Y, Rotstein Z. Fetal aortic arch measurements between 14 and 38 weeks' gestation: *in-utero* ultrasonographic study. Ultrasound Obstet Gynecol 2000; 15(3): 226-30.
[http://dx.doi.org/10.1046/j.1469-0705.2000.00068.x] [PMID: 10846779]

[23]   Achiron R, Zimand S, Hegesh J, Lipitz S, Zalel Y, Rotstein Z. Fetal aortic arch measurements between 14 and 38 weeks' gestation: *in-utero* ultrasonographic study. Ultrasound Obstet Gynecol 2000; 15(3): 226-30.
[http://dx.doi.org/10.1046/j.1469-0705.2000.00068.x] [PMID: 10846779]

[24]   Pasquini L, Mellander M, Seale A, *et al.* Z-scores of the fetal aortic isthmus and duct: an aid to assessing arch hypoplasia. Ultrasound Obstet Gynecol 2007; 29(6): 628-33.
[http://dx.doi.org/10.1002/uog.4021] [PMID: 17476706]

[25]   Head CE, Jowett VC, Sharland GK, Simpson JM. Timing of presentation and postnatal outcome of infants suspected of having coarctation of the aorta during fetal life. Heart 2005; 91(8): 1070-4.
[http://dx.doi.org/10.1136/hrt.2003.033027] [PMID: 16020599]

[26]   Hornberger LK, Weintraub RG, Pesonen E, *et al.* Echocardiographic study of the morphology and growth of the aortic arch in the human fetus. Observations related to the prenatal diagnosis of coarctation. Circulation 1992; 86(3): 741-7.
[http://dx.doi.org/10.1161/01.CIR.86.3.741] [PMID: 1516185]

[27]   Rizzo G, Arduini D, Capponi A. Use of 4-dimensional sonography in the measurement of fetal great vessels in mediastinum to distinguish true-from false-positive coarctation of the aorta. J Ultrasound Med 2010; 29(2): 325-6.
[http://dx.doi.org/10.7863/jum.2010.29.2.325] [PMID: 20103809]

[28]   Slodki M, Rychik J, Moszura T, Janiak K, Respondek-Liberska M. Measurement of the great vessels in the mediastinum could help distinguish true from false-positive coarctation of the aorta in the third trimester. J Ultrasound Med 2009; 28(10): 1313-7.
[http://dx.doi.org/10.7863/jum.2009.28.10.1313] [PMID: 19778876]

[29]   Nyberg DA, McGahan JP, Pretorius D, Pilu G. Diagnostic Imaging of Fetal Anomalies. Philadephia, PA: Lippincot Williams & Wilkins 2003; pp. 467-72.

[30]   Hornberger LK, Sanders SP, Rein AJ, Spevak PJ, Parness IA, Colan SD. Left heart obstructive lesions and left ventricular growth in the midtrimester fetus. A longitudinal study. Circulation 1995; 92(6): 1531-8.
[http://dx.doi.org/10.1161/01.CIR.92.6.1531] [PMID: 7664437]

[31]   Shone JD, Sellers RD, Anderson RC, Adams P Jr, Lillehei CW, Edwards JE. The developmental complex of "parachute mitral valve," supravalvular ring of left atrium, subaortic stenosis, and coarctation of aorta. Am J Cardiol 1963; 11: 714-25.
[http://dx.doi.org/10.1016/0002-9149(63)90098-5] [PMID: 13988650]

[32]   Gardiner HM, Kovacevic A, Tulzer G, *et al.* Natural history of 107 cases of fetal aortic stenosis from a European multicenter retrospective study. Ultrasound Obstet Gynecol 2016; 48(3): 373-81.
[http://dx.doi.org/10.1002/uog.15876] [PMID: 26843026]

[33]   Freud LR, McElhinney DB, Marshall AC, *et al.* Fetal aortic valvuloplasty for evolving hypoplastic left heart syndrome: postnatal outcomes of the first 100 patients. Circulation 2014; 130(8): 638-45.
[http://dx.doi.org/10.1161/CIRCULATIONAHA.114.009032] [PMID: 25052401]

[34]   Mäkikallio K, McElhinney DB, Levine JC, *et al.* Fetal aortic valve stenosis and the evolution of hypoplastic left heart syndrome: patient selection for fetal intervention. Circulation 2006; 113(11): 1401-5.
[http://dx.doi.org/10.1161/CIRCULATIONAHA.105.588194] [PMID: 16534003]

[35]   Tworetzky W, Wilkins-Haug L, Jennings RW, *et al.* Balloon dilation of severe aortic stenosis in the fetus: potential for prevention of hypoplastic left heart syndrome: candidate selection, technique, and results of successful intervention. Circulation 2004; 110(15): 2125-31.
[http://dx.doi.org/10.1161/01.CIR.0000144357.29279.54] [PMID: 15466631]

[36]   Selamet Tierney ES, Wald RM, McElhinney DB, *et al.* Changes in left heart hemodynamics after technically successful *in-utero* aortic valvuloplasty. Ultrasound Obstet Gynecol 2007; 30(5): 715-20.
[http://dx.doi.org/10.1002/uog.5132] [PMID: 17764106]

[37]   McElhinney DB, Marshall AC, Wilkins-Haug LE, *et al.* Predictors of technical success and postnatal biventricular outcome after *in utero* aortic valvuloplasty for aortic stenosis with evolving hypoplastic left heart syndrome. Circulation 2009; 120(15): 1482-90.
[http://dx.doi.org/10.1161/CIRCULATIONAHA.109.848994] [PMID: 19786635]

[38]   Arzt W, Wertaschnigg D, Veit I, Klement F, Gitter R, Tulzer G. Intrauterine aortic valvuloplasty in fetuses with critical aortic stenosis: experience and results of 24 procedures. Ultrasound Obstet Gynecol 2011; 37(6): 689-95.
[http://dx.doi.org/10.1002/uog.8927] [PMID: 21229549]

[39]   Marshall AC, Tworetzky W, Bergersen L, *et al.* Aortic valvuloplasty in the fetus: technical characteristics of successful balloon dilation. J Pediatr 2005; 147(4): 535-9.
[http://dx.doi.org/10.1016/j.jpeds.2005.04.055] [PMID: 16227042]

[40]   Isaaz K. Tissue Doppler imaging for the assessment of left ventricular systolic and diastolic functions. Curr Opin Cardiol 2002; 17(5): 431-42.
[http://dx.doi.org/10.1097/00001573-200209000-00001] [PMID: 12357118]

[41]   McMahon CJ, Nagueh SF, Pignatelli RH, *et al.* Characterization of left ventricular diastolic function by tissue Doppler imaging and clinical status in children with hypertrophic cardiomyopathy. Circulation 2004; 109(14): 1756-62.
[http://dx.doi.org/10.1161/01.CIR.0000124723.16433.31] [PMID: 15023880]

[42]   Comas M, Crispi F. Assessment of fetal cardiac function using tissue Doppler techniques. Fetal Diagn Ther 2012; 32(1-2): 30-8.
[http://dx.doi.org/10.1159/000335028] [PMID: 22626950]

[43]   Ichizuka K, Matsuoka R, Hasegawa J, *et al.* The Tei index for evaluation of fetal myocardial performance in sick fetuses. Early Hum Dev 2005; 81(3): 273-9.
[http://dx.doi.org/10.1016/j.earlhumdev.2004.07.003] [PMID: 15814209]

[44]   Steinhard J, Heinig J, Schmitz R, Breithardt OA, Kiesel L, Klockenbusch W. [Tissue Doppler imaging of the fetal heart--a new parametric ultrasound technique in prenatal medicine]. Ultraschall Med 2007; 28(6): 578-83.
[http://dx.doi.org/10.1055/s-2007-963643] [PMID: 18008214]

[45]   Gardiner HM, Pasquini L, Wolfenden J, *et al.* Myocardial tissue Doppler and long axis function in the fetal heart. Int J Cardiol 2006; 113(1): 39-47.
[http://dx.doi.org/10.1016/j.ijcard.2005.10.029] [PMID: 16360223]

[46] Paladini D, Lamberti A, Teodoro A, Arienzo M, Tartaglione A, Martinelli P. Tissue Doppler imaging of the fetal heart. Ultrasound Obstet Gynecol 2000; 16(6): 530-5.
[http://dx.doi.org/10.1046/j.1469-0705.2000.00251.x] [PMID: 11169346]

[47] Watanabe S, Hashimoto I, Saito K, *et al.* Characterization of ventricular myocardial performance in the fetus by tissue Doppler imaging. Circ J 2009; 73(5): 943-7.
[http://dx.doi.org/10.1253/circj.CJ-08-0529] [PMID: 19276611]

[48] Bui YK, Kipps AK, Brook MM, Moon-Grady AJ. Tissue Doppler is more sensitive and reproducible than spectral pulsed-wave Doppler for fetal right ventricle myocardial performance index determination in normal and diabetic pregnancies. J Am Soc Echocardiogr 2013; 26(5): 507-14.
[http://dx.doi.org/10.1016/j.echo.2013.02.006] [PMID: 23498900]

[49] Comas M, Crispi F, Gómez O, Puerto B, Figueras F, Gratacós E. Gestational age- and estimated fetal weight-adjusted reference ranges for myocardial tissue Doppler indices at 24-41 weeks' gestation. Ultrasound Obstet Gynecol 2011; 37(1): 57-64.
[http://dx.doi.org/10.1002/uog.8870] [PMID: 21046540]

[50] Friedman KG, Schidlow D, Freud L, Escobar-Diaz M, Tworetzky W. Left ventricular diastolic function and characteristics in fetal aortic stenosis. Am J Cardiol 2014; 114(1): 122-7.
[http://dx.doi.org/10.1016/j.amjcard.2014.04.013] [PMID: 24819899]

[51] Wohlmuth C, Wertaschnigg D, Wieser I, Arzt W, Tulzer G. Tissue Doppler imaging in fetuses with aortic stenosis and evolving hypoplastic left heart syndrome before and after fetal aortic valvuloplasty. Ultrasound Obstet Gynecol 2016; 47(5): 608-15.
[http://dx.doi.org/10.1002/uog.14885] [PMID: 25914144]

[52] Simpson JM, Sharland GK. Natural history and outcome of aortic stenosis diagnosed prenatally. Heart 1997; 77(3): 205-10.
[http://dx.doi.org/10.1136/hrt.77.3.205] [PMID: 9093035]

[53] Gerboni S, Sabatino G, Mingarelli R, Dallapiccola B. Coarctation of the aorta, interrupted aortic arch, and hypoplastic left heart syndrome in three generations. J Med Genet 1993; 30(4): 328-9.
[http://dx.doi.org/10.1136/jmg.30.4.328] [PMID: 8487284]

[54] Celoria GC, Patton RB. Congenital absence of the aortic arch. Am Heart J 1959; 58: 407-13.
[http://dx.doi.org/10.1016/0002-8703(59)90157-7] [PMID: 13808756]

[55] Hirano Y, Masuyama H, Hayata K, Eto E, Nobumoto E, Hiramatsu Y. Prenatal diagnosis of interrupted aortic arch: usefulness of three-vessel and four-chamber views. Acta Med Okayama 2016; 70(6): 485-91.
[PMID: 28003674]

[56] Bennasar M, Martinez JM. Interruption of the Aortic Arch. In: Copel JA, D'Alton ME, Gratacos E, et al Eds. 1ˢᵗ Eds. Philadelphia, PA: Elsevier Saunders 2012; pp. 429-30.

[57] Lewin MB, Lindsay EA, Jurecic V, Goytia V, Towbin JA, Baldini A. A genetic etiology for interruption of the aortic arch type B. Am J Cardiol 1997; 80(4): 493-7.
[http://dx.doi.org/10.1016/S0002-9149(97)00401-3] [PMID: 9285664]

[58] Goldmuntz E, Clark BJ, Mitchell LE, *et al.* Frequency of 22q11 deletions in patients with conotruncal defects. J Am Coll Cardiol 1998; 32(2): 492-8.
[http://dx.doi.org/10.1016/S0735-1097(98)00259-9] [PMID: 9708481]

[59] Rauch A, Hofbeck M, Leipold G, *et al.* Incidence and significance of 22q11.2 hemizygosity in patients with interrupted aortic arch. Am J Med Genet 1998; 78(4): 322-31.
[http://dx.doi.org/10.1002/(SICI)1096-8628(19980724)78:4<322::AID-AJMG4>3.0.CO;2-N] [PMID: 9714433]

[60] Reardon MJ, Hallman GL, Cooley DA. Interrupted aortic arch: brief review and summary of an eighteen-year experience. Tex Heart Inst J 1984; 11(3): 250-9.
[PMID: 15227058]

[61]   Volpe P, Tuo G, De Robertis V, *et al*. Fetal interrupted aortic arch: 2D-4D echocardiography, associations and outcome. Ultrasound Obstet Gynecol 2010; 35(3): 302-9.
[http://dx.doi.org/10.1002/uog.7530] [PMID: 20069674]

[62]   Vogel M, Vernon MM, McElhinney DB, Brown DW, Colan SD, Tworetzky W. Fetal diagnosis of interrupted aortic arch. Am J Cardiol 2010; 105(5): 727-34.
[http://dx.doi.org/10.1016/j.amjcard.2009.10.053] [PMID: 20185024]

[63]   Slodki M, Moszura T, Janiak K, *et al*. The three-vessel view in the fetal mediastinum in the diagnosis of interrupted aortic arch. Ultrasound Med Biol 2011; 37(11): 1808-13.
[http://dx.doi.org/10.1016/j.ultrasmedbio.2011.06.002] [PMID: 21840641]

[64]   Feit LR, Copel JA, Kleinman CS. Foramen ovale size in the normal and abnormal human fetal heart: an indicator of transatrial flow physiology. Ultrasound Obstet Gynecol 1991; 1(5): 313-9.
[http://dx.doi.org/10.1046/j.1469-0705.1991.01050313.x] [PMID: 12797035]

[65]   Chin AJ, Weinberg PM, Barber G. Subcostal two-dimensional echocardiographic identification of anomalous attachment of septum primum in patients with left atrioventricular valve underdevelopment. J Am Coll Cardiol 1990; 15(3): 678-81.
[http://dx.doi.org/10.1016/0735-1097(90)90645-6] [PMID: 2303638]

[66]   Lurie PR. Changing concepts of endocardial fibroelastosis. Cardiol Young 2010; 20(2): 115-23.
[http://dx.doi.org/10.1017/S1047951110000181] [PMID: 20346203]

[67]   Noonan JA, Nadas AS. The hypoplastic left heart syndrome; an analysis of 101 cases. Pediatr Clin North Am 1958; 5(4): 1029-56.
[http://dx.doi.org/10.1016/S0031-3955(16)30727-1] [PMID: 13600906]

[68]   Jiang Y, Xu Y, Tang J, Xia H. Assessment of structural and functional abnormalities of the myocardium and the ascending aorta in fetus with hypoplastic left heart syndrome. BioMed Res Int 2016; 20162616729
[http://dx.doi.org/10.1155/2016/2616729] [PMID: 26981527]

[69]   Hickey EJ, Caldarone CA, McCrindle BW. Left ventricular hypoplasia: a spectrum of disease involving the left ventricular outflow tract, aortic valve, and aorta. J Am Coll Cardiol 2012; 59(1) (Suppl.): S43-54.
[http://dx.doi.org/10.1016/j.jacc.2011.04.046] [PMID: 22192721]

[70]   Allan LD, Sharland G, Tynan MJ. The natural history of the hypoplastic left heart syndrome. Int J Cardiol 1989; 25(3): 341-3.
[http://dx.doi.org/10.1016/0167-5273(89)90226-X] [PMID: 2613383]

[71]   Frommelt MA. Challenges and controversies in fetal diagnosis and treatment: hypoplastic left heart syndrome. Clin Perinatol 2014; 41(4): 787-98.
[http://dx.doi.org/10.1016/j.clp.2014.08.004] [PMID: 25459774]

[72]   Danford DA, Cronican P. Hypoplastic left heart syndrome: progression of left ventricular dilation and dysfunction to left ventricular hypoplasia *in utero*. Am Heart J 1992; 123(6): 1712-3.
[http://dx.doi.org/10.1016/0002-8703(92)90834-I] [PMID: 1595559]

[73]   Norwood WI, Lang P, Hansen DD. Physiologic repair of aortic atresia-hypoplastic left heart syndrome. N Engl J Med 1983; 308(1): 23-6.
[http://dx.doi.org/10.1056/NEJM198301063080106] [PMID: 6847920]

[74]   Feinstein JA, Benson DW, Dubin AM, *et al*. Hypoplastic left heart syndrome: current considerations and expectations. J Am Coll Cardiol 2012; 59(1) (Suppl.): S1-S42.
[http://dx.doi.org/10.1016/j.jacc.2011.09.022] [PMID: 22192720]

[75]   Goldberg DJ, Shaddy RE, Ravishankar C, Rychik J. The failing Fontan: etiology, diagnosis and management. Expert Rev Cardiovasc Ther 2011; 9(6): 785-93.
[http://dx.doi.org/10.1586/erc.11.75] [PMID: 21714609]

[76]   Ye M, Coldren C, Liang X, *et al.* Deletion of ETS-1, a gene in the Jacobsen syndrome critical region, causes ventricular septal defects and abnormal ventricular morphology in mice. Hum Mol Genet 2010; 19(4): 648-56.
[http://dx.doi.org/10.1093/hmg/ddp532] [PMID: 19942620]

[77]   Natowicz M, Chatten J, Clancy R, *et al.* Genetic disorders and major extracardiac anomalies associated with the hypoplastic left heart syndrome. Pediatrics 1988; 82(5): 698-706.
[PMID: 3186348]

[78]   Atz AM, Travison TG, Williams IA, *et al.* Prenatal diagnosis and risk factors for preoperative death in neonates with single right ventricle and systemic outflow obstruction: screening data from the pediatric heart network single ventricle reconstruction trial. J Thorac Cardiovasc Surg 2010; 140(6): 1245-50.
[http://dx.doi.org/10.1016/j.jtcvs.2010.05.022] [PMID: 20561642]

[79]   Gaynor JW, Mahle WT, Cohen MI, *et al.* Risk factors for mortality after the Norwood procedure. Eur J Cardiothorac Surg 2002; 22(1): 82-9.
[http://dx.doi.org/10.1016/S1010-7940(02)00198-7] [PMID: 12103378]

[80]   Jones HN, Olbrych SK, Smith KL, *et al.* Hypoplastic left heart syndrome is associated with structural and vascular placental abnormalities and leptin dysregulation. Placenta 2015; 36(10): 1078-86.
[http://dx.doi.org/10.1016/j.placenta.2015.08.003] [PMID: 26278057]

[81]   Vlahos AP, Lock JE, McElhinney DB, van der Velde ME. Hypoplastic left heart syndrome with intact or highly restrictive atrial septum: outcome after neonatal transcatheter atrial septostomy. Circulation 2004; 109(19): 2326-30.
[http://dx.doi.org/10.1161/01.CIR.0000128690.35860.C5] [PMID: 15136496]

[82]   Glatz JA, Tabbutt S, Gaynor JW, *et al.* Hypoplastic left heart syndrome with atrial level restriction in the era of prenatal diagnosis. Ann Thorac Surg 2007; 84(5): 1633-8.
[http://dx.doi.org/10.1016/j.athoracsur.2007.06.061] [PMID: 17954074]

[83]   Rychik J, Rome JJ, Collins MH, DeCampli WM, Spray TL. The hypoplastic left heart syndrome with intact atrial septum: atrial morphology, pulmonary vascular histopathology and outcome. J Am Coll Cardiol 1999; 34(2): 554-60.
[http://dx.doi.org/10.1016/S0735-1097(99)00225-9] [PMID: 10440172]

[84]   Marshall AC, van der Velde ME, Tworetzky W, *et al.* Creation of an atrial septal defect *in utero* for fetuses with hypoplastic left heart syndrome and intact or highly restrictive atrial septum. Circulation 2004; 110(3): 253-8.
[http://dx.doi.org/10.1161/01.CIR.0000135471.17922.17] [PMID: 15226215]

[85]   Olivieri L, Ratnayaka K, Levy RJ, Berger J, Wessel D, Donofrio M. Hypoplastic left heart syndrome with intact atrial septum sequelae of left atrial hypertension *in utero.* J Am Coll Cardiol 2011; 57(20)e369
[http://dx.doi.org/10.1016/j.jacc.2010.10.064] [PMID: 21565633]

[86]   Schidlow DN, Freud L, Friedman K, Tworetzky W. Fetal interventions for structural heart disease. Echocardiography 2017; 34(12): 1834-41.
[http://dx.doi.org/10.1111/echo.13667] [PMID: 29287139]

[87]   Jantzen DW, Moon-Grady AJ, Morris SA, *et al.* Hypoplastic left heart syndrome with intact or restrictive atrial septum: a report from the international fetal cardiac intervention registry. Circulation 2017; 136(14): 1346-9.
[http://dx.doi.org/10.1161/CIRCULATIONAHA.116.025873] [PMID: 28864444]

[88]   Moon-Grady AJ, Morris SA, Belfort M, *et al.* International fetal cardiac intervention registry: a worldwide collaborative description and preliminary outcomes. J Am Coll Cardiol 2015; 66(4): 388-99.
[http://dx.doi.org/10.1016/j.jacc.2015.05.037] [PMID: 26205597]

[89]   Chaturvedi RR, Ryan G, Seed M, van Arsdell G, Jaeggi ET. Fetal stenting of the atrial septum: technique and initial results in cardiac lesions with left atrial hypertension. Int J Cardiol 2013; 168(3): 2029-36.
[http://dx.doi.org/10.1016/j.ijcard.2013.01.173] [PMID: 23481911]

[90]   Kalish BT, Tworetzky W, Benson CB, *et al.* Technical challenges of atrial septal stent placement in fetuses with hypoplastic left heart syndrome and intact atrial septum. Catheter Cardiovasc Interv 2014; 84(1): 77-85.
[http://dx.doi.org/10.1002/ccd.25098] [PMID: 23804575]

[91]   Pedra SR, Peralta CF, Crema L, Jatene IB, da Costa RN, Pedra CA. Fetal interventions for congenital heart disease in Brazil. Pediatr Cardiol 2014; 35(3): 399-405.
[http://dx.doi.org/10.1007/s00246-013-0792-3] [PMID: 24030590]

[92]   Quintero RA, Huhta J, Suh E, Chmait R, Romero R, Angel J. *In utero* cardiac fetal surgery: laser atrial septotomy in the treatment of hypoplastic left heart syndrome with intact atrial septum. Am J Obstet Gynecol 2005; 193(4): 1424-8.
[http://dx.doi.org/10.1016/j.ajog.2005.02.126] [PMID: 16202736]

[93]   Friedman KG, Sleeper LA, Freud LR, *et al.* Improved technical success, postnatal outcome and refined predictors of outcome for fetal aortic valvuloplasty. Ultrasound Obstet Gynecol 2018; 52(2): 212-20.
[http://dx.doi.org/10.1002/uog.17530] [PMID: 28543953]

[94]   Allan LD, Maxwell DJ, Carminati M, Tynan MJ. Survival after fetal aortic balloon valvoplasty. Ultrasound Obstet Gynecol 1995; 5(2): 90-1.
[http://dx.doi.org/10.1046/j.1469-0705.1995.05020090.x] [PMID: 7719873]

[95]   Maxwell D, Allan L, Tynan MJ. Balloon dilatation of the aortic valve in the fetus: a report of two cases. Br Heart J 1991; 65(5): 256-8.
[http://dx.doi.org/10.1136/hrt.65.5.256] [PMID: 2039669]

[96]   Kohl T, Sharland G, Allan LD, *et al.* World experience of percutaneous ultrasound-guided balloon valvuloplasty in human fetuses with severe aortic valve obstruction. Am J Cardiol 2000; 85(10): 1230-3.
[http://dx.doi.org/10.1016/S0002-9149(00)00733-5] [PMID: 10802006]

[97]   Galindo A, Nieto O, Villagrá S, Grañeras A, Herraiz I, Mendoza A. Hypoplastic left heart syndrome diagnosed in fetal life: associated findings, pregnancy outcome and results of palliative surgery. Ultrasound Obstet Gynecol 2009; 33(5): 560-6.
[http://dx.doi.org/10.1002/uog.6355] [PMID: 19367583]

[98]   Forbess JM, Cook N, Roth SJ, Serraf A, Mayer JE Jr, Jonas RA. Ten-year institutional experience with palliative surgery for hypoplastic left heart syndrome. Risk factors related to stage I mortality. Circulation 1995; 92(9) (Suppl.): II262-6.
[http://dx.doi.org/10.1161/01.CIR.92.9.262] [PMID: 7586421]

[99]   Vida VL, Bacha EA, Larrazabal A, *et al.* Hypoplastic left heart syndrome with intact or highly restrictive atrial septum: surgical experience from a single center. Ann Thorac Surg 2007; 84(2): 581-5.
[http://dx.doi.org/10.1016/j.athoracsur.2007.04.017] [PMID: 17643639]

[100] Gellis L, Drogosz M, Lu M, *et al.* Echocardiographic predictors of neonatal illness severity in fetuses with critical left heart obstruction with intact or restrictive atrial septum. Prenat Diagn 2018; 38(10): 788-94.
[http://dx.doi.org/10.1002/pd.5322] [PMID: 29956347]

[101] Vlahos AP, Lock JE, McElhinney DB, van der Velde ME. Hypoplastic left heart syndrome with intact or highly restrictive atrial septum: outcome after neonatal transcatheter atrial septostomy. Circulation 2004; 109(19): 2326-30.
[http://dx.doi.org/10.1161/01.CIR.0000128690.35860.C5] [PMID: 15136496]

[102] Bravo C, Gámez F, Pérez R, Álvarez T, De León-Luis J. Fetal Aortic Arch Anomalies: Key Sonographic Views for Their Differential Diagnosis and Clinical Implications Using the Cardiovascular System Sonographic Evaluation Protocol. J Ultrasound Med 2016; 35(2): 237-51.
[http://dx.doi.org/10.7863/ultra.15.02063] [PMID: 26715656]

[103] De León-Luis J, Gámez F, Bravo C, *et al*. Second-trimester fetal aberrant right subclavian artery: original study, systematic review and meta-analysis of performance in detection of Down syndrome. Ultrasound Obstet Gynecol 2014; 44(2): 147-53.
[http://dx.doi.org/10.1002/uog.13336] [PMID: 24585513]

[104] Yoo SJ, Min JY, Lee YH, Roman K, Jaeggi E, Smallhorn J. Fetal sonographic diagnosis of aortic arch anomalies. Ultrasound Obstet Gynecol 2003; 22(5): 535-46.
[http://dx.doi.org/10.1002/uog.897] [PMID: 14618670]

[105] Peng R, Xie HN, Zheng J, Zhou Y, Lin MF. Fetal right aortic arch: associated anomalies, genetic anomalies with chromosomal microarray analysis, and postnatal outcome. Prenat Diagn 2017; 37(4): 329-35.
[http://dx.doi.org/10.1002/pd.5015] [PMID: 28165153]

[106] Miranda JO, Callaghan N, Miller O, Simpson J, Sharland G. Right aortic arch diagnosed antenatally: associations and outcome in 98 fetuses. Heart 2014; 100(1): 54-9.
[http://dx.doi.org/10.1136/heartjnl-2013-304860] [PMID: 24192976]

[107] Berg C, Bender F, Soukup M, *et al*. Right aortic arch detected in fetal life. Ultrasound Obstet Gynecol 2006; 28(7): 882-9.
[http://dx.doi.org/10.1002/uog.3883] [PMID: 17086578]

[108] Zidere V, Tsapakis EG, Huggon IC, Allan LD. Right aortic arch in the fetus. Ultrasound Obstet Gynecol 2006; 28(7): 876-81.
[http://dx.doi.org/10.1002/uog.3841] [PMID: 17066500]

[109] McElhinney DB, Clark BJ III, Weinberg PM, *et al*. Association of chromosome 22q11 deletion with isolated anomalies of aortic arch laterality and branching. J Am Coll Cardiol 2001; 37(8): 2114-9.
[http://dx.doi.org/10.1016/S0735-1097(01)01286-4] [PMID: 11419896]

[110] Achiron R, Rotstein Z, Heggesh J, *et al*. Anomalies of the fetal aortic arch: a novel sonographic approach to *in-utero* diagnosis. Ultrasound Obstet Gynecol 2002; 20(6): 553-7.
[http://dx.doi.org/10.1046/j.1469-0705.2002.00850.x] [PMID: 12493043]

[111] Tuo G, Volpe P, Bava GL, *et al*. Prenatal diagnosis and outcome of isolated vascular rings. Am J Cardiol 2009; 103(3): 416-9.
[http://dx.doi.org/10.1016/j.amjcard.2008.09.100] [PMID: 19166700]

[112] Galindo A, Nieto O, Nieto MT, *et al*. Prenatal diagnosis of right aortic arch: associated findings, pregnancy outcome, and clinical significance of vascular rings. Prenat Diagn 2009; 29(10): 975-81.
[http://dx.doi.org/10.1002/pd.2327] [PMID: 19603384]

[113] Razon Y, Berant M, Fogelman R, Amir G, Birk E. Prenatal diagnosis and outcome of right aortic arch without significant intracardiac anomaly. J Am Soc Echocardiogr 2014; 27(12): 1352-8.
[http://dx.doi.org/10.1016/j.echo.2014.08.003] [PMID: 25240492]

[114] Rauch R, Rauch A, Koch A, *et al*. Laterality of the aortic arch and anomalies of the subclavian artery-reliable indicators for 22q11.2 deletion syndromes? Eur J Pediatr 2004; 163(11): 642-5.
[http://dx.doi.org/10.1007/s00431-004-1518-6] [PMID: 15300432]

[115] D'Antonio F, Khalil A, Zidere V, Carvalho JS. Fetuses with right aortic arch: a multicenter cohort study and meta-analysis. Ultrasound Obstet Gynecol 2016; 47(4): 423-32.
[http://dx.doi.org/10.1002/uog.15805] [PMID: 26643657]

[116] McLaren CA, Elliott MJ, Roebuck DJ. Vascular compression of the airway in children. Paediatr Respir Rev 2008; 9(2): 85-94.
[http://dx.doi.org/10.1016/j.prrv.2007.12.008] [PMID: 18513668]

[117] Bonnard A, Auber F, Fourcade L, Marchac V, Emond S, Révillon Y. Vascular ring abnormalities: a retrospective study of 62 cases. J Pediatr Surg 2003; 38(4): 539-43.
[http://dx.doi.org/10.1053/jpsu.2003.50117] [PMID: 12677561]

[118] Bronshtein M, Lorber A, Berant M, Auslander R, Zimmer EZ. Sonographic diagnosis of fetal vascular rings in early pregnancy. Am J Cardiol 1998; 81(1): 101-3.
[http://dx.doi.org/10.1016/S0002-9149(97)00864-3] [PMID: 9462619]

[119] Chaoui R, Kalache KD, Heling KS, Tennstedt C, Bommer C, Körner H. Absent or hypoplastic thymus on ultrasound: a marker for deletion 22q11.2 in fetal cardiac defects. Ultrasound Obstet Gynecol 2002; 20(6): 546-52.
[http://dx.doi.org/10.1046/j.1469-0705.2002.00864.x] [PMID: 12493042]

[120] Tonni G, Rosignoli L, Cariati E, *et al.* Fetal thymus: visualization rate and volume by integrating 2D- and 3D-ultrasound during 2nd trimester echocardiography. J Matern Fetal Neonatal Med 2016; 29(14): 2223-8.
[http://dx.doi.org/10.3109/14767058.2015.1081892] [PMID: 26365654]

[121] Kau T, Sinzig M, Gasser J, *et al.* Aortic development and anomalies. Semin Intervent Radiol 2007; 24(2): 141-52.
[http://dx.doi.org/10.1055/s-2007-980040] [PMID: 21326792]

[122] Naidu DP, Wohlmuth C, Gardiner HM. Prenatal diagnosis of double aortic arch: can we predict airway obstruction (pseudo-CHAOS) and need for airway EXIT? Ultrasound Obstet Gynecol 2017; 49(5): 660-1.
[http://dx.doi.org/10.1002/uog.17212] [PMID: 27486072]

[123] Patel CR, Lane JR, Spector ML, Smith PC. Fetal echocardiographic diagnosis of vascular rings. J Ultrasound Med 2006; 25(2): 251-7.
[http://dx.doi.org/10.7863/jum.2006.25.2.251] [PMID: 16439790]

[124] Yagel S, Arbel R, Anteby EY, Raveh D, Achiron R. The three vessels and trachea view (3VT) in fetal cardiac scanning. Ultrasound Obstet Gynecol 2002; 20(4): 340-5.
[http://dx.doi.org/10.1046/j.1469-0705.2002.00801.x] [PMID: 12383314]

[125] Turan S, Turan OM, Maisel P, Gaskin P, Harman CR, Baschat AA. Three-dimensional sonography in the prenatal diagnosis of aortic arch abnormalities. J Clin Ultrasound 2009; 37(5): 253-7.
[http://dx.doi.org/10.1002/jcu.20559] [PMID: 19253354]

[126] Mogra R, Kesby G, Sholler G, Hyett J. Identification and management of fetal isolated right-sided aortic arch in an unselected population. Ultrasound Obstet Gynecol 2016; 48(6): 739-43.
[http://dx.doi.org/10.1002/uog.15892] [PMID: 26918379]

[127] McElhinney DB, Hoydu AK, Gaynor JW, Spray TL, Goldmuntz E, Weinberg PM. Patterns of right aortic arch and mirror-image branching of the brachiocephalic vessels without associated anomalies. Pediatr Cardiol 2001; 22(4): 285-91.
[http://dx.doi.org/10.1007/s002460010231] [PMID: 11455394]

[128] Chaoui R, Schneider MBE, Kalache KD. Right aortic arch with vascular ring and aberrant left subclavian artery: prenatal diagnosis assisted by three-dimensional power Doppler ultrasound. Ultrasound Obstet Gynecol 2003; 22(6): 661-3.
[http://dx.doi.org/10.1002/uog.933] [PMID: 14689548]

[129] Valletta EA, Pregarz M, Bergamo-Andreis IA, Boner AL. Tracheoesophageal compression due to congenital vascular anomalies (vascular rings). Pediatr Pulmonol 1997; 24(2): 93-105.
[http://dx.doi.org/10.1002/(SICI)1099-0496(199708)24:2<93::AID-PPUL4>3.0.CO;2-J] [PMID: 9292900]

[130] Horváth P, Hucin B, Hruda J, *et al.* Intermediate to late results of surgical relief of vascular tracheobronchial compression. Eur J Cardiothorac Surg 1992; 6(7): 366-71.
[http://dx.doi.org/10.1016/1010-7940(92)90174-V] [PMID: 1497929]

[131]   Evans WN, Acherman RJ, Berthoty D, *et al.* Right aortic arch with situs solitus. Congenit Heart Dis 2018; 13(4): 624-7.
[http://dx.doi.org/10.1111/chd.12623] [PMID: 30033669]

[132]   Jhaveri S, Komarlu R. Fetal diagnosis of a rare finding: right-sided cervical aortic arch with aberrant left subclavian artery and absent ductus arteriosus in tetralogy of Fallot. Ultrasound Obstet Gynecol 2018; Epub ahead of print
[http://dx.doi.org/10.1002/uog.20151] [PMID: 30338597]

[133]   Patel CR, Smith GL, Lane JR, Robinson HB. Prenatal echocardiographic diagnosis of a right aortic arch and bilateral arterial duct with isolation of the left subclavian artery from the left pulmonary artery. J Ultrasound Med 2007; 26(8): 1107-10.
[http://dx.doi.org/10.7863/jum.2007.26.8.1107] [PMID: 17646375]

[134]   Cordisco A, Murzi B, Chiappa E. Right aortic arch with bilateral arterial duct and nonconfluent pulmonary arteries without associated cardiac defects: Prenatal diagnosis and successful postnatal treatment. J Obstet Gynaecol Res 2018; 44(9): 1828-31.
[http://dx.doi.org/10.1111/jog.13709] [PMID: 29978531]

[135]   Tonni G, Lituania M, Chitayat D, *et al.* Complete trisomy 9 with unusual phenotypic associations: Dandy-Walker malformation, cleft lip and cleft palate, cardiovascular abnormalities. Taiwan J Obstet Gynecol 2014; 53(4): 592-7.
[http://dx.doi.org/10.1016/j.tjog.2014.01.005] [PMID: 25510707]

[136]   Shum DJ, Clifton MS, Coakley FV, *et al.* Prenatal tracheal obstruction due to double aortic arch: a potential mimic of congenital high airway obstruction syndrome. AJR Am J Roentgenol 2007; 188(1): W82-5.
[http://dx.doi.org/10.2214/AJR.05.0356] [PMID: 17179331]

[137]   Edwards JE. Vascular rings related to anomalies of the aortic arches. Mod Concepts Cardiovasc Dis 1948; 17(8): 1.
[PMID: 18873268]

[138]   Trobo D, Bravo C, Alvarez T, Pérez R, Gámez F, De León-Luis J. Prenatal sonographic features of a double aortic arch: literature review and perinatal management. J Ultrasound Med 2015; 34(11): 1921-7.
[http://dx.doi.org/10.7863/ultra.14.12076] [PMID: 26446822]

[139]   Trobo Marina D, Bravo C, Lancharro Á, Gámez Alderete F, Marín C, de León-Luis J. Neonatal magnetic resonance imaging in double aortic arch diagnosed prenatally by ultrasound. J Obstet Gynaecol 2016; 36(4): 526-8.
[http://dx.doi.org/10.3109/01443615.2015.1110125] [PMID: 26979672]

[140]   Xiong Y, Chen M, Chan LW, *et al.* A novel way of visualizing the ductal and aortic arches by real-time three-dimensional ultrasound with live xPlane imaging. Ultrasound Obstet Gynecol 2012; 39(3): 316-21.
[http://dx.doi.org/10.1002/uog.9081] [PMID: 21710662]

[141]   Dell'Oro S, Verderio M, Incerti M, Mastrolia SA, Cozzolino S, Vergani P. 2D *versus* 3D real time ultrasound with live xPlane imaging to visualize aortic and ductal arches: comparison between methods. PeerJ 2018; 6e4561
[http://dx.doi.org/10.7717/peerj.4561] [PMID: 29637020]

[142]   Anuwutnavin S, Satou G, Finn P, Lee L, Sklansky M. Fetal diagnosis of d-transposition of the great arteries associated with a double aortic arch. J Ultrasound Med 2015; 34(9): 1701-6.
[http://dx.doi.org/10.7863/ultra.15.14.10012] [PMID: 26269298]

[143]   Yao WM, Wang JM, Huang HF, Ye YH. Prenatal diagnosis of double aortic arch and D-transposition of the great arteries: a case report. Prenat Diagn 2010; 30(4): 382-3.
[http://dx.doi.org/10.1002/pd.2472] [PMID: 20155782]

[144] Seo HK, Je HG, Kang IS, Lim KA. Prenatal double aortic arch presenting with a right aortic arch and an anomalous artery arising from the ascending aorta. Int J Cardiovasc Imaging 2010; 26 (Suppl. 1): 165-8.
[http://dx.doi.org/10.1007/s10554-009-9553-z] [PMID: 20033491]

[145] Hauck A, da Cruz EM, Jaggers J, Jone PN. Tricuspid atresia associated with truncus arteriosus *versus* aortopulmonary window: combining fetal and postnatal echocardiography to make the diagnosis. Echocardiography 2013; 30(10): E336-9.
[http://dx.doi.org/10.1111/echo.12354] [PMID: 24033694]

[146] Respondek-Liberska M, Gradecka M, Czichos E. Significant fetal pulmonary regurgitation as a possible prenatal sign of aorto-pulmonary window in the fetus with intrauterine growth retardation. A case report. Fetal Diagn Ther 2004; 19(1): 72-4.
[http://dx.doi.org/10.1159/000074264] [PMID: 14646422]

CHAPTER 12

Fetal Conotruncal Anomalies

Maria Virgina Lima Machado[*]

CardioFetal Clinic – Centro de Cardiologia e Ecocardiografia Fetal, Pediátrica e Adulto, São Paulo – SP, Brazil

Abstract: Conotruncal anomalies are characterized by abnormalities of the great vessels of the heart. There are five types of conotruncal anomalies named as tetralogy of Fallot, double outlet of the right ventricle, transposition of the great arteries, truncus arteriosus and corrected transposition of the great arteries. These lesions known as "conotruncal anomalies" are caused by aberrant development of the conotruncal region of the embryonic heart. Prenatal diagnosis of congenital heart disease optimizes obstetric and neonatal care. Identification of these anomalies in prenatal life allows a variety of treatment with options to be considered, including delivery at a tertiary center, termination of pregnancy in some cases and *in utero* therapy. Majority of fetuses with conotruncal anomalies will undergo surgery in the neonatal period or in the first year of life. This chapter will discuss the fetal echocardiographic findings, extracardiac and chromosomal anomalies associations, prenatal and postnatal outcomes of conotruncal anomalies.

Keywords: Conotruncal anomalies, Corrected transposition of the great arteries, Double outlet right ventricle, Tetralogy of Fallot, Truncus arteriosus, Transposition of the great arteries.

INTRODUCTION

Congenital heart disease (CHD) is the most common abnormality found amongst live birth [1 - 3]. It has been reported to occur in approximately 1 in 100 live birth [4 - 8]. Conotruncal anomalies accounts for 25-30% of CHD in infants [9, 10]. Tetralogy of Fallot and complete transposition are the two most common conotruncal anomalies, each occurring in 8-12% of infants with cardiac defects. Double outlet ventricles, truncus arteriosus, and corrected transposition of the great arteries are less common. The incidence of CHD rated on live births underestimate considerably, the incidence of cardiac defect in the fetus [1, 2, 7, 11]. Stillbirth and fetal loss in the first trimester are often the result of complex

---

[*] **Corresponding author Maria Virginia Lima Machado:** CardioFetal Clinic – Centro de Cardiologia e Ecocardiografia Fetal, Pediátrica e Adulto, Rua Itapeva, 518 – conj. 1307 - 13º andar - Bela Vista, CEP 01332-000, São Paulo – SP, E-mail: v.machado2009@live.com

Edward Araujo Júnior, Nathalie Jeanne M. Bravo-Valenzuela and Alberto Borges Peixoto (Eds.)

heart defects or chromosomal abnormalities or a combination of both. Therefore, the incidence of CHD in the fetus has been reported as much higher than that found in postnatal life [12].

The development of the heart is an interaction of genes, environment and chance. An abnormal interaction of any of these processes may lead to a congenital heart defect. Majority of cases of CHD have a multifactorial cause. The tissue that forms the outflow tract of the heart originates in the neural crest and branchial arch mesenchyme. These cells migrate along an undefined pathway to specific locations in the conotruncus and conotruncal septum. Interference with this migration results in a spectrum of conotruncal malformations [13 - 15].

A screening program for the detection of fetal cardiac anomalies has been widely established over the last twenty years [16 - 18]. Obstetric ultrasound includes the four-chamber view of the fetal heart as a standard part of every examination [16, 19]. The four-chamber view has been reported to have a sensitivity and specificity respectively in the detection of CHD [20, 21]. Nonetheless, four-chamber view alone does not identify conotruncal abnormalities such as Tetralogy of Fallot (TOF) or truncus arteriosus [22]. That is why conotruncal anomalies have a lower prevalence in fetal series than in pediatric series [23, 24]. It has been advocated to include the aortic and pulmonary outflow tract views, as part of every routine obstetric examination of the fetal heart [25, 26] and the three-vessel view of the upper mediastinum [27 - 29]. With more complete examination of the fetal heart, there has been a significant improvement in the detection rates of conotruncal anomalies. As conotruncal anomalies often require care and treatment immediately after delivery, prenatal detection is critically important.

TETRALOGY OF FALLOT

Tetralogy of Fallot (TOF) is described as an anomaly consisting of four anatomical features: a ventricular septal defect (VSD) (subaortic), overriding aorta, an infundibular and valvar pulmonary stenosis and right ventricular hypertrophy (Fig. **1**). This latter characteristic is not typically present in the fetus. These features are the consequence of anterior, superior and leftward deviation of the outlet septum from the rest of the ventricular septum, which is considered the major cause of problem in the pathology of TOF [30, 31].

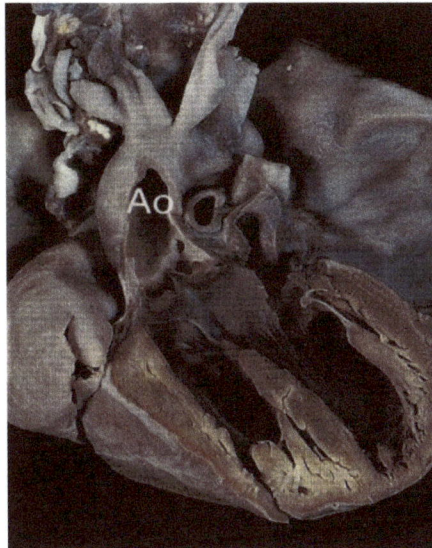

Fig. (1). Simulated view of the left outflow tract in fetal specimen demonstrating aorta arising astride an outlet ventricular septal defect. Ao: aorta

There is a variety of spectrum of TOF where there is minimal obstruction to the right ventricle until severe forms such as pulmonary atresia with VSD and absent pulmonary valve (Fig. **2**). TOF is the most common form of cyanotic CHD, which accounts for 10% of infants with CHD [32]. The newborns with classic form of TOF and pulmonary stenosis accounts for 80% in postnatal life [33]. In prenatal series, TOF accounted for 7.2% of all cases of fetal CHD [34].

ECHOCARDIOGRAPHIC FINDINGS

In TOF, the situs is solitus and there is levocardia in the majority of fetuses. The axis of the fetal heart may be abnormal in some cases and the cardiac apex is deviated leftward [30, 31]. The four-chamber view appears normal in most cases. However, a large VSD can be visible in this plane. The ventricular septal defect involves the outlet part of the ventricular septum [32, 33]. A perimembranous VSD, the tricuspid valve is in direct contact with the aortic valve and is seen immediately below the overriding aortic valve in the left ventricular outflow tract view. A muscular outlet ventricular septal defect is less frequent.

TOF is detected in the five-chamber view imaging a subaortic VSD and an overriding aortic root. The diagnosis of TOF is made by assessing of the outflow tract of the ventricles [32, 34, 35]. Long axis views of the left ventricle will demonstrate the ventricular septal defect and the aorta overriding the crest of the ventricular septum (Fig. **3**).

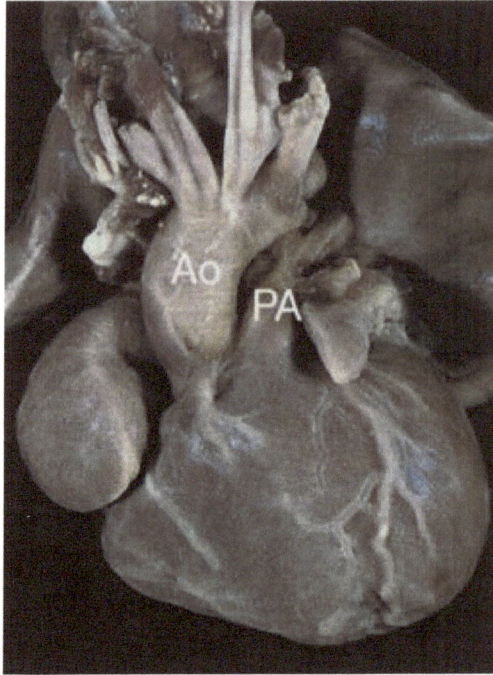

Fig. (2). External view of the heart the of a fetal specimen with Tetralogy of Fallot showing the pulmonary trunk smaller than the aorta. Ao: aorta; PA: pulmonary artery.

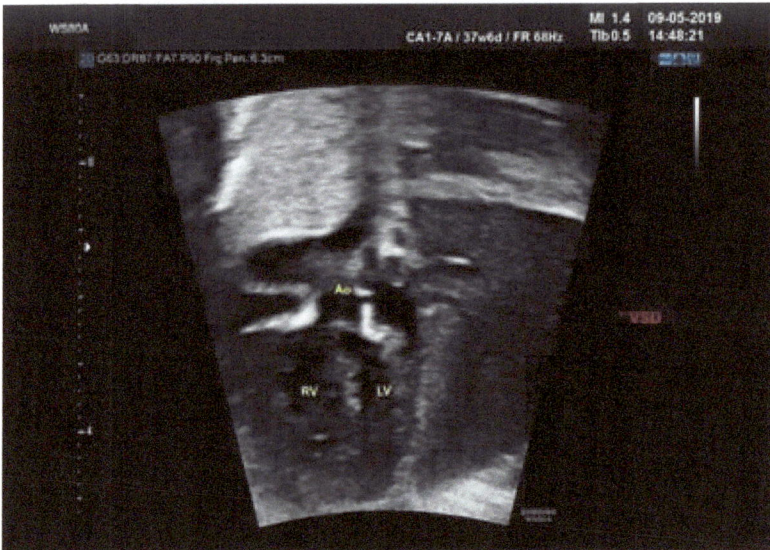

Fig. (3). Long axis views of the left ventricle of a mid-trimester fetus showing the ventricular septal defect and the aorta overriding the crest of the ventricular septum. Ao: aorta; RV: right ventricle; LV: left ventricle; *VSD: ventricular septal defect.

The override of the aorta is caused by a discontinuity between the interventricular septum and the medial aortic wall connecting the aorta to the right ventricle. The aorta is shifted to the right, a condition termed aortic dextroposition and receives blood from both the right and the left ventricles. Color Doppler mapping will show flow into the aorta from both the left and right ventricles (Fig. **4A**). The aortic valve overrides the ventricular septal defect (Fig. **4B**).

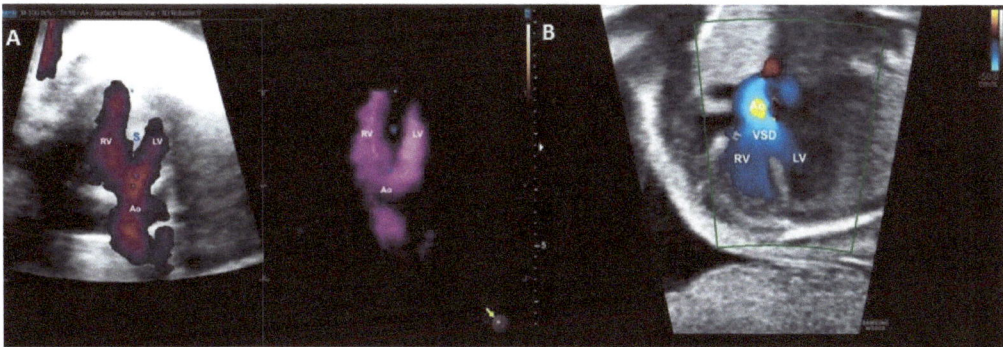

Fig. (4). Tetralogy of Fallot – Color Doppler mapping of outflow tract of the left ventricle showing flow into the aorta from the left and right ventricles (**A**) and the aortic valve overrides the ventricular septal defect (**B**). S: interventricular septum; Ao: aorta; RV: right ventricle; LV: left ventricle; VSD: ventricular septal defect.

The diagnosis of TOF also requires a detection of a small main pulmonary artery visualized in short axis view of the right ventricle or the three-vessel view of the upper mediastinum. Hypoplasia of pulmonary artery is caused by the deviation of the outlet septum. A small pulmonary artery indicates some degree of right ventricular outflow obstruction (Fig. **5**). Pulsed Doppler will show increased velocity across the pulmonary valve.

The ductus arteriosus is a small channel arising from the aortic arch and often difficult to identify in tetralogy [35, 36]. The blood flow through the ductus arteriosus varies considerably according to the severity of subpulmonary stenosis [37]. The ductus arteriosus flow can be right to left, bidirectional, or left to right. Flow across the ductus arteriosus is anterograde in mild TOF especially in mid gestation but in severe pulmonary outflow tract obstruction and hypoplastic pulmonary artery a left to right shunt through the ductus arteriosus from the aorta to the pulmonary artery (reversal flow) may be detected. This is a predictive sign of severe disease that may require prostaglandin therapy immediately after birth and surgical correction in neonatal period. The ductus arteriosus is absent in TOF with absent pulmonary valve syndrome [38] and patent when absent pulmonary valve syndrome occurs with an intact ventricular septum or a simple ventricular septal defect [39 - 41].

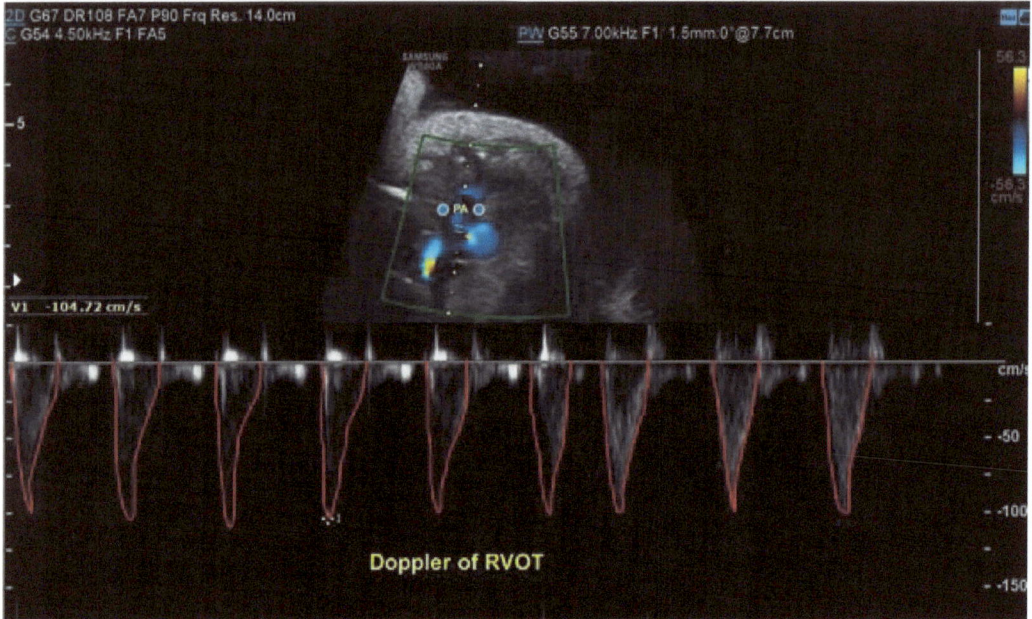

Fig. (5). Tetralogy of Fallot - Short axis view of the right ventricle of a 35-week gestation fetus with small pulmonary artery (RV outflow obstruction). Pulsed Doppler of RV outflow tract show increased velocity across the pulmonary valve (peak velocity= 104.7cm/s). PA: pulmonary artery; RVOT: right ventricle outflow tract.

A right aortic arch is associated with some cases in TOF. This finding can be easily identified in the three-vessel view with descending aorta seen on the right anteriorly of the spine. The three-vessel trachea view is also suitable to demonstrate the size and alignment of dilated aorta displaced anteriorly and the small main pulmonary artery posteriorly. Color flow mapping at this plane view can also demonstrate a small pulmonary artery. Conversely to the small size of the main pulmonary artery, the sizes of the branch pulmonary arteries are usually normal [36]. Pulmonary arterial growth during fetal life is variable and unpredictable [34]. Progression of the outflow tract obstruction may occur in some cases and small branch pulmonary arteries at mid-gestation suggest severe disease. Doppler velocities across the narrowed right ventricular outflow tract are typically normal or only mildly increased comparing to postnatal findings [32, 36].

In the first trimester, the diagnosis of TOF is possible but more difficult due to small size of the heart and fetal movements [42]. Diagnostic features of TOF include a large aortic root and or a small pulmonary artery. Color flow mapping of five-chamber view will show anterograde flow in both vessels and a discrepancy in size. In early gestation that is an important sign because the aortic overriding may not be easily detected. Increased nuchal translucency measurement showed to be associated with TOF, even in the absence of chromosomal abnormalities [35].

In some milder forms of TOF, especially in mid gestation, the discrepancy in size between the pulmonary artery and the aorta may be insignificant and becomes more evident in the third trimester.

In three-dimensional (3D) ultrasound, the tomographic ultrasound imaging mode applied to a 3D volume acquired at the level of the four-chamber view allows the demonstration of the VSD, aortic overriding, and the stenosis pulmonary artery in a single view of multiple planes. Spatio-temporal image correlation (STIC) and Fetal Intelligent Navigation Echocardiography (FINE) with color Doppler displayed in glass body mode provides a clear demonstration of the lesion in the three-vessel-trachea view [43, 44] (Fig. **6**).

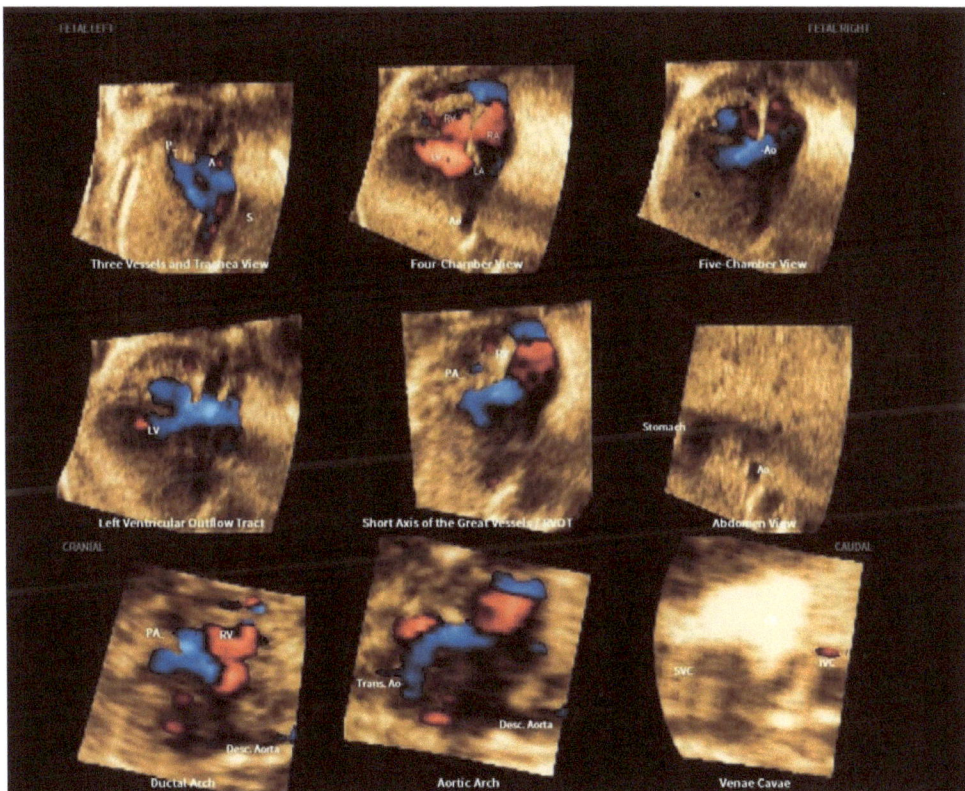

Fig. (6). Fetal Intelligent Navigation Echocardiography of a case of tetralogy of Fallot at 37 weeks and 6 days. Color Doppler showing overriding of aorta and misaligned ventricular septal defect. RA: right atrium; RV: right ventricle; LA: left atrium; LV: left ventricle; PA: pulmonary artery; Ao: aorta.

ASSOCIATED CARDIAC AND EXTRACARDIAC ANOMALIES

TOF can be associated with other cardiac anomalies such as atrioventricular septal defect, multiple ventricular septal defects, total anomalous pulmonary venous drainage, and coronary artery fistula. The presence of a right sided aortic arch to the right of the trachea, is seen in 25% of cases with TOF [45].

A secundum type of atrial septal defect may be present in postnatal life but cannot be diagnosed in the fetus. It has been reported that patent forame ovale or an atrial septal defect was found in 83% and a persistent left superior vena cava in 11% of newborns with TOF [46]. Anomaly of the pulmonary artery such as one pulmonary artery (left) disconnected from the main pulmonary artery and connected to the ipsilateral ductus arteriosus. Anatomical variations of coronary artery are occasionally seen, and this may have an impact on the surgical approach to repair [47]. Occasionally an atrioventricular septal defect associated with TOF increases the risk of chromosomal abnormalities [48].

TOF is usually associated with either chromosomal anomalies, syndromes or structural extracardiac malformations. Associated extracardiac congenital anomalies are fairly common with no specific organ involvement. A higher incidence of extracardiac malformations, chromosomal anomalies, and genetic syndromes is seen in the fetus with TOF when compared to the neonates. The risk of deletion 22q11 in cases of TOF increases when thymus is hypoplastic, the aortic arch is right sided, extracardiac anomalies or polyhydramnios is found [49, 50]. Other defects can be found such as midline defects, omphalocele, pentalogy of Cantrell, central nervous abnormalities, diaphragmatic hernia and renal malformations. Vactrel or Charge syndromes with multiple lesions associated are less common. It has been reported in a large fetal series that TOF was associated with chromosomal abnormalities in 21% of cases. Of these, 32% were trisomy, and 23% were 22q11 deletion. The most common trisomy 18 (19%), 6% (trisomy 13) and 13% had various other chromosomal abnormalities including unbalanced translocations and deletions, a case of 47XXY, a case of 69XXX and a case of 92XXYY [51].

TRUNCUS ARTERIOSUS

Truncus arteriosus (TA) is a conotruncal anomaly characterized by a single arterial trunk which arises from the base of the heart giving origin to the systemic, coronary, and pulmonary arteries (Fig. 7) [52].

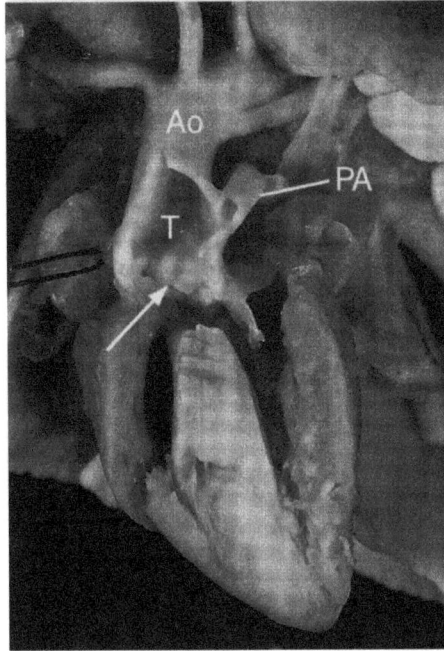

Fig. (7). Simulated view of the left ventricular outflow in a 21-week fetal specimen showing the truncal valve (arrow) overriding the crest of the ventricular septum. Ao: aorta; PA: pulmonary artery; T: truncal valve.

A large VSD is always present in this anomaly and is located immediately underneath the truncal valve, which overrides the ventricular septum [53, 54]. The truncal valve is almost in fibrous continuity with the mitral valve. TA results from the failure of the truncus swellings, which normally divide the truncus arteriosus into the aorta and pulmonary arteries during embryogenesis to fuse resulting in a persistent common trunk [55].

The spectrum of the disease is mainly related to the anatomic origin of the right and left pulmonary arteries, which may arise from the origin of the trunk or as direct branches from the TA or the descending aorta (Fig. **8**). TA is classified into four types by Collet and Edwards based on the anatomic origin of the pulmonary arteries [56, 57]. The most common diagnosed type in the fetus is type 1. TA is found in 1.6% of all newborns with congenital heart disease [58] and is reported to occur in about 1.07 of 10,000 births [59]. Is found equally in boys and girls and is more prevalent in fetal series [60]. Association with chromosomal anomalies and microdeletion 22q11 are common.

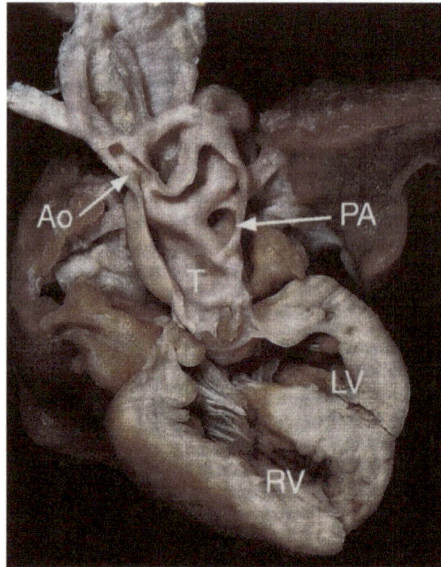

Fig. (8). In the anatomic specimen, viewed from the front, a single artery arises from the ventricular mass and gives rise to the right and left pulmonary arterial branches and the aortic arch. Ao: aorta; PA: pulmonary artery; LV: left ventricle; RV: right ventricle; T: truncal valve.

FETAL ECHOCARDIOGRAPHIC FINDINGS

The heart position may be abnormal with the apex directed more towards to the left as in TOF. The four-chamber view appears normal in TA unless the VSD is large and visible in this plane (Fig. **9**). Occasionally one of the ventricular chambers may be more dominant and rarely there may atresia of either atrioventricular valve.

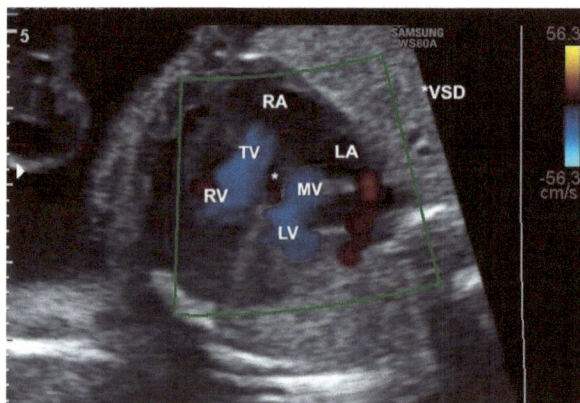

Fig. (9). Four-chamber view in a 27-week-old fetus with truncus arteriosus showing a ventricular septal defect with color Doppler. RA: right atrium; RV: right ventricle; LA: left atrium; LV: left ventricle; TV: tricuspid valve; MV: mitral valve; *VSD: ventricular septal defect.

Left ventricular outflow tract view demonstrates the ventricular septum defect and a single arterial trunk arising from the heart giving rise to the aortic arch and the pulmonary arteries (Fig. **10**). The diagnosis can be also achieved on five-chamber view by imaging the left outflow tract to identify the mal-aligned VSD with an overriding large vessel (Fig. **11**).

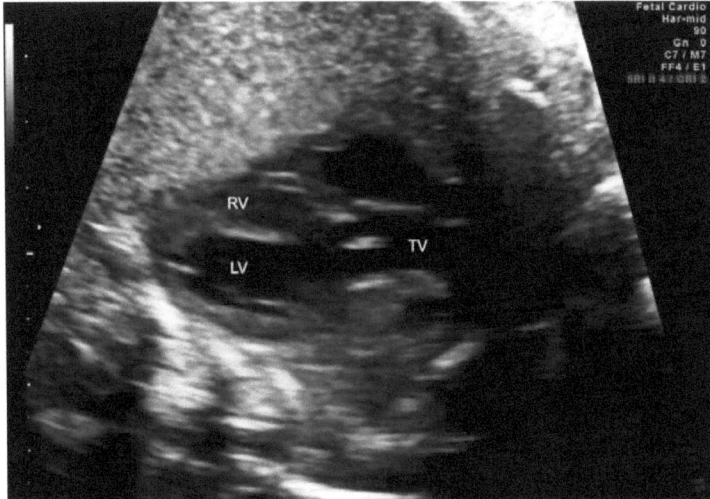

Fig. (10). Outflow tract of the ventricles showing a single arterial trunk arising from both ventricles (Truncus Arteriosus Type I). RV; right ventricle; LV: left ventricle; TV: truncal valve.

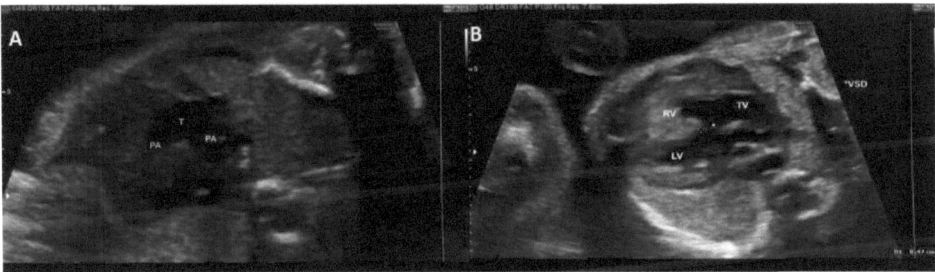

Fig. (11). Truncus arteriosus type 2, both pulmonary arteries arise separately from the truncus arteriosus. PA: pulmonary artery; RV: right ventricle; LV: left ventricle; *VSD: ventricular septal defect; TV: truncal valve.

Absent pulmonary artery and valve arising from the right ventricle or identifying the main pulmonary artery or pulmonary arteries directly arising from the arterial trunk confirms the diagnosis and differentiates this abnormality from TOF. The truncal valve is often thickened and dysplastic and often associated with stenosis or regurgitation. The truncal valve can have two to five cusps and it may be regurgitant and less commonly stenotic. Color Doppler mapping is useful to show turbulent flow across the truncal valve and an increase velocity indicates truncal valve stenosis. A regurgitant flow in the left ventricle identify truncal valve regurgitation.

The 3-vessel-trachea view shows a single large vessel (the aortic arch) in the case of an absent arterial ductus found in 50% of the cases [61, 62]. There is an inverse relationship between development of the aortic arch and ductus arteriosus. The 3-vessel-trachea view shows, in the majority of cases, the aortic arch to the left of the trachea (left aortic arch) and to the right (right aortic arch) and in 30% (Fig. **12**). The thymus gland is seen in this view between the transverse aortic arch and the anterior thorax wall. When it is small or absent, it is a sign of possible association with 22q11 microdeletion that occurs in about one third of cases [63, 64].

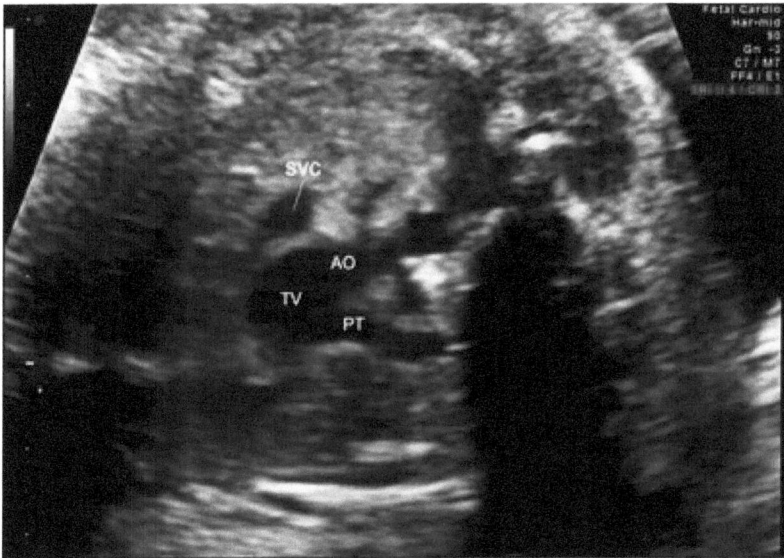

Fig. (12). The three vessels and trachea view shows relationship of the aortic arch to the left of the trachea (left aortic arch). AO: aorta; PT: pulmonary trunk; TV: truncal valve; SVC: superior vena cava.

THREE-DIMENSIONAL ULTRASOUND

Tomographic ultrasound imaging allows for the demonstration of the anatomic characteristics of TA in different planes [65]. Three-dimensional ultrasound in the rendering mode, especially with power Doppler, inversion mode, or B-flow, it helps to identify TA, its bifurcations and the small pulmonary branches mainly in TA type 2 and 3.

CARDIAC AND EXTRACARDIAC ASSOCIATIONS

Association with cardiac malformations are common with TA. VSD is always seen as part of the cardiac malformation. The ductus arteriosus is absent in 50% of the cases, and it remains patent postnatally in about two thirds of patients [61, 62]. Right-sided aortic arch has been reported in 30% of cases and interrupted arch in 15% of cases. Other anomalies of the aortic arch such as hypoplasia of the arch or persistence of double aortic arch are rare [60, 65, 66]. Abnormal origin of the coronary arteries is found in third of TA cases and this information is relevant for surgical planning [67]. Truncal valve dysplasia occurs with incompetence or stenosis. Other cardiac anomalies are rather such as atrioventricular septal defect, single ventricle and tricuspid atresia with VSD. Chromosomal anomalies have been found in about 4.5% of the cases such as trisomies 21, 18, and 13 [68]. It has been reported trisomy 9, triploidy and an unbalanced translocation. Microdeletion of chromosome 22q11, Di George or Shprintzen syndromes are frequent associated in 30% to 40% of cases [69 - 72]. TA has been reported in 21% of infants with DiGeorge syndrome [73].

Fetal karyotype should be offered when TA is diagnosed. TA and double outlet right ventricle are the most common cardiac abnormalities reported in fetuses of diabetic mothers [58]. Extracardiac structural malformations are seen in up to 40% of TA cases and are typically nonspecific such as absent arm cleft lip, dolichocephaly, exomphalos and renal abnormalities [69, 70].

FETAL ECHOCARDIOGRAPHIC FINDINGS OF TRUNCUS ARTERIOSUS

1. Leftward deviation of cardiac axis.
2. Four-chamber view appears normal.
3. Large subtruncal ventricular septal defect.
4. Single arterial trunk usually arising astride a ventricular septal defect.
5. Large TA root with biventricular origin.
6. Main pulmonary artery or branch pulmonary arteries arise from the main trunk.
7. TA valve has usually three leaflets (tricuspid) but can have four to five leaflets and two leaflets (bicuspid).
8. TA dysplastic truncal valve stenotic or regurgitation.
9. Aortic arch may be right-sided.
10. Three-vessel-trachea - single large vessel (aortic arch).
11. Confirmation of the diagnosis by identifying the pulmonary trunk (or arteries) directly arising from the overriding large vessel.

DOUBLE-OUTLET RIGHT VENTRICLE

Double-outlet right ventricle (DORV) is a type of a heterogeneous group of cardiac anomalies where the aorta and pulmonary artery arise predominately from the morphological right ventricle (Fig. **13**) [74 - 76]. By defining the ventriculoarterial connections, a great artery is considered to be connected to a ventricle when more than half of its valve is committed to that ventricle. The definition of DORV by the Congenital Heart Surgery Nomenclature and Database Project, stated that "DORV is a type of ventriculoarterial connection in which both great vessels arise either entirely or predominately from the right ventricle" [77]. Both great arteries arise primarily from the morphological right ventricle but differ with regard to the variable spatial relationship of the great arteries, the location of the ventricular septal defect, the presence or absence of pulmonary and aortic outflow obstruction.

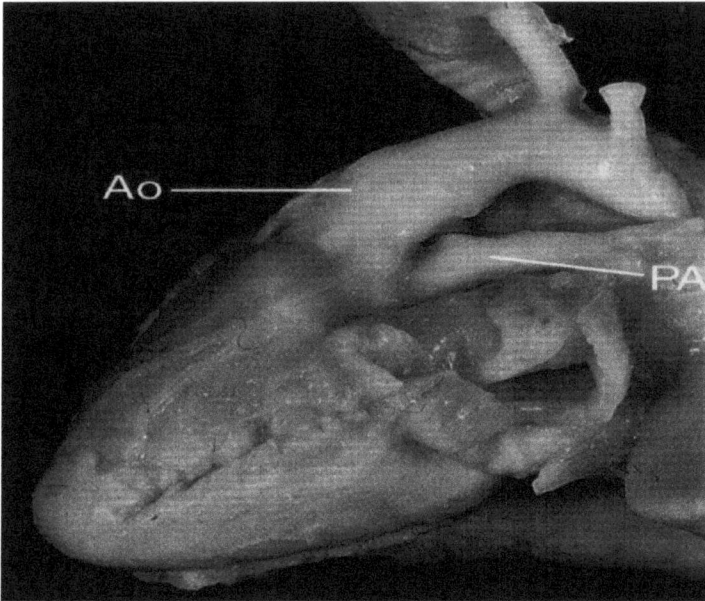

Fig. (13). View from the left side of a fetal heart specimen showing the aorta anterior to the pulmonary trunk. Ao: aorta; PA: pulmonary artery.

There are four types of DORV with different anatomic relationships of the aorta to the pulmonary artery such as right posterior aorta, a right anterior aorta, a left anterior aorta, and a right lateral aorta. The VSD associated with DORV has been described in four anatomical locations: subaortic type; subpulmonary type; subaortic and subpulmonary type (doubly committed); and nonrelated to both arteries (Figs. **14** and **15**). The subtype of DORV is difficult to identify prenatally as the position of the VSD is difficult to establish with accuracy in fetal echocardiography.

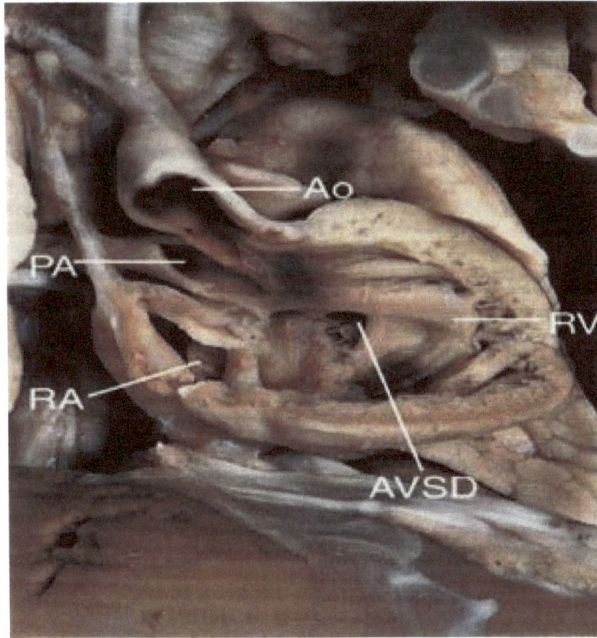

Fig. (14). Pathological specimen of the fetal heart with double-outlet right ventricle (DORV) showing anteriorly positioned aorta and posterior and hypoplastic pulmonary artery - DORV type transposition of the great arteries (TGA). Ao: aorta; PA: pulmonary artery; RA: right atrium; RV: right ventricle; AVSD: atrioventricular septal defect.

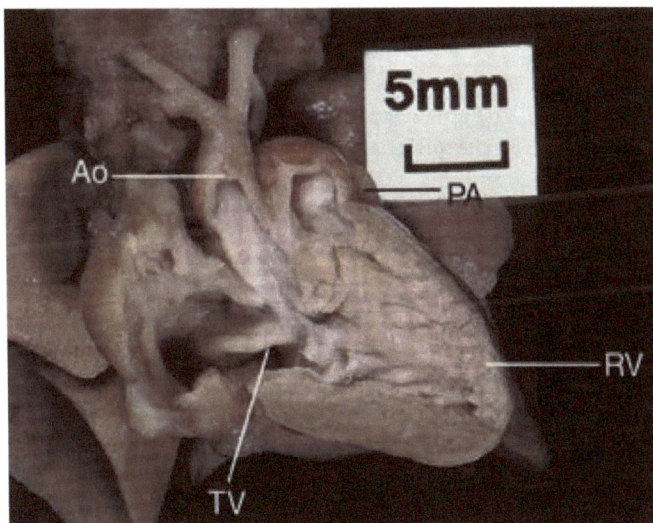

Fig. (15). View of the heart showing the both arterial valves taking origin from the morphologic right ventricle with aorta posterior and pulmonary artery anterior – DORV type tetralogy of Fallot (TOF). Ao: aorta; PA: pulmonary artery; RV: right ventricle; TV: tricuspid valve.

DORV occurs in about 1.5% of children born with CHD and has an incidence of approximately 0.09 per 1,000 live births [1]. It is found equally in boys and girls. DORV is more common in fetal series and has been reported in up to 6% of CHD [23]. The prevalence of DORV is increased in diabetic pregnancies [58].

FETAL ECHOCARDIOGRAPHIC FINDINGS

Echocardiographic diagnosis of DORV consists of a detection of aorta and pulmonary artery arise predominately from the morphological right ventricle, the anatomic relationship of the great vessels and the location of the VSD when present (Fig. **16**). The ventricular septal defect is most commonly subaortic, less frequently subpulmonary, and least commonly doubly committed or non-committed.

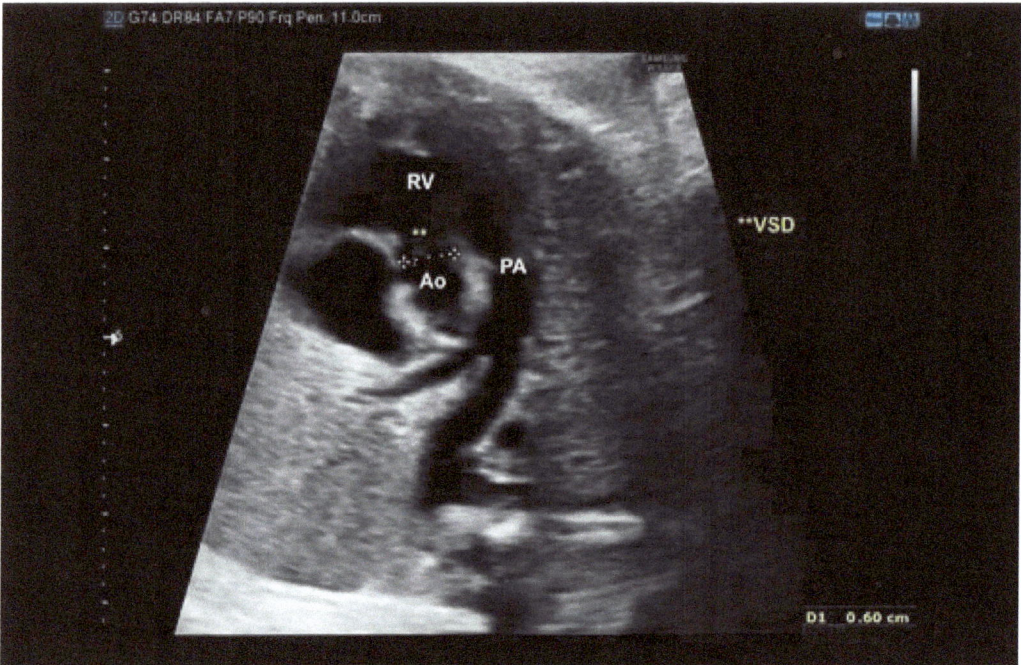

Fig. (16). Five chamber view of a 35-week fetus showing aorta and pulmonary artery arising from the right ventricle (DORV). Ao: aorta; RV: right ventricle; PA: pulmonary artery; **VSD: ventricular septal defect.

The fetal echocardiographic features will depend on the type of double outlet right ventricle, the position of the great arteries and associated cardiac lesions.

DROV can occur with any atrial situs and any atrioventricular connection. It often occurs in heterotaxy syndrome. However, it most commonly occurs with situs solitus and concordant atrioventricular connection.

In situs solitus the aorta is usually located to the right of the pulmonary artery. They tend to have a side-by-side relationship. However, any great artery relationship can be found. Both arterial trunks tend to have a parallel orientation. In many cases, both great arteries valves are supported by a completely muscular infundibulum. The four-chamber view may appear normal in the first and second trimester though the ventricular, septal defect may sometimes be seen in this view. If there is a dilated right ventricular chamber this will be detectable in the four-chamber view. The left ventricle becomes diminutive with advancing gestation, which may result in an abnormal four-chamber view later in pregnancy. Cardiac lesion associated such as abnormalities of the atrioventricular valves atrioventricular septal defect, double inlet ventricle, mitral atresia, the four-chamber view will appear abnormal. Five-chamber view is abnormal, and it shows VSD, the lack of continuity of the of the aorta with the ventricular septum, and the origin of both great arteries from the anterior chamber (right ventricle), the location and position of the VSD in relation to the great arteries. In five-chamber view and the 3-vessel-trachea view, the parallel arrangement of the great vessels is demonstrated. Views of the great arteries will be abnormal with both great arteries arising predominantly from the right ventricle. When the aorta is in a right posterior position to the pulmonary artery, the great vessels still assume a parallel course to each other [78, 79]. When the pulmonary artery is small a pulmonary stenosis is associated. When the aortic arch is small, coarctation of the aorta, or an interrupted aortic arch is present. Pulmonary artery atresia or stenosis is more common than aortic atresia or aortic coarctation in DORV.

Color Doppler mapping shows flow across the VSD from the left to the right ventricle and flow from the right ventricle into both arteries. A turbulent flow will demonstrate the presence of stenosis or reverse flow in the corresponding vessel. The anatomic relationship of the great arteries is visualized by color Doppler.

DROV with a subaortic ventricular septal defect is often associated with subpulmonary obstruction and infundibular morphology similar to TOF. On the other hand, DROV with a subpulmonary ventricular septal defect is often associated with subaortic obstruction [74]. Where there is subaortic obstruction, an obstructive lesion of the aortic arch is common. The obstruction is caused by deviation of the outlet septum and may be associated with arterial valve stenosis. Subpulmonary or subaortic obstruction can be suspected when one great artery is significantly smaller that the other at the three-vessel view. The 3-vessel-trachea view also shows a right-sided aortic arch.

Three-dimensional ultrasound can be used with tomographic ultrasound imaging to demonstrate DORV findings in one display [14, 80]. Three-dimensional rendering using surface, minimum (transparent), inversion, or color modes, can demonstrate the type of spatial arrangements of the great arteries and the anatomic relationship of the VSD to the great arteries (Fig. **17**).

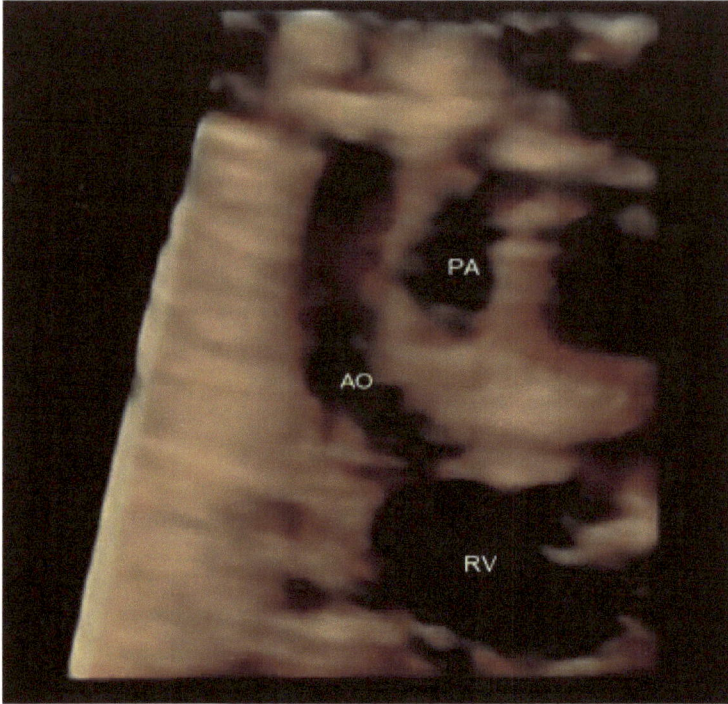

Fig. (17). Three-dimensional ultrasound rendering mode demonstrates double-outlet right ventricle (DORV) transposition of the great arteries (TGA) type, aorta anterior arising from the right ventricle and pulmonary artery posteriorly. AO: aorta; PA: pulmonary artery; RV: right ventricle.

CARDIAC AND EXTRACARDIAC ASSOCIATIONS

Cardiac findings are common, and the spectrum of cardiac lesions varies from malformations of the atrioventricular valves, atrial and ventricular septae. Mitral atresia, a cleft anterior mitral leaflet, atrial septal defects, atrioventricular septal defects, subaortic stenosis, aortic coarctation, right aortic arch, persistent left superior vena cava, and anomalous pulmonary venous return, among others. Pulmonary stenosis is the most common associated malformation and occurs in about 70% of cases [81]. DORV can be part of left or right isomerism, and this combination increases the likelihood of associated venous anomalies [82]. In isomerism, DORV may be combined with an unbalanced atrioventricular septal defect or with a double inlet single ventricle with commonly associated pulmonary obstruction. DORV can also be found in corrected transposition, where the right ventricle is left-sided.

The association of DORV with anomalies of the atrioventricular valves increase the risk of abnormalities, and the association of DORV with isomerism practically excludes the presence of chromosomal abnormalities [83, 84]. DORV can be associated with chromosomal anomalies such as trisomies 13 and 18 more rarely trisomy 21. It has also been reported with 22q11 deletion and trisomy 9 [85, 86]. Extracardiac anomalies are very common and are nonspecific organs [87]. DROV can also occur with extracardiac anomaly, which included cleft lip and palate, cystic hygroma, dextrocardia, congenital diaphragmatic hernia, duodenal atresia, exomphalos, limb, renal and spinal abnormalities and ventriculomegaly.

FETAL ECHOCARDIOGRAPHIC FINDINGS

1. Four chamber view may be normal.
2. Five-chamber view is abnormal, shows the ventricular septal defect and the origin of both great arteries from the anterior chamber (right ventricle).
3. The right ventricle is dilated.
4. Both great arteries arise predominantly from the right ventricle.
5. VSD is subaortic - Aortic override
6. VSD is subpulmonar - Pulmonary override and parallel great arteries.
7. Small pulmonary artery if pulmonary stenosis.
8. Small aorta if aortic obstruction (coarctation or interrupted aortic arch).
9. Associated cardiac lesions – atrioventricular septal defect, mitral atresia, isomerism, anomalous venous drainage.
10. Tetralogy of Fallot and transposition of great arteries are the two main differential diagnoses for DORV.

COMPLETE TRANSPOSITION OF THE GREAT ARTERIES

Complete transposition of the great arteries (TGA) is a conotruncal abnormality where there is a concordant atrioventricular connection and a discordant ventriculoarterial connection. The right atrium connects to right ventricle and the left atrium to the left ventricle and the aorta arises from the right ventricle and the pulmonary artery from the left ventricle. This condition is called complete transposition of great arteries (Fig. **18**). Both great arteries display parallel course with the aorta anterior and to the right of the pulmonary artery, thus the term D-TGA (D for dexter).

D-TGA is a frequent cardiac anomaly occurring in 5% of all congenital cardiac malformations with an incidence of 0.315 cases per 1,000 live births and 2:1 male preponderance [88, 89]. D-TGA can be an isolated cardiac malformation, termed simple D-TGA, or associated with other cardiac anomalies. Ventricular septal defects and pulmonary stenosis (left ventricular tract outflow obstruction) are common associations with D-TGA and may be present either alone or in combination in up to 30% to 40% of cases [90]. Associated extracardiac malformations are rare.

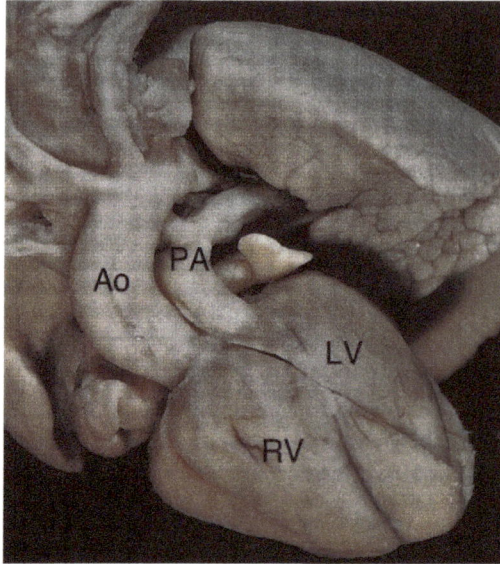

Fig. (18). External view of a fetal heart with transposition of the great arteries. The pulmonary trunk is smaller than the aorta due to subpulmonary stenosis. Ao: aorta; PA: pulmonary artery; RV: right ventricle; LV: left ventricle.

Prenatal screening policy for CHD to diagnose D-TGA will focus on the views of outflow tract of the ventricles. Four-chamber view alone, will undoubtedly fail in detecting TGA. Prenatal screening for CHD at a population level reports from 12.5% to 72.5% [91]. The decrease in neonatal morbidity and mortality in prenatally detected TGA is due to assessment of the great vessels as part of the extended basic cardiac examination of the fetus [91 - 93].

FETAL ECHOCARDIOGRAPHIC FINDING

Usually in TGA, the situs is solitus and there is levocardia. The right ventricle is the right sided and anterior ventricle and the left ventricle is left sided and posterior and the great arteries relationship is abnormal, with the pulmonary artery arising from the left ventricle and the aorta from the right ventricle. The four-chamber view appears normal except for an associated ventricular septal defect (Fig. **19**). In simple TGA, the interventricular septum is intact. The diagnosis can only be made if views of great arteries are examined. The great arteries arise from the heart in a parallel orientation and there is a loss of the normal cross-over of the great arteries (Fig. **20**). From the four-chamber view, moving cranially the first vessel to be seen in transposition is the pulmonary artery whereas in the normal heart the first vessel seen is the aorta.

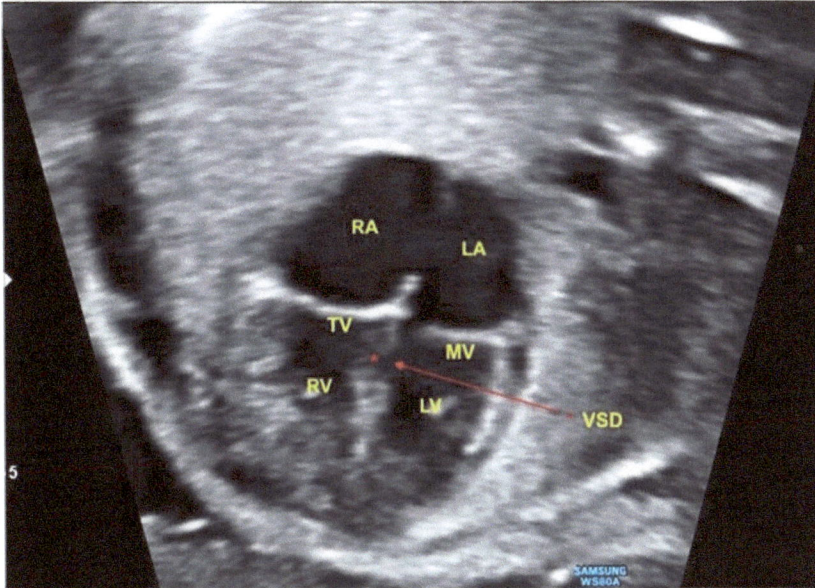

Fig. (19). Four-chamber view of a 30-week-old fetus with transposition of the great arteries (TGA) showing normal atrioventricular connection and a ventricular septal defect (VSD) (arrow). RA: right atrium; LA: left atrium; RV: right ventricle; LV: left ventricle; TV: tricuspid valve; MV: mitral valve; VSD: ventricular septal defect.

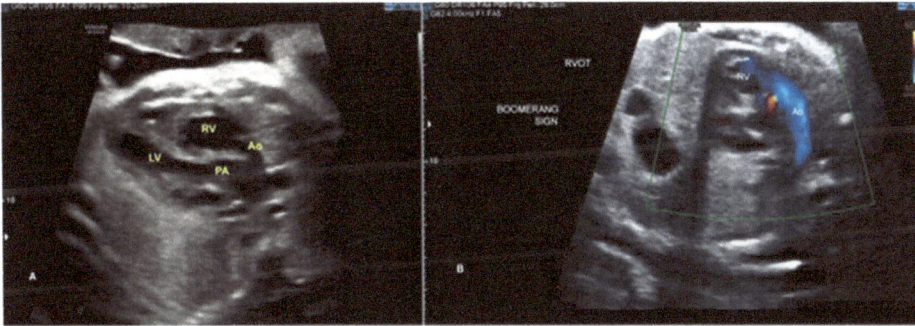

Fig. (20). (**A**) The great arteries arise from the heart in a parallel orientation and there is a loss of the normal cross-over of the great arteries. (**B**) The pulmonary artery arising from the left ventricle and the aorta from the right ventricle (boomerang shaped RVOT). Ao: aorta; PA: pulmonary artery; RV: right ventricle; LV: left ventricle; RVOT: right ventricle outflow tract.

Five-chamber view will show the pulmonary artery arising from the left ventricle and bifurcating in right and left pulmonary arteries. The aorta arises from the right ventricle in an anterior and parallel course to the pulmonary artery. This parallel orientation of the great arteries in D-TGA is best obtained in an oblique plane of the heart. The three-vessel-trachea view will show a single large vessel (the transverse aortic arch) with a superior vena cava to its right. The large vessel noted in the three-vessel-trachea view is the aorta, which is positioned anteriorly and superiorly to the pulmonary artery. To complete the examination of the heart the longitudinal views, such as the sagittal view will show the aortic arch seen arising from the anterior right ventricle and giving rise to head and neck vessels (Fig. **21**).

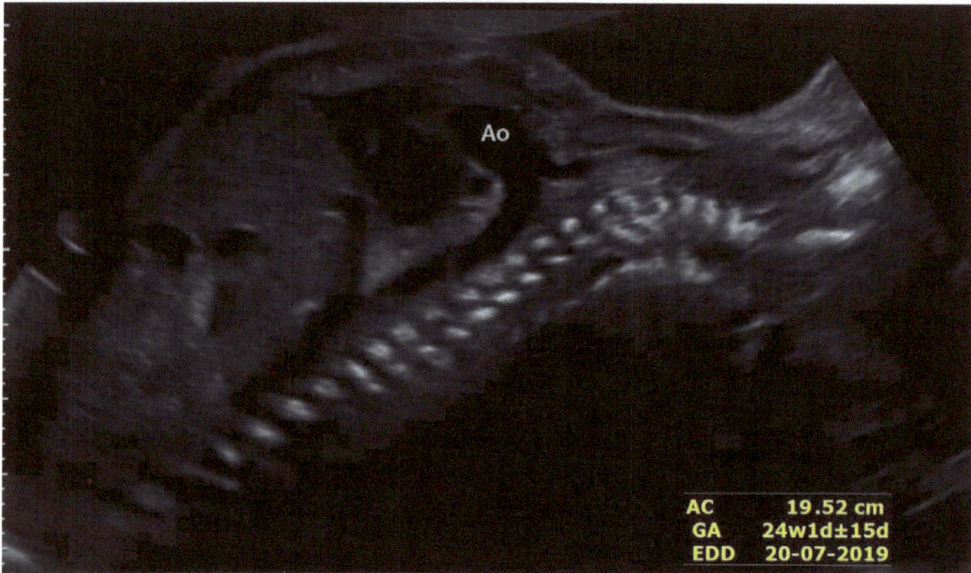

Fig. (21). Sagittal view showing the aorta anteriorly arising from the right ventricle. Ao: aorta.

Color Doppler mapping will demonstrate flow into both great arteries in a parallel orientation from five-chamber view. In the three-vessel view, the aorta and superior vena cava will be seen but the pulmonary artery is not visualized. Visualization of an associated ventricular septal defect, patency of the foramen ovale and assessment left ventricular outflow (pulmonary artery) can be enhanced by color Doppler [94]. The assessment of flow and size of forame oval and pulmonary veins is important to plan the postnatal management. In this situation color flow mapping is helpful showing the patency of forame oval and high velocities flow in pulmonary veins.

Three dimensional ultrasound will focus on rotations along different axes and color display of rendering volumes, emphasizing the diagnosis of D-TGA tomographic ultrasound imaging, glass body mode, inversion mode and other three-dimensional rendering displays have the ability to enhance visualization of the spatial relationship of the great vessels as the arise from their respective cardiac chambers (Fig. 22).

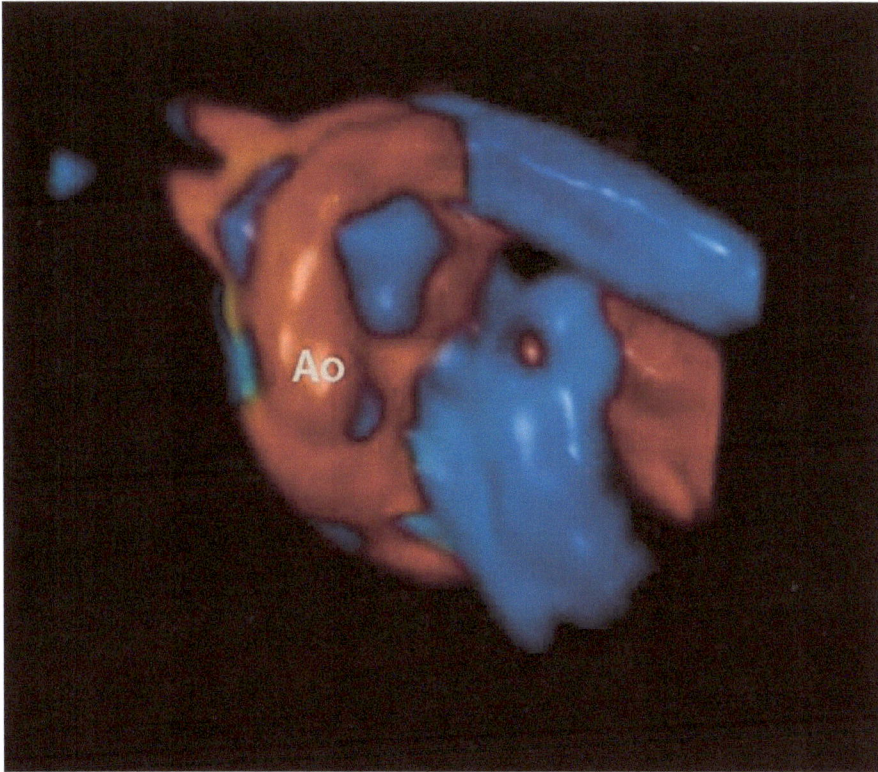

Fig. (22). Transposition of the great arteries (TGA) by three-dimensional ultrasound in the rendering mode with color Doppler demonstrates aorta (Ao) anterior arising from the right ventricle. Visualization of the spatial relationship of the great vessels.

CARDIAC AND EXTRACARDIAC ANOMALIES ASSOCIATED

Ventricular septal defect and pulmonary stenosis are the two most common associated cardiac findings in D-TGA [20]. The VSD can be of variable size and anatomic location and in the pulmonary stenosis the pulmonary valve is thickened and pulmonary artery small. Color flow mapping will show a turbulent flow across the pulmonary valve. The other lesion that can occur is coarctation of the aorta. In this condition, the aorta is small, and the arch appears hypoplastic and there may be association with sub-aortic narrowing.

Abnormal course and bifurcation of coronary arteries are found in patients with a D-TGA, and its prevalence in more than 50% when the great vessels are side by side or when the aorta is posterior and to the right of the pulmonary artery [95, 96]. Other associated complex cardiac anomalies are rare and can involve the atrioventricular valves or either ventricular chamber that may be rudimentary or small. TGA usually occurs in isolation and is rarely associated with chromosomal abnormalities, though extracardiac abnormalities can sometimes be associated. It has been reported that none of the cases of simple TGA had a chromosomal abnormality, but 5% had an extracardiac abnormality including dextrocardia and hemivertebrae [51]. Microdeletion of 22q11 could be present and should be ruled out especially when extracardiac malformations or a complex D-TGA is present.

FETAL ECHOCARDIOGRAPHIC FINDINGS

1. Normal four-chamber view except if there is a VSD.
2. Five-chamber view and outflow tract view abnormal. Atrioventricular concordance and ventriculoarterial discordance. Pulmonary artery arises from the left ventricle and aorta arises from the right ventricle.
3. Parallel arrangement of the great arteries course with the aorta anterior and to the right of the pulmonary artery.
4. Aortic arch with wide sweeping and arising the neck vessels.
5. Abnormal three – vessel view, only seen two vessels.
6. Association with pulmonary stenosis will show an increased Doppler velocity across the pulmonary valve and coarctation of aorta, a small aortic arch.

CONGENITALLY CORRECTED TRANSPOSITION OF GREAT ARTERIES

Congenitally corrected transposition (c-TGA) is a rare conotruncal anomaly characterized by atrioventricular and ventriculoarterial discordance. Because of discordant connections at two levels, the atrioventricular and ventriculoarterial connection and the is congenitally "corrected".

In this cardiac anomaly, the morphologic right atrium (right sided) is connected to the morphologic left ventricle (right sided) by the mitral valve and morphologic left atrium (left sided) is connected to the morphologic right ventricle (left sided) by the tricuspid valve. The great vessels are also transposed and discordantly connected to the ventricles; the pulmonary artery is connected to the morphologic left ventricle and the aorta is connected to the morphologic right ventricle. The aorta is located anteriorly and to the left of the pulmonary artery. Discordance at both the atrioventricular and ventriculoarterial levels results in hemodynamic compensation where the systemic venous blood reaches the pulmonary artery and the pulmonary venous return blood reaches to the aorta, so the circulation is anatomically corrected.

This is a rare and complex anomaly accounting for approximately 1% of CHD in postnatal series and for 1.6% in fetal series [97, 98]. It is more frequent in males as it is DTGA. It is thought to result from abnormal left-looping of the bulboventricular cardiac tube during embryogenesis [99]. The spectrum of disease is wide and c-TGA is isolated in only 9% to 16% of cases [100, 101].

FETAL ECHOCARDIOGRAPHIC FINDINGS

The first step to assess a fetus with a c-TGA is to determine the situs and the position of the heart in the chest. The latter is often abnormal in this condition, though it may be normal in some cases. The heart may lie more centrally in the chest, with the ventricular septum in a more anteroposterior position than normal. Situs inversus is noted in 5% of c-TGA cases [102] and dextrocardia/mesocardiac is present in about 25% of c-TGA cases [103]. The four-chamber view allows the assessment of typical ventricular morphology and it helps to diagnose atrioventricular discordance (Fig. 23). The diagnosis of c-TGA is primarily based on the recognition of atrioventricular discordance by the analysis of anatomic characteristics of ventricular morphology.

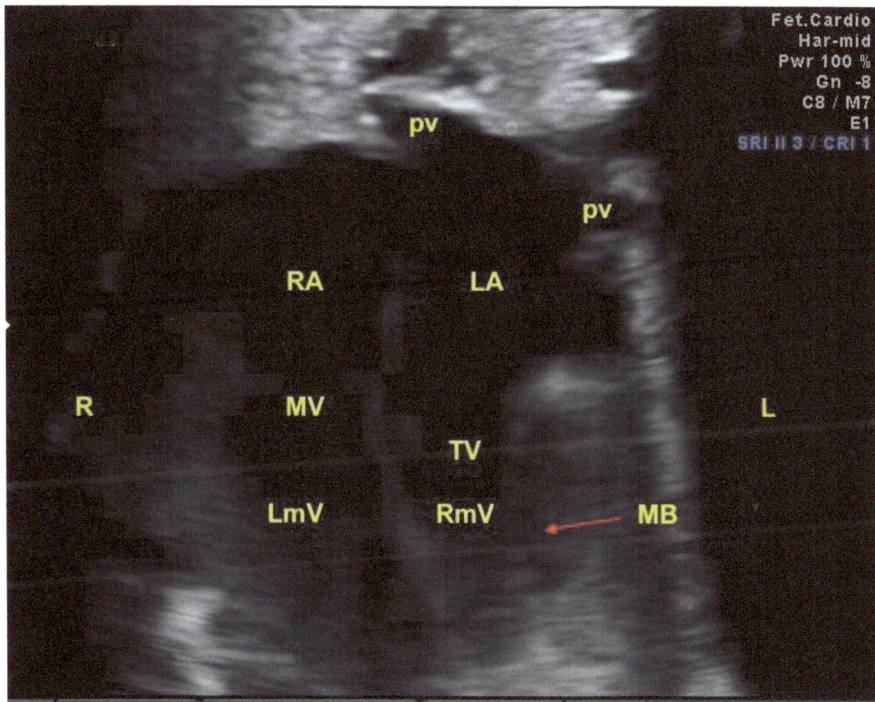

Fig. (23). Four-chamber view of a mid trimester fetus showing the right atrium connected to the morphologic left ventricle (right sided) by the mitral valve and left atrium connected to the morphologic right ventricle (left sided) by the tricuspid valve. RA: right atrium; MV: mitral valve; LmV: morphologic left ventricle; pv: pulmonary vein; LA: left atrium; TV: tricuspid valve; RmV: morphologic right ventricle; MB: moderator band; R: right side; L: left side.

The morphological right ventricle (left side) in c-TGA is found posterior connected to the left atrium and it is important to assess morphological characteristics of right ventricle such as the presence of moderator band, an apical attachment of the atrioventricular valve, chordal attachment of the atrioventricular valve directly to the wall should be assessed. The morphological left ventricle (right side) in c-TGA is found anterior connected to the right atrium, a more elongated appearance. A ventricular septal defect may be evident in the four-chamber view. Assessment of the outflow tracts shows the great arteries usually arise in a parallel orientation, with the aorta arising from the left-sided morphologically right ventricle and the pulmonary artery more rightwards from the morphologically left ventricle. In cases associated with other intracardiac anomalies, the four-chamber view will generally appear abnormal and is commonly the primary reason for fetal echocardiography referral in c-TGA fetuses [100, 101].

Color Doppler is important for the detection of the presence of VSD, pulmonary stenosis, and tricuspid valve regurgitation. Also, it helps in confirming the parallel course of the great vessels, especially if either the aorta or the pulmonary artery shows severe obstruction.

CARDIAC AND EXTRACARDIAC ANOMALIES ASSOCIATION

Congenitally corrected transposition of great arteries (c-TGA) can occur as an isolated lesion, but are frequently associated with other cardiac abnormalities, include ventricular septal defects, pulmonary stenosis or atresia, Ebstein anomaly and dextrocardia/mesocardiac. Complete heart block is also a well-recognized association [100 - 104]. Other cardiac abnormalities such as absent left-sided connection (tricuspid atresia) or aortic stenosis or atresia and abnormalities of the aortic arch (coarctation and interrupted aortic arch) can be found. Extracardiac abnormalities and chromosomal anomalies are very rare in this condition. Screening for 22q11 microdeletion is recommended especially when c-TGA is associated with other cardiac and extracardiac abnormalities.

FETAL ECHOCARDIOGRAPHIC FINDINGS

1. c-TGA is characterized by atrioventricular and ventriculoarterial discordance.
2. Abnormal four-chamber view. The morphologic right atrium is connected with the morphologic left ventricle and the morphologic left atrium is connected with the morphologic right ventricle.
3. Abnormal outflow tracts view. The pulmonary artery is connected to the morphologic left ventricle and the aorta is connected to the morphologic right ventricle.
4. Great vessels are parallel with the aorta commonly located anteriorly and to the

left of the pulmonary artery.

5. There is hemodynamic compensation where the systemic venous blood leads to the pulmonary artery and the pulmonary venous blood leads to the aorta.
6. Centrally positioned heart.
7. Normal pulmonary venous drainage. Pulmonary veins drain to the atrium (left atrium) that is connected to the right ventricle.
8. Associated cardiac abnormalities such as ventricular septal defect, pulmonary obstruction, and tricuspid valve abnormalities (Ebstein anomaly).

PROGNOSIS AND OUTCOME OF FETAL CONOTRUNCAL ANOMALIES

The prognosis and outcome of fetuses with conotruncal anomalies is affected by multifactorial variables, such as the severity of the cardiac anomaly, association with extracardiac abnormalities, gestational age at delivery, perinatal care, timing and suitability for corrective surgery. All these aspects are also dependent on institutional experience in managing a neonate with a critical cardiac care. That why is advisable to deliver these babies at a tertiary center with surgical and clinical experience in managing complex CHD in the neonatal period.

There is a wide spectrum of pathology associated with conotruncal lesions that affect the morbidity and mortality of each fetus. A more severe spectrum of cardiac lesion is found in fetal life comparing to CHD diagnosed postnatally. Prenatal diagnosis allows to plan individual care with choice from the available options, which include tailored neonatal treatment and termination of pregnancy.

When the diagnosis of conotruncal anomaly is made during the first and second trimesters, some parents will choose termination of pregnancy [5, 7]. The main reason for the termination of pregnancy is the frequent association with chromosomal and extracardiac anomalies. Stillborn and fetal demise often occur with the conotruncal anomalies.

Prenatal screening chromosomal and other noncardiac anomalies is recommended for those fetuses with TOF, DROV, truncus arteriosus, and aortic arch interruption. Fetal diagnosis will optimize the neonatal care directing those patients, who need a surgical procedure immediately after birth to tertiary centers. Also, it is important to plan the time and mode of delivery, and initiation of appropriate perinatal treatment mainly in those babies who have a ductal dependent cardiac anomaly.

There is some evidence of increased morbidity and mortality associated with the delayed postnatal diagnosis of specific critical lesions that require urgent medical care and surgical intervention early after delivery. Assessment of flow at the level of the foramen ovale and ductus arteriosus with color and spectral Doppler should be given close attention closer to term in fetuses with TGA and obstructive right and left lesions. Premature closure or narrowing of the foramen ovale and/or the ductus arteriosus is associated with worsening neonatal outcome and may require emergency postnatal procedures [23, 24].

Complete TGA in fetal life is well tolerated but is a life-threatening malformation in neonates and it is amenable to complete repair with excellent long-term results. Prognosis of a neonate with D-TGA is excellent provided the child is born at a tertiary institution with pediatric cardiac intensive services [6, 9]. Prenatal detection of D-TGA and/or neonatal treatment before cyanosis appears to improve outcome [6, 9]. Newborns with isolated complete transposition will develop severe cyanosis, metabolic acidosis and multiorgan failure unless the ductus arteriosus is maintained patent by the intravenous administration of prostaglandin. Some newborns with a restrictive foramen oval (obstructed flow through foramen), will need a balloon atrial septostomy within a few hours after birth. Thus, the importance to delivery these newborns at a center equipped with cardiac catheterization to perform these procedures [9, 23, 24]. Corrective surgery involves an arterial switch operation where the aorta and pulmonary artery are transacted above the semilunar valves and switched with reimplantation of the coronary circulation.

Delay in diagnosis and treatment of neonates with conotruncal anomalies and severe pulmonary or aortic stenosis or atresia or interrupted aortic arch will increase significantly the morbidity and mortality. Intravenous prostaglandin infusion to maintain patency of the ductus arteriosus is important to maintain ductus patency. Closure of the arterial ductus would result in lower cardiac output, acidosis, hypoxia and death. These cardiac anomalies are called 'ductus dependent' [25, 27]. Intravenous prostaglandin infusion allows arterial duct patency for days and or even weeks in order to wait to a palliative surgery Blalock-Taussig shunt operation or catheter cardiac intervention.

The prenatal diagnosis of absent ductus arteriosus in truncus arteriosus, absent pulmonary valve syndrome, and pulmonary atresia is also important because these lesions will not respond to prostaglandin.

The majority of conotruncal anomalies will need a corrective surgery with good immediate and long-term outcomes [62]. The exception is TA with aortic arch obstruction which carries a high early mortality [63]. Most infants with DROV, TA and severe TOF who underwent to a corrective surgery will require further surgery or cardiac catheterization interventions later in life, *e.g.* replacement of the conduits, implantation of valves, dilation of narrowed vessels and grafts, *etc.*

CONSENT FOR PUBLICATION

Not applicable.

CONFLICT OF INTEREST

The authors confirm that the contents of this chapter have no conflict of interest.

ACKNOWLEDGEMENTS

Declare none.

REFERENCES

[1]   Mitchell SC, Korones SB, Berendes HW. Congenital heart disease in 56,109 births. Incidence and natural history. Circulation 1971; 43(3): 323-32.
[http://dx.doi.org/10.1161/01.CIR.43.3.323] [PMID: 5102136]

[2]   Hoffman JI, Christianson R. Congenital heart disease in a cohort of 19,502 births with long-term follow-up. Am J Cardiol 1978; 42(4): 641-7.
[http://dx.doi.org/10.1016/0002-9149(78)90635-5] [PMID: 696646]

[3]   Ferencz C, Rubin JD, McCarter RJ, *et al.* Congenital heart disease: prevalence at livebirth. The Baltimore-Washington Infant Study. Am J Epidemiol 1985; 121(1): 31-6.
[http://dx.doi.org/10.1093/oxfordjournals.aje.a113979] [PMID: 3964990]

[4]   Jones KL. Smith's Recognizable Patterns of Human Malformation. 4th ed., Philadelphia: WB Saunders 1988.

[5]   Nora JJ, Fraser FC. Cardiovascular disease: Medical Genetics: Principles and Practice. 3rd ed. Philadelphia: Lea & Febiger 1989; pp. 321-37.

[6]   Stamm ER, Drose A, Thickmann D. The Fetal Heart. Diagnostic Ultrasound of Fetal Anomalies. St Louis: Mosby-Year Book 1991; pp. 800-27.

[7]   Hoffman JI. Incidence of congenital heart disease: II. Prenatal incidence. Pediatr Cardiol 1995; 16(4): 155-65.
[http://dx.doi.org/10.1007/BF00801907] [PMID: 7567659]

[8]   Hoffman JI. Incidence of congenital heart disease: I. Postnatal incidence. Pediatr Cardiol 1995; 16(3): 103-13.
[http://dx.doi.org/10.1007/BF00801907] [PMID: 7617503]

[9]   Fyler DC, Buckley LP, Hellenbrand WE, Cohn HE. Report of the New England Regional Infant Cardiac Program. Pediatrics 1980; 65(2 Pt 2): 375-461.
[PMID: 7355042]

[10]   Scott DJ, Rigby ML, Miller GA, Shinebourne EA. The presentation of symptomatic heart disease in infancy based on 10 years' experience (1973-82). Implications for the provision of services. Br Heart J 1984; 52(3): 248-57.
[http://dx.doi.org/10.1136/hrt.52.3.248] [PMID: 6466510]

[11]   Allan LD, Crawford DC, Anderson RH, *et al.* Echocardiographic and anatomic correlation in fetal congenital heart disease. Br Heart J 1984; 52: 548-8.
[http://dx.doi.org/10.1136/hrt.52.5.542]

[12]   Nyberg DA, Emerson DS. Cardiac malformations.Diagnostic ultrasound of fetal anomalies. St Louis: Mosby-Year Book 1990; pp. 300-41.

[13]   Kirby ML, Gale TF, Stewart DE. Neural crest cells contribute to normal aorticopulmonary septation. Science 1983; 220(4601): 1059-61.
[http://dx.doi.org/10.1126/science.6844926] [PMID: 6844926]

[14]   Kirby ML, Turnage KL III, Hays BM. Characterization of conotruncal malformations following ablation of "cardiac" neural crest. Anat Rec 1985; 213(1): 87-93.
[http://dx.doi.org/10.1002/ar.1092130112] [PMID: 4073565]

[15]   Restivo A, Piacentini G, Placidi S, Saffirio C, Marino B. Cardiac outflow tract: a review of some embryogenetic aspects of the conotruncal region of the heart. Anat Rec A Discov Mol Cell Evol Biol 2006; 288(9): 936-43.
[http://dx.doi.org/10.1002/ar.a.20367] [PMID: 16892424]

[16]   Allan LD, Crawford DC, Chita SK, Tynan MJ. Prenatal screening for congenital heart disease. Br Med J (Clin Res Ed) 1986; 292(6537): 1717-9.
[http://dx.doi.org/10.1136/bmj.292.6537.1717] [PMID: 3089369]

[17]   Cardiac screening examination of the fetus guidelines for performing the 'basic' and 'extended basic' cardia scan. Ultrasound Obstet Gynecol 2013; 41: 348-59.

[18]   AIUM practice guideline for the performance of obstetric ultrasound examinations. J Ultrasound Med 2010; 29(1): 157-66.
[http://dx.doi.org/10.7863/jum.2010.29.1.157] [PMID: 20040792]

[19]   Ott WJ. The accuracy of antenatal fetal echocardiography screening in high-and low-risk patients. Am J Obstet Gynecol 1997; 89: 227-32.
[PMID: 7778627]

[20]   Sharland GK, Allan LD. Screening for congenital heart disease prenatally. Results of a 2 1/2-year study in the South East Thames Region. Br J Obstet Gynaecol 1992; 99(3): 220-5.
[http://dx.doi.org/10.1111/j.1471-0528.1992.tb14503.x] [PMID: 1606121]

[21]   Shultz SM, Pretorius DH, Budorick NE. Four-chamber view of the fetal heart: demonstration related to menstrual age. J Ultrasound Med 1994; 13(4): 285-9.
[http://dx.doi.org/10.7863/jum.1994.13.4.285] [PMID: 7932993]

[22]   Paladini D, Rustico M, Todros T, *et al.* Conotruncal anomalies in prenatal life. Ultrasound Obstet Gynecol 1996; 8(4): 241-6.
[http://dx.doi.org/10.1046/j.1469-0705.1996.08040241.x] [PMID: 8916376]

[23]   Allan LD, Sharland GK, Milburn A, *et al.* Prospective diagnosis of 1,006 consecutive cases of congenital heart disease in the fetus. J Am Coll Cardiol 1994; 23(6): 1452-8.
[http://dx.doi.org/10.1016/0735-1097(94)90391-3] [PMID: 8176106]

[24]   Tegnander E, Williams W, Johansen OJ, Blaas HG, Eik-Nes SH. Prenatal detection of heart defects in a non-selected population of 30,149 fetuses-detection rates and outcome. Ultrasound Obstet Gynecol 2006; 27(3): 252-65.
[http://dx.doi.org/10.1002/uog.2710] [PMID: 16456842]

[25]   Tometzki AJ, Suda K, Kohl T, Kovalchin JP, Silverman NH. Accuracy of prenatal echocardiographic diagnosis and prognosis of fetuses with conotruncal anomalies. J Am Coll Cardiol 1999; 33(6): 1696-701.
[http://dx.doi.org/10.1016/S0735-1097(99)00049-2] [PMID: 10334445]

[26]   Sivanandam S, Glickstein JS, Printz BF, *et al.* Prenatal diagnosis of conotruncal malformations: diagnostic accuracy, outcome, chromosomal abnormalities, and extracardiac anomalies. Am J Perinatol 2006; 23(4): 241-5.
[http://dx.doi.org/10.1055/s-2006-939535] [PMID: 16625498]

[27]   Yoo SJ, Lee YH, Kim ES, *et al.* Three-vessel view of the fetal upper mediastinum: an easy means of detecting abnormalities of the ventricular outflow tracts and great arteries during obstetric screening. Ultrasound Obstet Gynecol 1997; 9(3): 173-82.

[http://dx.doi.org/10.1046/j.1469-0705.1997.09030173.x] [PMID: 9165680]

[28]   Yoo SJ, Lee YH, Cho KS. Abnormal three-vessel view on sonography: a clue to the diagnosis of congenital heart disease in the fetus. AJR Am J Roentgenol 1999; 172(3): 825-30.
[http://dx.doi.org/10.2214/ajr.172.3.10063890] [PMID: 10063890]

[29]   Viñals F, Heredia F, Giuliano A. The role of the three vessels and trachea view (3VT) in the diagnosis of congenital heart defects. Ultrasound Obstet Gynecol 2003; 22(4): 358-67.
[http://dx.doi.org/10.1002/uog.882] [PMID: 14528470]

[30]   Shipp TD, Bromley B, Hornberger LK, Nadel A, Benacerraf BR. Levorotation of the fetal cardiac axis: a clue for the presence of congenital heart disease. Obstet Gynecol 1995; 85(1): 97-102.
[http://dx.doi.org/10.1016/0029-7844(94)00328-B] [PMID: 7800334]

[31]   Smith RS, Comstock CH, Kirk JS, Lee W. Ultrasonographic left cardiac axis deviation: a marker for fetal anomalies. Obstet Gynecol 1995; 85(2): 187-91.
[http://dx.doi.org/10.1016/0029-7844(94)00350-M] [PMID: 7824228]

[32]   Shinebourne EA, Babu-Narayan SV, Carvalho JS. Tetralogy of Fallot: from fetus to adult. Heart 2006; 92(9): 1353-9.
[http://dx.doi.org/10.1136/hrt.2005.061143] [PMID: 16908723]

[33]   Fyler DC. Tetralogy of Fallot.Nadas' pediatric cardiology. 4th ed. Philadelphia: Hanley & Belfus 1992; pp. 471-91.

[34]   Pepas LP, Savis A, Jones A, Sharland GK, Tulloh RM, Simpson JM. An echocardiographic study of tetralogy of Fallot in the fetus and infant. Cardiol Young 2003; 13(3): 240-7.
[http://dx.doi.org/10.1017/S1047951103000477] [PMID: 12903870]

[35]   Poon LCY, Huggon IC, Zidere V, Allan LD. Tetralogy of Fallot in the fetus in the current era. Ultrasound Obstet Gynecol 2007; 29(6): 625-7.
[http://dx.doi.org/10.1002/uog.3971] [PMID: 17405110]

[36]   Hornberger LK, Sanders SP, Sahn DJ, *et al. In utero* pulmonary artery and aortic growth and potential for progression of pulmonary outflow tract obstruction in tetralogy of Fallot. J Am Coll Cardiol 1995; 25(3): 739-45.
[http://dx.doi.org/10.1016/0735-1097(94)00422-M] [PMID: 7860923]

[37]   Mielke G, Steil E, Kendziorra H, Goelz R. Ductus arteriosus-dependent pulmonary circulation secondary to cardiac malformations in fetal life. Ultrasound Obstet Gynecol 1997; 9(1): 25-9.
[http://dx.doi.org/10.1046/j.1469-0705.1997.09010025.x] [PMID: 9060126]

[38]   Moon-Grady AJ, Tacy TA, Brook MM, Hanley FL, Silverman NH. Value of clinical and echocardiographic features in predicting outcome in the fetus, infant, and child with tetralogy of Fallot with absent pulmonary valve complex. Am J Cardiol 2002; 89(11): 1280-5.
[http://dx.doi.org/10.1016/S0002-9149(02)02326-3] [PMID: 12031728]

[39]   Razavi RS, Sharland GK, Simpson JM. Prenatal diagnosis by echocardiogram and outcome of absent pulmonary valve syndrome. Am J Cardiol 2003; 91(4): 429-32.
[http://dx.doi.org/10.1016/S0002-9149(02)03238-1] [PMID: 12586257]

[40]   Volpe P, Paladini D, Marasini M, *et al.* Characteristics, associations and outcome of absent pulmonary valve syndrome in the fetus. Ultrasound Obstet Gynecol 2004; 24(6): 623-8.
[http://dx.doi.org/10.1002/uog.1729] [PMID: 15386602]

[41]   Galindo A, Gutiérrez-Larraya F, Martínez JM, *et al.* Prenatal diagnosis and outcome for fetuses with congenital absence of the pulmonary valve. Ultrasound Obstet Gynecol 2006; 28(1): 32-9.
[http://dx.doi.org/10.1002/uog.2807] [PMID: 16795129]

[42]   Achiron R, Rotstein Z, Lipitz S, Mashiach S, Hegesh J. First-trimester diagnosis of fetal congenital heart disease by transvaginal ultrasonography. Obstet Gynecol 1994; 84(1): 69-72.
[PMID: 8008327]

[43]   Hartge D, Hoffmann U, Schröer A, Weichert J. Three- and four-dimensional ultrasound in the diagnosis of fetal tetralogy of fallot with absent pulmonary valve and microdeletion 22q11. Pediatr Cardiol 2010; 31(7): 1100-3.
[http://dx.doi.org/10.1007/s00246-010-9748-z] [PMID: 20552182]

[44]   Hongmei W, Ying Z, Ailu C, Wei S. Novel application of four-dimensional sonography with B-flow imaging and spatiotemporal image correlation in the assessment of fetal congenital heart defects. Echocardiography 2012; 29(5): 614-9.
[http://dx.doi.org/10.1111/j.1540-8175.2011.01639.x] [PMID: 22404098]

[45]   Silverman N, Sinder A. Conditions with override of the ventricular septum by the systemic artery.Two-dimensional echocardiography in congenital heart disease. Norwalk, CT: Appleton-Century-Crofts 1982; pp. 149-55.

[46]   Rao BN, Anderson RC, Edwards JE. Anatomic variations in the tetralogy of Fallot. Am Heart J 1971; 81(3): 361-71.
[http://dx.doi.org/10.1016/0002-8703(71)90106-2] [PMID: 5547435]

[47]   Need LR, Powell AJ, del Nido P, Geva T. Coronary echocardiography in tetralogy of fallot: diagnostic accuracy, resource utilization and surgical implications over 13 years. J Am Coll Cardiol 2000; 36(4): 1371-7.
[http://dx.doi.org/10.1016/S0735-1097(00)00862-7] [PMID: 11028497]

[48]   Uretzky G, Puga FJ, Danielson GK, *et al.* Complete atrioventricular canal associated with tetralogy of Fallot. Morphologic and surgical considerations. J Thorac Cardiovasc Surg 1984; 87(5): 756-66.
[http://dx.doi.org/10.1016/S0022-5223(19)38458-2] [PMID: 6232431]

[49]   Goldmuntz E, Clark BJ, Mitchell LE, *et al.* Frequency of 22q11 deletions in patients with conotruncal defects. J Am Coll Cardiol 1998; 32(2): 492-8.
[http://dx.doi.org/10.1016/S0735-1097(98)00259-9] [PMID: 9708481]

[50]   Momma K, Kondo C, Matsuoka R. Tetralogy of Fallot with pulmonary atresia associated with chromosome 22q11 deletion. J Am Coll Cardiol 1996; 27(1): 198-202.
[http://dx.doi.org/10.1016/0735-1097(95)00415-7] [PMID: 8522695]

[51]   Sharland G. Fetal Cardiology Simplified: a practice manual. Shrewsbury, UK: Tfm Pub. Ltd 2013; pp. 203-37.

[52]   Freedom RM, Mawson JB, Yoo SJ, Benson LN. Truncus arteriosus or common arterial trunk Congenital Heart Disease: Textbook of Angiocardiography. Armonk, NY: Futura 1997; pp. 219-41.

[53]   Duke C, Sharland GK, Jones AM, Simpson JM. Echocardiographic features and outcome of truncus arteriosus diagnosed during fetal life. Am J Cardiol 2001; 88(12): 1379-84.
[http://dx.doi.org/10.1016/S0002-9149(01)02117-8] [PMID: 11741556]

[54]   Volpe P, Paladini D, Marasini M, *et al.* Common arterial trunk in the fetus: characteristics, associations, and outcome in a multicentre series of 23 cases. Heart 2003; 89(12): 1437-41.
[http://dx.doi.org/10.1136/heart.89.12.1437] [PMID: 14617557]

[55]   Van Mierop LH, Patterson DF, Schnarr WR. Pathogenesis of persistent truncus arteriosus in light of observations made in a dog embryo with the anomaly. Am J Cardiol 1978; 41(4): 755-62.
[http://dx.doi.org/10.1016/0002-9149(78)90828-7] [PMID: 645581]

[56]   Collett RW, Edwards JE. Persistent truncus arteriosus; a classification according to anatomic types. Surg Clin North Am 1949; 29(4): 1245-70.
[http://dx.doi.org/10.1016/S0039-6109(16)32803-1] [PMID: 18141293]

[57]   Van Praagh R, Van Praagh S. The anatomy of common aorticopulmonary trunk (truncus arteriosus communis) and its embryologic implications. A study of 57 necropsy cases. Am J Cardiol 1965; 16(3): 406-25.
[http://dx.doi.org/10.1016/0002-9149(65)90732-0] [PMID: 5828135]

[58] Ferencz C, Rubin JD, McCarter RJ, Clark EB. Maternal diabetes and cardiovascular malformations: predominance of double outlet right ventricle and truncus arteriosus. Teratology 1990; 41(3): 319-26.
[http://dx.doi.org/10.1002/tera.1420410309] [PMID: 2326756]

[59] Hoffman JI, Kaplan S. The incidence of congenital heart disease. J Am Coll Cardiol 2002; 39(12): 1890-900.
[http://dx.doi.org/10.1016/S0735-1097(02)01886-7] [PMID: 12084585]

[60] Sharland GK. Common arterial trunk Fetal Cardiology Simplified: a practice manual. Shrewsbury, UK: Tfm Pub. Ltd 2013; pp. 222-8.

[61] Van Praagh R, Van Praagh S. The anatomy of common aorticopulmonary trunk (truncus arteriosus communis) and its embryologic implications. A study of 57 necropsy cases. Am J Cardiol 1965; 16(3): 406-25.
[http://dx.doi.org/10.1016/0002-9149(65)90732-0] [PMID: 5828135]

[62] Calder L, Van Praagh R, Van Praagh S, *et al.* Truncus arteriosus communis. Clinical, angiocardiographic, and pathologic findings in 100 patients. Am Heart J 1976; 92(1): 23-38.
[http://dx.doi.org/10.1016/S0002-8703(76)80400-0] [PMID: 985630]

[63] Machlitt A, Tennstedt C, Körner H, Bommer C, Chaoui R. Prenatal diagnosis of 22q11 microdeletion in an early second-trimester fetus with conotruncal anomaly presenting with increased nuchal translucency and bilateral intracardiac echogenic foci. Ultrasound Obstet Gynecol 2002; 19(5): 510-3.
[http://dx.doi.org/10.1046/j.1469-0705.2002.00688.x] [PMID: 11982988]

[64] Chaoui R, Kalache KD, Heling KS, Tennstedt C, Bommer C, Körner H. Absent or hypoplastic thymus on ultrasound: a marker for deletion 22q11.2 in fetal cardiac defects. Ultrasound Obstet Gynecol 2002; 20(6): 546-52.
[http://dx.doi.org/10.1046/j.1469-0705.2002.00864.x] [PMID: 12493042]

[65] Butto F, Lucas RV Jr, Edwards JE. Persistent truncus arteriosus: pathologic anatomy in 54 cases. Pediatr Cardiol 1986; 7(2): 95-101.
[http://dx.doi.org/10.1007/BF02328958] [PMID: 3797293]

[66] Nath PH, Zollikofer C, Castaneda-Zuniga W, Formanek A, Amplatz K. Persistent truncus arteriosis associated with interruption of the aortic arch. Br J Radiol 1980; 53(633): 853-9.
[http://dx.doi.org/10.1259/0007-1285-53-633-853] [PMID: 7437705]

[67] Marcelletti C, McGoon DC, Danielson GK, Wallace RB, Mair DD. Early and late results of surgical repair of truncus arteriosus. Circulation 1977; 55(4): 636-41.
[http://dx.doi.org/10.1161/01.CIR.55.4.636] [PMID: 837509]

[68] Harris JA, Francannet C, Pradat P, Robert E. The epidemiology of cardiovascular defects, part 2: a study based on data from three large registries of congenital malformations. Pediatr Cardiol 2003; 24(3): 222-35.
[http://dx.doi.org/10.1007/s00246-002-9402-5] [PMID: 12632214]

[69] Volpe P, Paladini D, Marasini M, *et al.* Common arterial trunk in the fetus: characteristics, associations, and outcome in a multicentre series of 23 cases. Heart 2003; 89(12): 1437-41.
[http://dx.doi.org/10.1136/heart.89.12.1437] [PMID: 14617557]

[70] Fyler DC, Buckley LP, Hellenbrand WE, *et al.* Report of the New England Regional Infant Cardiac Program. Pediatrics 1980; 65(2 Pt 2): 375-461.
[PMID: 7355042]

[71] Harris JA, Francannet C, Pradat P, Robert E. The epidemiology of cardiovascular defects, part 2: a study based on data from three large registries of congenital malformations. Pediatr Cardiol 2003; 24(3): 222-35.
[http://dx.doi.org/10.1007/s00246-002-9402-5] [PMID: 12632214]

[72] Boudjemline Y, Fermont L, Le Bidois J, Lyonnet S, Sidi D, Bonnet D. Prevalence of 22q11 deletion in fetuses with conotruncal cardiac defects: a 6-year prospective study. J Pediatr 2001; 138(4): 520-4.

[http://dx.doi.org/10.1067/mpd.2001.112174] [PMID: 11295715]

[73]   Van Mierop LH, Kutsche LM. Cardiovascular anomalies in DiGeorge syndrome and importance of neural crest as a possible pathogenetic factor. Am J Cardiol 1986; 58(1): 133-7.
[http://dx.doi.org/10.1016/0002-9149(86)90256-0] [PMID: 3728313]

[74]   Freedom RM, Mawson JB, Yoo SJ, Benson LN. Double outlet right ventricle Congenital Heart Disease: Textbook of Angiocardiography. Armonk, NY: Futura 1997; pp. 1163-9.

[75]   Smith RS, Comstock CH, Kirk JS, Lee W, Riggs T, Weinhouse E. Double-outlet right ventricle: an antenatal diagnostic dilemma. Ultrasound Obstet Gynecol 1999; 14(5): 315-9.
[http://dx.doi.org/10.1046/j.1469-0705.1999.14050315.x] [PMID: 10623990]

[76]   Kim N, Friedberg MK, Silverman NH. Diagnosis and prognosis of fetuses with double outlet right ventricle. Prenat Diagn 2006; 26(8): 740-5.
[http://dx.doi.org/10.1002/pd.1500] [PMID: 16807954]

[77]   Walters HL III, Mavroudis C, Tchervenkov CI, Jacobs JP, Lacour-Gayet F, Jacobs ML. Congenital Heart Surgery Nomenclature and Database Project: double outlet right ventricle. Ann Thorac Surg 2000; 69(4) (Suppl.): S249-63.
[http://dx.doi.org/10.1016/S0003-4975(99)01247-3] [PMID: 10798433]

[78]   Hornberger L. Double outlet right ventricle.Textbook of fetal cardiology. London: Greenwich Medical Media 2000; pp. 274-87.

[79]   Allan LD. Sonographic detection of parallel great arteries in the fetus. AJR Am J Roentgenol 1997; 168(5): 1283-6.
[http://dx.doi.org/10.2214/ajr.168.5.9129427] [PMID: 9129427]

[80]   Paladini D, Vassallo M, Sglavo G, Lapadula C, Martinelli P. The role of spatio-temporal image correlation (STIC) with tomographic ultrasound imaging (TUI) in the sequential analysis of fetal congenital heart disease. Ultrasound Obstet Gynecol 2006; 27(5): 555-61.
[http://dx.doi.org/10.1002/uog.2749] [PMID: 16619376]

[81]   Bradley TJ, Karamlou T, Kulik A, et al. Determinants of repair type, reintervention, and mortality in 393 children with double-outlet right ventricle. J Thorac Cardiovasc Surg 2007; 134(4): 967-973.e6.
[http://dx.doi.org/10.1016/j.jtcvs.2007.05.061] [PMID: 17903515]

[82]   Berg C, Geipel A, Kamil D, et al. The syndrome of right isomerism -- prenatal diagnosis and outcome. Ultraschall Med 2006; 27(3): 225-33.
[http://dx.doi.org/10.1055/s-2005-858639] [PMID: 16703488]

[83]   Dadvand P, Rankin J, Shirley MD, Rushton S, Pless-Mulloli T. Descriptive epidemiology of congenital heart disease in Northern England. Paediatr Perinat Epidemiol 2009; 23(1): 58-65.
[http://dx.doi.org/10.1111/j.1365-3016.2008.00987.x] [PMID: 19228315]

[84]   Machado MV, Crawford DC, Anderson RH, Allan LD. Atrioventricular septal defect in prenatal life. Br Heart J 1988; 59(3): 352-5.
[http://dx.doi.org/10.1136/hrt.59.3.352] [PMID: 3355725]

[85]   Obler D, Juraszek AL, Smoot LB, Natowicz MR. Double outlet right ventricle: aetiologies and associations. J Med Genet 2008; 45(8): 481-97.
[http://dx.doi.org/10.1136/jmg.2008.057984] [PMID: 18456715]

[86]   Chaoui R, Körner H, Bommer C, Göldner B, Bierlich A, Bollmann R. Prenatal diagnosis of heart defects and associated chromosomal aberrations. Ultraschall Med 1999; 20(5): 177-84.
[PMID: 10595385]

[87]   Gedikbasi A, Oztarhan K, Gul A, Sargin A, Ceylan Y. Diagnosis and prognosis in double-outlet right ventricle. Am J Perinatol 2008; 25(7): 427-34.
[http://dx.doi.org/10.1055/s-0028-1083840] [PMID: 18720325]

[88]   Webb GD, McLaughlin PR, Gow RM, Liu PP, Williams WG. Transposition complexes. Cardiol Clin

1993; 11(4): 651-64.
[http://dx.doi.org/10.1016/S0733-8651(18)30144-9] [PMID: 8252565]

[89]   Allan LD, Crawford DC, Anderson RH, Tynan M. Spectrum of congenital heart disease detected echocardiographically in prenatal life. Br Heart J 1985; 54(5): 523-6.
[http://dx.doi.org/10.1136/hrt.54.5.523] [PMID: 4052293]

[90]   Kirklin JW, Barratt-Boyes BG. Complete transposition of the great arteries.Cardiac surgery. New York: Churchill Livingston 1993; pp. 1383-467.

[91]   Khoshnood B, De Vigan C, Vodovar V, *et al.* Trends in prenatal diagnosis, pregnancy termination, and perinatal mortality of newborns with congenital heart disease in France, 1983-2000: a population-based evaluation. Pediatrics 2005; 115(1): 95-101.
[http://dx.doi.org/10.1542/peds.2004-0516] [PMID: 15629987]

[92]   Bonnet D, Coltri A, Butera G, *et al.* Detection of transposition of the great arteries in fetuses reduces neonatal morbidity and mortality. Circulation 1999; 99(7): 916-8.
[http://dx.doi.org/10.1161/01.CIR.99.7.916] [PMID: 10027815]

[93]   Cardiac screening examination of the fetus: guidelines for performing the 'basic' and 'extended basic' cardiac scan. Ultrasound Obstet Gynecol 2006; 27(1): 107-13.
[PMID: 16374757]

[94]   Chaoui R, McEwing R. Three cross-sectional planes for fetal color Doppler echocardiography. Ultrasound Obstet Gynecol 2003; 21(1): 81-93.
[http://dx.doi.org/10.1002/uog.5] [PMID: 12528169]

[95]   Massoudy P, Baltalarli A, de Leval MR, *et al.* Anatomic variability in coronary arterial distribution with regard to the arterial switch procedure. Circulation 2002; 106(15): 1980-4.
[http://dx.doi.org/10.1161/01.CIR.0000033518.61709.56] [PMID: 12370223]

[96]   Pasquini L, Sanders SP, Parness IA, *et al.* Coronary echocardiography in 406 patients with d-loop transposition of the great arteries. J Am Coll Cardiol 1994; 24(3): 763-8.
[http://dx.doi.org/10.1016/0735-1097(94)90026-4] [PMID: 8077550]

[97]   Ferencz C, Rubin JD, McCarter RJ, *et al.* Congenital heart disease: prevalence at livebirth. The Baltimore-Washington Infant Study. Am J Epidemiol 1985; 121(1): 31-6.
[http://dx.doi.org/10.1093/oxfordjournals.aje.a113979] [PMID: 3964990]

[98]   Samánek M, Vorísková M. Congenital heart disease among 815,569 children born between 1980 and 1990 and their 15-year survival: a prospective Bohemia survival study. Pediatr Cardiol 1999; 20(6): 411-7.
[http://dx.doi.org/10.1007/s002469900502] [PMID: 10556387]

[99]   Stending G, Seidl W. Contribution to the development of the heart. Part 2: morphogenesis of congenital heart diseases. Thorac Cardiovasc Surg 1981; 29: 1-16.
[http://dx.doi.org/10.1055/s-2007-1023435]

[100]   Sharland G, Tingay R, Jones A, Simpson J. Atrioventricular and ventriculoarterial discordance (congenitally corrected transposition of the great arteries): echocardiographic features, associations, and outcome in 34 fetuses. Heart 2005; 91(11): 1453-8.
[http://dx.doi.org/10.1136/hrt.2004.052548] [PMID: 15761049]

[101]   Paladini D, Volpe P, Marasini M, *et al.* Diagnosis, characterization and outcome of congenitally corrected transposition of the great arteries in the fetus: a multicenter series of 30 cases. Ultrasound Obstet Gynecol 2006; 27(3): 281-5.
[http://dx.doi.org/10.1002/uog.2715] [PMID: 16485324]

[102]   Witham AC. Double outlet right ventricle; a partial transposition complex. Am Heart J 1957; 53(6): 928-39.
[http://dx.doi.org/10.1016/0002-8703(57)90329-0] [PMID: 13424473]

[103]   Losekoot TG, Becker AE. Discordant atrioventricular connection and congenitally corrected

transposition.Pediatric cardiology. Edinburgh: Churchill Livingstone 1987; pp. 867-88.

[104] Allan L. Atrioventricular discordance.Textbook of fetal cardiology. London: Greenwich Medical Media Limited 2000; pp. 183-92.

CHAPTER 13

Fetal Aortic Arch Anomalies

Oliver Graupner, Aline Wolter and Roland Axt-Fliedner[*]

Division of Prenatal Medicine & Fetal Therapy, Justus-Liebig University Giessen, Giessen, Germany

Abstract: The normal left aortic arch courses from the ascending aorta to the left, upwards and backwards in relation to the trachea. The aortic arch branches into the right innominate, left common carotid and the left subclavian artery in sequence. The aortic arch is divided into the proximal transverse arch and the distal transverse arch and the aortic isthmus. Abnormalities of the aortic arch involve obstructive lesions, *e.g.* coarctation of the aorta, and abnormalities of branching and position of the aortic arch and the latter are topic of this article. Branching and position abnormalities of the aortic arch have clinical meanings: mechanical compression of airway and esophagus by forming a vascular ring or sling, association with cardiac abnormalities, and association with chromosomal abnormalities. This chapter describes anatomical, genetical and echocardiographic features as well as clinical postnatal implications of abnormalities of branching and position of the aortic arch.

Keywords: Aortic arch, Echocardiography, Fetus, Prenatal diagnosis, Vascular ring.

INTRODUCTION

Aortic arch anomalies (AAA) include anomalies (isolated or combined) of the position or branching pattern of the aortic arch. Many of the AAA are characterized by a disruption of embryogenesis that results in either abnormal persistence or abnormal regression of single or multiple portions of aortic arch. Some AAA do not cause fetal or neonatal symptoms and may even remain undetected. However, there are certain AAA that cause different grades of compression of the trachea and/or esophagus due to complete (vascular ring) or partial (vascular sling) encirclement [1]. There is a frequent association of AAA with other congenital heart disease (CHD) forms or chromosomal aberrations, such as chromosome 22q11 deletion [2, 3].

---

[*] **Corresponding author Roland Axt-Fliedner:** Division of Prenatal Medicine & Fetal Therapy, Department of Obstetrics and Gynecology, Justus-Liebig University Giessen, Klinikstrasse 32, 35392 Gießen, Germany; E-mail: roland.axt-fliedner@gyn.med.uni-giessen.de

Edward Araujo Júnior, Nathalie Jeanne M. Bravo-Valenzuela and Alberto Borges Peixoto (Eds.)

ANATOMY

The aortic arch (AA) describes the section between the ascending and descending aorta. In the transverse part it comes to the diversion of the head and neck arteries (in the anatomical order: right brachiocephalic, left common carotid, and left subclavian artery). The AA extends to the left of the trachea and esophagus and above the proximal portion of the left main bronchus. It is divided into two parts (proximal – distal) by the origin of left common carotid artery. The small section between the origin of left common carotid artery and the insertion of the ductus arteriosus is called the aortic isthmus [2].

EMBRYOLOGY

The double aortic arch model established from Edwards in 1948 facilitates understanding of the pathophysiology of AAA [4, 5]. The aortic sac is divided into the ascending aorta and the pulmonary artery trunk. Two AAs build the transition from the ascending to the descending aorta shaping a vascular ring, which encircles trachea and esophagus. Each AA has three branches: ipsilateral common carotid artery and subclavian artery as well as the arterial duct, which marks the transition from the distal AA to the associated branch pulmonary artery. The left AA and the left arterial duct persist and the right AA distal to the origin of the right subclavian artery and the right arterial duct involute, physiologically. Consequently, the proximal part of the right AA is converted to the right brachiocephalic artery, which is bisected into the right common carotid and subclavian arteries.

FREQUENCY, GENETICS AND ASSOCIATED ABNORMALITIES

AAA occur in 1% to 2% of the general population [6, 7]. Most of AAA (approximately 50%) go along with CHD. Hence, isolated vascular rings are rare (1–1.6 per 1,000 pregnancies) [8 - 10]. The most frequent type of AAA is a left aortic arch with an aberrant right subclavian artery, followed by a right aortic arch anomaly with an aberrant left subclavian artery, a right aortic arch anomaly with mirror image branching, and a double aortic arch anomaly [10 - 13]. AAA are markers for fetal CHD and chromosomal defects, especially 22q11 microdeletion [3] and - specifically in the case of an aberrant right subclavian artery - Down syndrome [14]. The incidence of 22q11 deletion syndrome in fetuses with right aortic arch as an isolated abnormality is approximately 8% and 46% if this is associated with CHDs [15]. Therefore, after diagnosing AAA, a detailed fetal echocardiography and scan is required to look for possible associated malformations. Prenatal testing including detection of 22q11 microdeletion is recommended and should be offered to parents especially when other related conditions (CHD, extracardiac malformations and/or increased nuchal translucency) are described [1, 15]. Table **1** shows our results of 53 consecutive cases of AAA.

Table 1. Associated intracardiac and genetic anomalies in 53 consecutive cases of aortic arch anomalies in our unit.

		ARSA	RAA+mirror	RAA+ALSA	DAA	all
		23	**11**	**16**	**3**	**53**
	Assisted reproduction	2 (8.7%)	3 (27.3%)	1 (6.3%)	1 (33.3%)	7 (13.2%)
	Twin pregnancy	4 (17.4%)	1 (9.1%)	1 (6.3%)	0	6 (10.0%)
Associated anomalies	Intracardiac anomalies	9 (39.1%)	10 (90.9%)	8 (50.0%)	0	27 (45.0%)
	Extracardiac anomalies	3 (13%)	3 (27.3%)	5 (31.3%)	2 (66.7%)	13 (21.7%)
	Chromosomal anomalies	9 (39.1%)	1 (9.1%)	1 (6.3%)	1 (33.3%)	12 (22.6%)
Outcome	TOP	4 (17.4%)	0	0	0	4 (6.7%)
	IUD/abortion	1 (4.3%)	1 (9.1%)	0	0	2 (3.8%)
	Lost for FU prenatally	1 (4.3%)	0	0	0	1 (1.7%)
	Livebirth, survival FU	14 (60.9%)	10 (90.9%)	13 (81.3%)	3 (100%)	40 (66.7%)
	Livebirth, death during FU	1 (4.3%)	0	2 (12.5%)	0	3 (5.0%)
	Lost for FU postnatally	2 (8.7%)	0	1 (6.3%)	0	3 (5.0%)
	Operation because of vascular ring/sling	0	0	1 (6.3%)	0	1 (1.9%)

Follow up (FU) time: in median 21 months, in mean 28.5 months.
ARSA: aberrant right subclavian artery; RAA: right aortic arch; ALSA: aberrant left subclavian artery; DAA: double aortic arch; TOP: termination of pregnancy; IUD: intrauterine demise.

ECHOCARDIOGRAPHIC KEY FEATURES

The fetal upper mediastinum is the area of interest, which should be assessed regarding AAA detection [16]. Color Doppler imaging with a low velocity range (10–15 cm/s) is required to see the vessels [16, 17]. Prenatal echocardiographic evaluation of AAA can be started from the axial 3-vessel and trachea view [1, 16]. This view allows identification of the pulmonary artery communicating with the ductus arteriosus, and to its right, identification of a transverse section of the aortic arch, the superior vena cava, and the trachea. The AA and the ductus arteriosus make a "V" shape confluence, which diverges toward the anterior thoracic wall and converges to the left of the trachea. Normally, no major vascular structure crosses the midline behind the trachea. If there is a vessel seen behind the trachea, it should be considered as an aberrant branch of the AA or the AA itself with an abnormal retroesophageal course or an aberrant left pulmonary artery in a pulmonary artery sling, which has an abnormal course between the trachea and esophagus [1]. Furthermore, axial 3-vessel and trachea view is essential for the identification of vascular rings [18, 19]. Complementarily, using a coronal view, an aberrant subclavian artery, either right or left, can be confirmed when the transverse view is not sufficient enough [16]. The coronal view allows the presentation of the origin and course of the anomalous artery in the same plane [20].

Generally, assessment of AAA should contain the following three basic components [1]:

1. Left or right-sidedness of the AA relative to the trachea;
2. Branching pattern of the head and neck arteries relative to the AA;
3. Left or right-sidedness of the ductus arteriosus.

TYPES OF AORTIC ARCH ANOMALIES, SONOGRAPHIC SIGNS AND CLINICAL SIGNIFICANCE

Left Aortic Arch with an Aberrant Right Subclavian Artery

Due to an abnormal involution of the right aortic arch between the origins of the right common carotid and right subclavian arteries, the right subclavian artery remains attached to the distal remnant of the left-sided aortic arch. The combination of these vessels builds a vascular sling around the left side of the trachea and esophagus. A vascular ring formation is a rare case, but possible when there is a right-sided ductus arteriosus between the aberrant right subclavian artery and the right pulmonary artery [21] (Fig. 1).

The 3-vessel and trachea view at the level of the aortic isthmus makes the aberrant right subclavian artery visible. It crosses the fetal chest posterior to the trachea toward the right upper limb. Left aortic arch with an aberrant right subclavian artery is frequently an incidental and isolated (46% of cases) asymptomatic anomaly [6, 16]. The prevalence is between 0.4% and 1.9% [6]. Despite the fact that left aortic arch with an aberrant right subclavian artery can occur in both euploid and aneuploid fetuses, it appears to be somewhat more frequent in the latter [22 - 25]. Especially the Down syndrome is associated to this anomaly. However, this relation depends on its association to other structural malformations, because when isolated, an aberrant right subclavian artery has not shown any association with Down syndrome recently [6]. Like in all AAA, an aberrant right subclavian artery is also associated with 22q11 microdeletion [3]. CHDs are often associated (approximately 20%) with this anomaly. Types of

CHD most commonly described in this condition are atrioventricular septal defects and a persistent left superior vena cava [22 - 25].

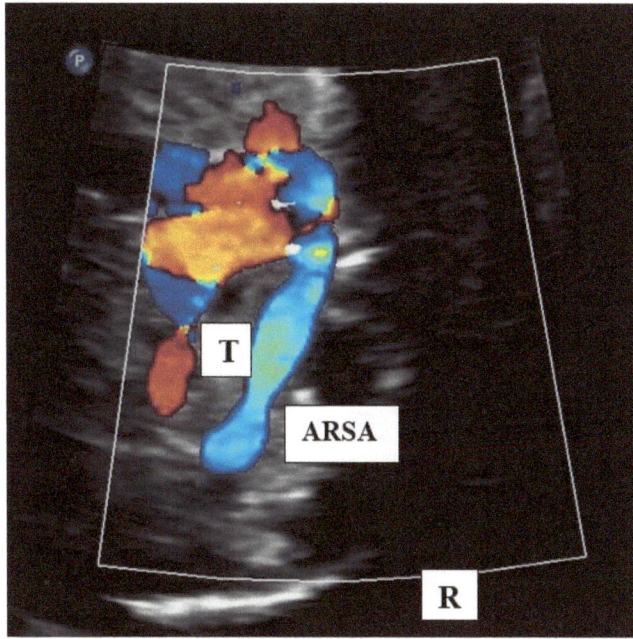

Fig. (1). Fetal transverse view in a case of left aortic arch with an aberrant right subclavian artery (ARSA). The aortic arch and the arterial duct appear to the left of the trachea in three-vessel-view forming a V-shaped structure. The right subclavian artery crosses the fetal chest posterior to the trachea (T) toward the right upper limb forming a vascular sling around trachea and esophagus. R: right side.

Right Aortic Arch with an Aberrant Left Subclavian Artery

This condition is the result of an abnormal persistence of the embryological right aortic arch and an abnormal regression of the left aortic arch between the origins of the left common carotid artery and the left subclavian artery [16]. The aberrant left subclavian artery can either have a course between the trachea and the esophagus (most collateral arteries) or a completely retroesophageal course [4] (Fig. **2**).

The left pulmonary artery is connected to the distal remnant of the left aortic arch by the usually left-sided ductus arteriosus. The combination of these vessels forms a vascular ring, which is the second most common type of vascular ring reported [16]. A rare variation is a right aortic arch with a right-sided ductus arteriosus and an aberrant left subclavian artery. The aberrant left subclavian artery runs behind the trachea to the left upper limb, forming a vascular sling [26]. Another rare variant is a right aortic arch with an aberrant origin of the left brachiocephalic artery [27]. In this condition, due to an abnormal regression of the left aortic arch proximal to the origin of the left common carotid artery, the persisting ductus arteriosus is usually left sided, completing a vascular ring [16].

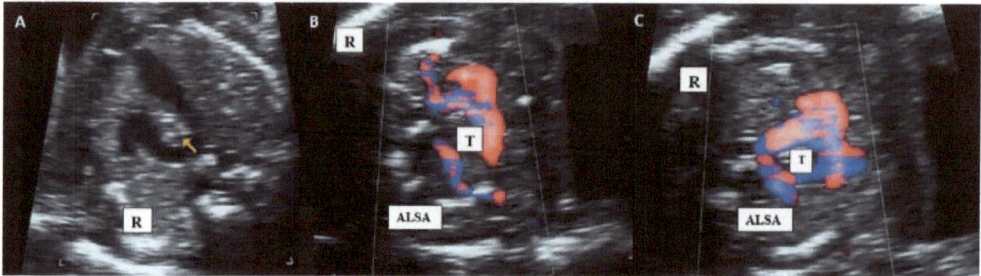

Fig. (2). Fetal transverse view in a case with right aortic arch and aberrant left subclavian artery (ALSA). The aortic arch is located to the right of the trachea in three vessel view forming a U-shaped structure with the arterial duct being left (arrow pointing towards the trachea) (**A**). The left subclavian artery crosses the fetal chest posterior to the trachea toward the left upper limb forming a vascular ring around trachea (T) and esophagus (**B** and **C**). R: rigth side.

The 3-vessel and trachea view depicts a shift of the aortic arch to the right of the trachea. Thus, a "U" shape instead of a "V" shape can be visualized. The aberrant left subclavian artery can be seen at the level of the aortic isthmus. It runs through the fetal chest posterior to the trachea toward the left upper limb.

The reported prevalence of a right aortic arch with an aberrant left subclavian artery is 1 to 1.7 per 1000 pregnancies [9, 12, 19, 28]. CHDs are associated with this anomaly in 6.6%–33.3%. Types of CHD most frequently described in this condition are ventricular septal defects, tetralogy of Fallot and pulmonary atresia with a ventricular septal defect [11, 12, 28, 29]. Chromosomal abnormalities, mainly 22q11 microdeletion, occur in 4.3% to 32% of cases despite the absence of CHD [3, 11 - 13, 15]. After birth, the distal remnant of the left aortic arch persists as the diverticulum of Kommerell. This vascular ring is usually not that tight (compared to the vascular ring formed by a double aortic arch) [16]. Hence, approximately 96% of cases are asymptomatic postnatally [13] and the degree of esophageal and/or tracheal compression depends on the size of the Kommerell diverticulum.

Right Aortic Arch with Mirror Image Branching

A right aortic arch with mirror image branching results by an abnormal involution of the left aortic arch distal to the origin of the left subclavian artery. In this condition, the ductus arteriosus is usually left-sided, connecting the origin of the left brachiocephalic artery or the descending aorta to the left pulmonary artery [16, 30] (Fig. **3**).

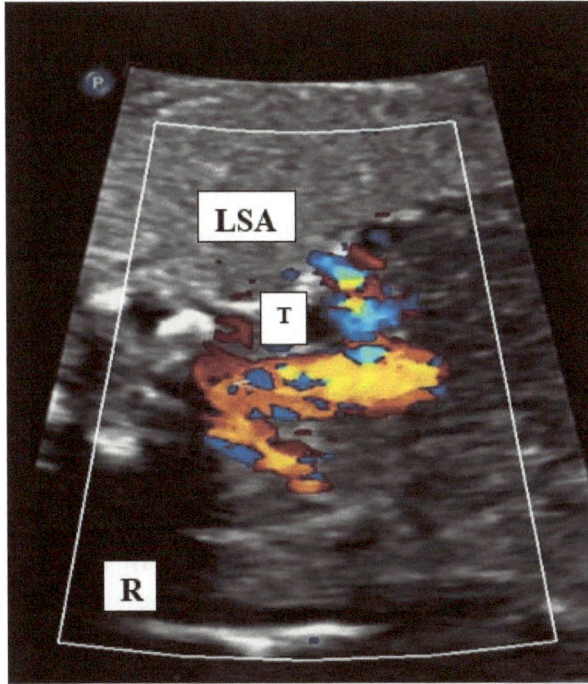

Fig. (3). Fetal transverse view in a case of right aortic arch with mirror imaging branching. The aortic arch is situated on the right of the trachea with a left ductus forming a U-shape structure. Both subclavian arteries can be seen in an ante tracheal position showing a mirror-imaging branching pattern. In case of left arterial duct there is mostly a vascular ring. LSA: left subclavian artery. R: right side; T: trachea.

In the 3-vessel and trachea view, the picture of a right aortic arch with mirror image branching depends significantly on the laterality of the ductus arteriosus [16]. There exist both variants for this condition, persistence of a left [3, 13, 26, 30] or right [8, 11] ductus arteriosus. However, left-sided ductus arteriosus is the one that is most reported, connecting the left pulmonary artery to the descending aorta (vascular ring) or to the left brachiocephalic artery (no vascular ring). In the condition of a right-sided ductus arteriosus, no vascular ring is formed. In the case of a connection between the ductus arteriosus and the descending aorta a "U" shape instead of a "V" shape can be visualized encircling the trachea. If there is a persistent right-sided ductus arteriosus a "V" shape formed by the right aortic arch and the right ductus arteriosus is observed on the right side of the trachea [16].

The reported prevalence of a right aortic arch with mirror image branching is approximately 3.5 per 1000 in high-risk pregnancies [12]. In this condition the incidence of associated CHD is high ranging from 91.5% to 100% [8, 11, 12, 28]. The most associated CHD is tetralogy of Fallot (41%–57%) [12], followed by a common arterial trunk (13%–36%), pulmonary atresia with a ventricular septal defect (10.3%–36%) and a double-outlet right ventricle (10.3%) [11, 12, 31, 32].

Furthermore, extracardiac anomalies are frequently observed (approximately 20%) [11, 12]. The incidence of 22q11 microdeletion ranges from 13.3% to 25%, especially in cases affected by conotruncal anomalies or extracardiac abnormalities [3, 11, 13]. Due to the high percentage of associated CHD and extracardiac malformations as well as the presence of chromosomal defects, the outcome of this type of AAA is mainly influenced by its comorbidities [16]. In most of the cases there is no vascular ring or sling reducing the risk of compressive symptoms postnatally [7, 8, 11].

Double Aortic Arch

As the tightest form of vascular ring [33] double aortic arch has its origin in the persistence of both the right and the left embryonic aortic arches on each side of the trachea and esophagus with common carotid and subclavian arteries arising separately from each arch. In most of the cases the left arterial duct persists, however a few cases with bilateral ducts have been reported [7, 34]. The proximal descending aorta is left sided in about two-thirds of cases [26]. Mostly, both arches are patent with a minority of cases in which an atretic segment exists [16]. In approximately 83% of patients the right arch is dominant [35] (Fig. **4**).

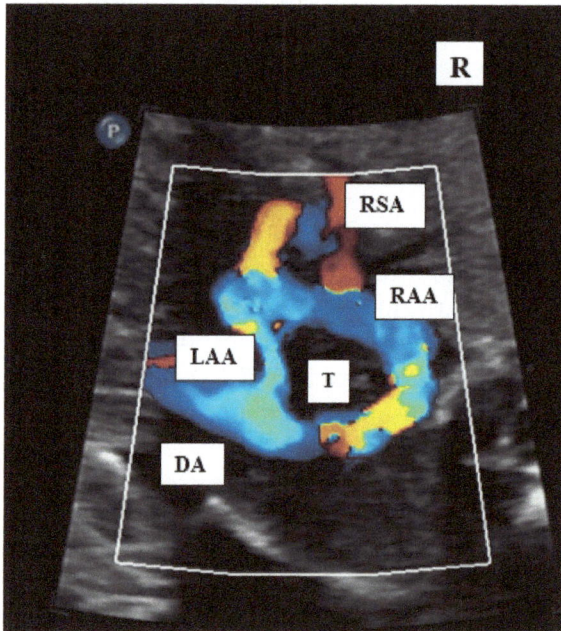

Fig. (4). Fetal transverse view in a case of double aortic arch. There are four instead of three vessels, with the vessels being right and left aortic arches, the ductus arteriosus (DA, left or right) and the superior vena cava. Typically, the left sided aortic arch is smaller (LAA) and left and right subclavian artery show (RSA) an ante tracheal course. Double aortic arch forms a tight vascular ring. R: right side; LAA: left aortic arch; RAA: right aortic arch; T: trachea.

In the 3-vessel and trachea view, a complete vascular ring encircling the trachea can be seen. In cephalic presentation, it may have the shape of number 6 (fetal spine on the right) or 9 (fetal spine on the left) instead of the classic V-shaped structure [16]. Anyway, a picture of four vessels instead of three is generated: the right and left aortic arch, the arterial duct (left or right sided), and the superior vena cava. This circumstance helps to identify double aortic arch in the complex of all aortic arch anomalies.

Double aortic arch is often added to a series of right aortic arch cases [8, 12, 18, 28]. In the majority of cases it is an isolated finding without further cardiac and extracardiac anomalies [16]. As a rare condition, double aortic arch cases are associated with CHD mainly ventricular septal defects and double outlet right ventricles [35]. Furthermore, the association with 22q11 microdeletion in the absence of CHD is low in double aortic arch cases [16].

Circumflex Retroesophageal Aortic Arch

In this condition, the proximal part of the descending aorta is located on the contralateral side of the aortic arch [36, 37]. In most of the cases there is a right-sided aortic arch and the branching pattern of the supra-aortic arteries varies. Most frequently, the left subclavian artery arises from the aorta through the diverticulum of Kommerell. As the left-sided ductus arteriosus connects the diverticulum to the left pulmonary artery, there is the shape of vascular ring [26].

In the 3-vessel and trachea view a D-shaped structure around the trachea can be illustrated. The D-shape is built by the right aortic arch with its retrotracheal segment and the left-sided ductus arteriosus on the opposite side forming the vascular ring [34]. Circumflex retroesophageal aortic arch is a rare anomaly, which is barely seen prenatally [16]. It is commonly associated with CHD and can lead to compressive symptoms in the newborn [38].

Postnatal Symptoms and Clinical Management

There is consensus that AAA do not require radiologic examinations with computed tomography or magnetic resonance imaging in all cases postnatally. These examinations should be reserved in particular for cases with symptomatic courses or those in which specific details on anatomy and circulation cannot be obtained by experienced postnatal echocardiography [8, 12, 28]. Postnatal echocardiography is sometimes difficult due to the shadowing of air bronchograms, which is why the detailed prenatal examination for the diagnosis of AAA gains importance [7].

There is a debate about the incidence of symptoms related to AAA depending on prenatal or postnatal series [16]. In prenatal series, most of the AAA are described as asymptomatic. However, some types of AAA forming a vascular ring like double aortic arch and some cases of a right aortic arch with an aberrant left subclavian artery can lead to compressive symptoms [13, 19]. In contrast, pediatric studies report that two thirds of AAA cases (most frequently double aortic arch) are symptomatic requiring surgery due to airway and/or esophageal compression [39, 40]. Typical symptoms may include stridor, cough, asthma, respiratory distress, apnea, recurrent pneumonia, dysphagia, and choking [41, 42]. As a simple rule, the worse the compression, the earlier the onset of symptoms [1]. Surgical strategies comprise the mechanical separation of the structures forming the vascular ring [43 - 46]. For instance, in symptomatic patients, performing a video-assisted thoracoscopy the aberrant left subclavian artery can be divided and connected to the ipsilateral common carotid artery [47 - 49].

CONCLUSION

AAA are rare conditions, which can be either isolated or, more commonly, associated with CHD or other anomalies, including chromosomal aberrations such as 22q11 deletion. Using the 3-vessel and trachea view can achieve diagnosis of fetal AAA. After diagnosing AAA, a detailed fetal echocardiography and scan is essential to detect possible associated malformations. Prenatal genetic testing including karyotyping and chromosomal microarray analysis should be offered to parents. The prognosis of AAA is influenced by associated abnormalities and the severity of tracheal and/or esophageal compression [16].

CONSENT FOR PUBLICATION

Not applicable.

CONFLICT OF INTEREST

The authors confirm that the contents of this chapter have no conflict of interest.

ACKNOWLEDGEMENTS

Declare none.

REFERENCES

[1]   Thakur V, Jaeggi ET, Yoo SJ. Aortic arch anomalies.Fetal Cardiology Embryology, Genetics, Physiology, Echocardiographic Evaluation, Diagnosis, and Perinatal Management of Cardiac Diseases. 3rd ed. New York, NY: Informa Healthcare 2018; pp. 401-12.

[2]   Moulaert AJ, Bruins CC, Oppenheimer-Dekker A. Anomalies of the aortic arch and ventricular septal defects. Circulation 1976; 53(6): 1011-5.
[http://dx.doi.org/10.1161/01.CIR.53.6.1011] [PMID: 1269116]

[3]   McElhinney DB, Clark BJ III, Weinberg PM, *et al.* Association of chromosome 22q11 deletion with isolated anomalies of aortic arch laterality and branching. J Am Coll Cardiol 2001; 37(8): 2114-9.
[http://dx.doi.org/10.1016/S0735-1097(01)01286-4] [PMID: 11419896]

[4]   Edwards JE. Anomalies of the derivatives of the aortic arch system. Med Clin North Am 1948; 32: 925-49.
[http://dx.doi.org/10.1016/S0025-7125(16)35662-0] [PMID: 18877614]

[5]   Edwards JE. Malformations of the aortic arch system manifested as vascular rings. Lab Invest 1953; 2(1): 56-75.
[PMID: 13036024]

[6]   De León-Luis J, Gámez F, Bravo C, *et al.* Second-trimester fetal aberrant right subclavian artery: original study, systematic review and meta-analysis of performance in detection of Down syndrome. Ultrasound Obstet Gynecol 2014; 44(2): 147-53.
[http://dx.doi.org/10.1002/uog.13336] [PMID: 24585513]

[7]   Yoo SJ, Min JY, Lee YH, Roman K, Jaeggi E, Smallhorn J. Fetal sonographic diagnosis of aortic arch anomalies. Ultrasound Obstet Gynecol 2003; 22(5): 535-46.
[http://dx.doi.org/10.1002/uog.897] [PMID: 14618670]

[8]   Achiron R, Rotstein Z, Heggesh J, *et al.* Anomalies of the fetal aortic arch: a novel sonographic approach to *in-utero* diagnosis. Ultrasound Obstet Gynecol 2002; 20(6): 553-7.
[http://dx.doi.org/10.1046/j.1469-0705.2002.00850.x] [PMID: 12493043]

[9]   Bronshtein M, Lorber A, Berant M, Auslander R, Zimmer EZ. Sonographic diagnosis of fetal vascular rings in early pregnancy. Am J Cardiol 1998; 81(1): 101-3.
[http://dx.doi.org/10.1016/S0002-9149(97)00864-3] [PMID: 9462619]

[10]   Tuo G, Volpe P, Bava GL, *et al.* Prenatal diagnosis and outcome of isolated vascular rings. Am J Cardiol 2009; 103(3): 416-9.
[http://dx.doi.org/10.1016/j.amjcard.2008.09.100] [PMID: 19166700]

[11]   Berg C, Bender F, Soukup M, *et al.* Right aortic arch detected in fetal life. Ultrasound Obstet Gynecol 2006; 28(7): 882-9.
[http://dx.doi.org/10.1002/uog.3883] [PMID: 17086578]

[12]   Galindo A, Nieto O, Nieto MT, *et al.* Prenatal diagnosis of right aortic arch: associated findings, pregnancy outcome, and clinical significance of vascular rings. Prenat Diagn 2009; 29(10): 975-81.
[http://dx.doi.org/10.1002/pd.2327] [PMID: 19603384]

[13]   Razon Y, Berant M, Fogelman R, Amir G, Birk E. Prenatal diagnosis and outcome of right aortic arch without significant intracardiac anomaly. J Am Soc Echocardiogr 2014; 27(12): 1352-8.
[http://dx.doi.org/10.1016/j.echo.2014.08.003] [PMID: 25240492]

[14]   Agathokleous M, Chaveeva P, Poon LC, Kosinski P, Nicolaides KH. Meta-analysis of second-trimester markers for trisomy 21. Ultrasound Obstet Gynecol 2013; 41(3): 247-61.
[http://dx.doi.org/10.1002/uog.12364] [PMID: 23208748]

[15]   Zidere V, Tsapakis EG, Huggon IC, Allan LD. Right aortic arch in the fetus. Ultrasound Obstet Gynecol 2006; 28(7): 876-81.
[http://dx.doi.org/10.1002/uog.3841] [PMID: 17066500]

[16]   Bravo C, Gámez F, Pérez R, Álvarez T, De León-Luis J. Fetal Aortic Arch Anomalies: Key Sonographic Views for Their Differential Diagnosis and Clinical Implications Using the Cardiovascular System Sonographic Evaluation Protocol. J Ultrasound Med 2016; 35(2): 237-51.
[http://dx.doi.org/10.7863/ultra.15.02063] [PMID: 26715656]

[17]   Chaoui R, Heling KS, Sarioglu N, Schwabe M, Dankof A, Bollmann R. Aberrant right subclavian artery as a new cardiac sign in second- and third-trimester fetuses with Down syndrome. Am J Obstet Gynecol 2005; 192(1): 257-63.
[http://dx.doi.org/10.1016/j.ajog.2004.06.080] [PMID: 15672034]

[18]   Jain S, Kleiner B, Moon-Grady A, Hornberger LK. Prenatal diagnosis of vascular rings. J Ultrasound Med 2010; 29(2): 287-94.
[http://dx.doi.org/10.7863/jum.2010.29.2.287] [PMID: 20103801]

[19]   Li S, Luo G, Norwitz ER, *et al.* Prenatal diagnosis of congenital vascular rings and slings: sonographic features and perinatal outcome in 81 consecutive cases. Prenat Diagn 2011; 31(4): 334-46.
[http://dx.doi.org/10.1002/pd.2678] [PMID: 21280058]

[20]   De León-Luis J, Bravo C, Gámez F, Ortiz-Quintana L. Coronal view as a complementary ultrasound approach for prenatal diagnosis of aberrant right subclavian artery. Ultrasound Obstet Gynecol 2012; 40(3): 370-1.
[http://dx.doi.org/10.1002/uog.11094] [PMID: 22262407]

[21]   Bakhtiary F, Dähnert I, Kostelka M. Aberrant right subclavian artery and right-sided ductus arteriosus. BMJ Case Rep 2010; 2010: bcr0420102937.
[http://dx.doi.org/10.1136/bcr.04.2010.2937] [PMID: 22778108]

[22]   Borenstein M, Cavoretto P, Allan L, Huggon I, Nicolaides KH. Aberrant right subclavian artery at 11 + 0 to 13 + 6 weeks of gestation in chromosomally normal and abnormal fetuses. Ultrasound Obstet Gynecol 2008; 31(1): 20-4.
[http://dx.doi.org/10.1002/uog.5226] [PMID: 18157795]

[23]   Borenstein M, Minekawa R, Zidere V, Nicolaides KH, Allan LD. Aberrant right subclavian artery at 16 to 23 + 6 weeks of gestation: a marker for chromosomal abnormality. Ultrasound Obstet Gynecol 2010; 36(5): 548-52.
[http://dx.doi.org/10.1002/uog.7683] [PMID: 20503237]

[24]   Zapata H, Edwards JE, Titus JL. Aberrant right subclavian artery with left aortic arch: associated cardiac anomalies. Pediatr Cardiol 1993; 14(3): 159-61.
[http://dx.doi.org/10.1007/BF00795645] [PMID: 8415218]

[25]   Fehmi Yazıcıoğlu H, Sevket O, Akın H, Aygün M, Özyurt ON, Karahasanoğlu A. Aberrant right subclavian artery in Down syndrome fetuses. Prenat Diagn 2013; 33(3): 209-13.
[http://dx.doi.org/10.1002/pd.4042] [PMID: 23319208]

[26]   Anderson R, Baker E, Redington A, *et al.* Vascular rings, pulmonary arterial sling and related conditions Paediatric Cardiology. London: Churchill Livingstone 2009; pp. 967-90.

[27]   Gandolfo F, Albanese SB, Secinaro AD, Carotti A. One-stage repair of aberrant left brachiocephalic artery and coarctation of the aorta in right aortic arch. Interact Cardiovasc Thorac Surg 2013; 17(2): 444-6.
[http://dx.doi.org/10.1093/icvts/ivt213] [PMID: 23667064]

[28]   Miranda JO, Callaghan N, Miller O, Simpson J, Sharland G. Right aortic arch diagnosed antenatally: associations and outcome in 98 fetuses. Heart 2014; 100(1): 54-9.
[http://dx.doi.org/10.1136/heartjnl-2013-304860] [PMID: 24192976]

[29]   Valletta EA, Pregarz M, Bergamo-Andreis IA, Boner AL. Tracheoesophageal compression due to congenital vascular anomalies (vascular rings). Pediatr Pulmonol 1997; 24(2): 93-105.
[http://dx.doi.org/10.1002/(SICI)1099-0496(199708)24:2<93::AID-PPUL4>3.0.CO;2-J]   [PMID: 9292900]

[30]   McElhinney DB, Hoydu AK, Gaynor JW, Spray TL, Goldmuntz E, Weinberg PM. Patterns of right aortic arch and mirror-image branching of the brachiocephalic vessels without associated anomalies. Pediatr Cardiol 2001; 22(4): 285-91.
[http://dx.doi.org/10.1007/s002460010231] [PMID: 11455394]

[31]   Hastreiter AR, D'Cruz IA, Cantez T, Namin EP, Licata R. Right-sided aorta. I. Occurrence of right aortic arch in various types of congenital heart disease. II. Right aortic arch, right descending aorta, and associated anomalies. Br Heart J 1966; 28(6): 722-39.
[http://dx.doi.org/10.1136/hrt.28.6.722] [PMID: 5332779]

[32] Glew D, Hartnell GG. The right aortic arch revisited. Clin Radiol 1991; 43(5): 305-7.
[http://dx.doi.org/10.1016/S0009-9260(05)80534-3] [PMID: 2036753]

[33] Edwards JE. Vascular rings related to anomalies of the aortic arches. Mod Concepts Cardiovasc Dis 1948; 17(8): 1.
[PMID: 18873268]

[34] Patel CR, Lane JR, Spector ML, Smith PC. Fetal echocardiographic diagnosis of vascular rings. J Ultrasound Med 2006; 25(2): 251-7.
[http://dx.doi.org/10.7863/jum.2006.25.2.251] [PMID: 16439790]

[35] Trobo D, Bravo C, Alvarez T, Pérez R, Gámez F, De León-Luis J. Prenatal sonographic features of a double aortic arch: literature review and perinatal management. J Ultrasound Med 2015; 34(11): 1921-7.
[http://dx.doi.org/10.7863/ultra.14.12076] [PMID: 26446822]

[36] Schneeweiss A, Blieden L, Shem-Tov A, Deutsch V, Neufeld HN. Retroesophageal right aortic arch. Pediatr Cardiol 1984; 5(3): 191-5.
[http://dx.doi.org/10.1007/BF02427044] [PMID: 6531261]

[37] Philip S, Chen SY, Wu MH, Wang JK, Lue HC. Retroesophageal aortic arch: diagnostic and therapeutic implications of a rare vascular ring. Int J Cardiol 2001; 79(2-3): 133-41.
[http://dx.doi.org/10.1016/S0167-5273(01)00402-8] [PMID: 11461734]

[38] Lee CH, Seo DJ, Bang JH, Goo HW, Park JJ. Translocation of the aortic arch with norwood procedure for hypoplastic left heart syndrome variant with circumflex retroesophageal aortic arch. Korean J Thorac Cardiovasc Surg 2014; 47(4): 389-93.
[http://dx.doi.org/10.5090/kjtcs.2014.47.4.389] [PMID: 25207249]

[39] Kir M, Saylam GS, Karadas U, *et al.* Vascular rings: presentation, imaging strategies, treatment, and outcome. Pediatr Cardiol 2012; 33(4): 607-17.
[http://dx.doi.org/10.1007/s00246-012-0187-x] [PMID: 22314366]

[40] Suh YJ, Kim GB, Kwon BS, *et al.* Clinical course of vascular rings and risk factors associated with mortality. Korean Circ J 2012; 42(4): 252-8.
[http://dx.doi.org/10.4070/kcj.2012.42.4.252] [PMID: 22563338]

[41] Licari A, Manca E, Rispoli GA, Mannarino S, Pelizzo G, Marseglia GL. Congenital vascular rings: a clinical challenge for the pediatrician. Pediatr Pulmonol 2015; 50(5): 511-24.
[http://dx.doi.org/10.1002/ppul.23152] [PMID: 25604054]

[42] Robson EA, Scott A, Chetcuti P, Crabbe D. Vascular ring diagnosis following respiratory arrest. BMJ Case Rep 2014; 2014: bcr2013202164.
[http://dx.doi.org/10.1136/bcr-2013-202164] [PMID: 24895385]

[43] van Son JA, Julsrud PR, Hagler DJ, *et al.* Surgical treatment of vascular rings: the Mayo Clinic experience. Mayo Clin Proc 1993; 68(11): 1056-63.
[http://dx.doi.org/10.1016/S0025-6196(12)60898-2] [PMID: 8231269]

[44] Chun K, Colombani PM, Dudgeon DL, Haller JA Jr. Diagnosis and management of congenital vascular rings: a 22-year experience. Ann Thorac Surg 1992; 53(4): 597-602.
[http://dx.doi.org/10.1016/0003-4975(92)90317-W] [PMID: 1554267]

[45] Kocis KC, Midgley FM, Ruckman RN. Aortic arch complex anomalies: 20-year experience with symptoms, diagnosis, associated cardiac defects, and surgical repair. Pediatr Cardiol 1997; 18(2): 127-32.
[http://dx.doi.org/10.1007/s002469900130] [PMID: 9049126]

[46] Alsenaidi K, Gurofsky R, Karamlou T, Williams WG, McCrindle BW. Management and outcomes of double aortic arch in 81 patients. Pediatrics 2006; 118(5): e1336-41.
[http://dx.doi.org/10.1542/peds.2006-1097] [PMID: 17000782]

[47] Koontz CS, Bhatia A, Forbess J, Wulkan ML. Video-assisted thoracoscopic division of vascular rings in pediatric patients. Am Surg 2005; 71(4): 289-91.
[PMID: 15943400]

[48] Slater BJ, Rothenberg SS. Thoracoscopic management of patent ductus arteriosus and vascular rings in infants and children. J Laparoendosc Adv Surg Tech A 2016; 26(1): 66-9.
[http://dx.doi.org/10.1089/lap.2015.0126] [PMID: 26312644]

[49] Lee JH, Yang JH, Jun TG. Video-assisted thoracoscopic division of vascular rings. Korean J Thorac Cardiovasc Surg 2015; 48(1): 78-81.
[http://dx.doi.org/10.5090/kjtcs.2015.48.1.78] [PMID: 25705605]

SUBJECT INDEX

M

N

www.ingramcontent.com/pod-product-compliance
Lightning Source LLC
Chambersburg PA
CBHW050808220326
41598CB00006B/154